OTOLARYNGOLOGY

Edited by **Balwant Singh Gendeh**

Otolaryngology
Edited by Balwant Singh Gendeh

Published by InTech

Janeza Trdine 9, 51000 Rijeka, Croatia

Publishing Process Manager Romina Skomersic

Technical Editor Teodora Smiljanic

Cover Designer InTech Design Team

Additional hard copies can be obtained from orders@intechopen.com

Otolaryngology, Edited by Balwant Singh Gendeh
p. cm.
ISBN 978-953-51-0624-1

For EU product safety concerns:
IN TECH d.o.o., Prolaz Marije Krucifikse Kozulić 3, 51000 Rijeka, Croatia,
info@intechopen.com or visit our website at intechopen.com.

Meet the editor

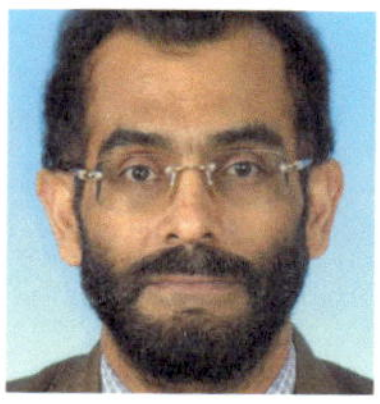

Dr Balwant Singh Gendeh is an ENT surgeon with sub-speciality interest in Rhinology, namely Allergy, Sinonasal diseases, Endoscopic sinus, anterior and ventral skull base surgery, and Functional and Cosmetic Nasal Surgery. He was a research registrar in ENT at the Royal Infirmary, Middlesborough, United Kingdom in 1993, and subsequently at Fulbright Scholar program, at the University of Pittsburgh Medical Center(UPMC), Pittsburgh. In 1997, he also worked at Hospital University of Pennsylvania (HUP), Philadelphia, USA, sub-specializing in Rhinology. Dr BS Gendeh has been a senior consultant ENT Surgeon at the National University of Malaysia Medical Center (UKMMC) and Professor at the Department of Otorhinolaryngology Head Neck surgery since 2000. He is involved in clinical activities, surgery, research, teaching medical students, residents and fellows. He has numerous publications in peer-reviewed journals, book chapters and edited books.

Contents

Preface

This book covers selected topics in Otolaryngology, providing a journey into the advancements in various aspects of the field. A collection of manuscripts of this nature involves extensive exposure and accumulation of knowledge from many experienced teaches over many years. It covers both basic and clinical concepts of otolaryngology. Each author contributed his/her own perspectives on each topic adding his/her own theories, future trends and research findings. I would like to dedicate this book to those of you who will pick up the torch and by continued research, close clinical observation and the highest quality of clinical care, as well as by publication and selfless teaching, further advance knowledge in otolaryngology from this point forward.

The chapters in this book are arranged systemically into four sections – Otology, Rhinology, Laryngology, and Head and Neck. This book is intended for general otolaryngologists, sub-specialists, researches, residents and fellows. Therefore, it should encourage researchers and clinicians to innovate new ideas for future basic research and clinical practice.

This book is the outcome of input from multi-national otolaryngologists from around the world with a common goal towards better human health care. Some of the authors are very experienced, while some are newcomers as researchers or clinicians.

This book is accessible online to allow free access to as many readers as possible. It is also available in print for those who do not have internet access or are interested in having their own hard copy. This will ultimately contribute to the global distribution of knowledge in otolaryngology between researchers and clinicians.

I would like to congratulate each and every one of the contributors for their excellent input on each chapter. Each author sacrificed their valuable time and effort to write a chapter resulting in the success of this book. I would like to sincerely thank Ms Martina Durovic and Ms Romina Skomersic, the book Publishing Process Managers for their expert assistance on all issues concerning this book, Ms Ana Nikolic, the Head of Editorial Consultants for her tireless assistance, and to all for choosing me to be the editor of this book. My kind gratitude to the technical editor for arranging the book in a uniform format and InTech – Open Access Publisher, for undertaking this novel mission. I wish that this book will be part of series of books in all sub-specialities of otolaryngology and that it will enhance global collaboration not only between physicians but also for betterment of humankind. I wish the reader an enjoyable journey and hope you will find this book interesting.

I would like to thank my teachers and students from whom I gained knowledge throughout the years. Lastly, I dedicate this book to my wife Dr Pritam Kaur Mangat, my daughter Dr Manvin Kaur Gendeh and my son Dr Hardip Singh Gendeh for all their patience and understanding.

Balwant Singh Gendeh, MBBS(Kashmir), MS (ORL-HNS) M'sia, AM(Mal),FAMM
Senior Consultant ENT Surgeon/Rhinology(Endoscopic Sinus/ Skull Base Surgery and Functional & Cosmetic Nasal Surgery), Department of Otorhinolaryngology-Head Neck Surgery(ORL-HNS)
National University Malaysia Medical Center(UKMMC)
Kuala Lumpur
Malaysia

Section 1

Otology

1

Proteins Involved in Otoconia Formation and Maintenance

Yunxia Wang Lundberg* and Yinfang Xu
Vestibular Neurogenetics Laboratory,
Boys Town National Research Hospital, Omaha, Nebraska
USA

1. Introduction

The vestibule of the inner ear senses head motion for spatial orientation and bodily balance. In vertebrates, the vestibular system consists of three fluid filled semicircular canals, which detect rotational acceleration, and two gravity receptor organs, the utricle and saccule, which respond to linear acceleration and gravity (**Figure 1**). The utricle and saccule are also referred to as the otolithic organs because they contain bio-crystals called otoconia (otolith in fish). These crystals are partially embedded in a honeycomb layer atop a fibrous meshwork, which are the otoconial complex altogether. This complex rests on the stereociliary bundles of hair cells in the utricular and saccular sensory epithelium (aka macula). When there is head motion, the otoconial complex is displaced against the macula, leading to deflection of the hair bundles. This mechanical stimulus is converted into electrical signals by the macular hair cells and transmitted into the central nervous system (CNS) through the afferent vestibular nerve. In the CNS, these electrical signals, combined with other proprioceptive inputs, are interpreted as position and motion data, which then initiate a series of corresponding neuronal responses to maintain the balance of the body. Electrophysiological and behavioral studies show that the size and density of these tiny biominerals determine the amount of stimulus input to the CNS (Anniko et al. 1988; Jones et al. 1999; Jones et al. 2004; Kozel et al. 1998; Simmler et al. 2000a; Trune and Lim 1983; Zhao et al. 2008b).

Otoconia dislocation, malformation and degeneration can result from congenital and environmental factors, including genetic mutation, aging, head trauma and ototoxic drugs, and can lead to various types of vestibular dysfunction such as dizziness/vertigo and imbalance. In humans, BPPV (benign paroxysmal positional vertigo), the most common cause of dizziness/vertigo, is believed to be caused by dislocation of otoconia from the utricle to the ampulla and further in the semicircular canals (Salvinelli et al. 2004; Schuknecht 1962; Schuknecht 1969; Squires et al. 2004). In animals, otoconial deficiency has been found to produce head tilting, swimming difficulty, and reduction or failure of the air-righting reflexes (Everett et al. 2001; Hurle et al. 2003; Nakano et al. 2008; Paffenholz et al. 2004; Simmler et al. 2000a; Zhao et al. 2008b).

Despite the importance of these biominerals, otoconial research is lagging far behind that of other biomineralized structures, such as bone and teeth, partly due to anatomical and

* Corresponding Author

methodological constraints. The mechanisms underlying otoconia formation and maintenance are not yet fully understood. In this review, we will summarize the current state of knowledge about otoconia, focusing on the identified compositions and regulatory proteins and their roles in bio-crystal formation and maintenance. Homologs and analogs of these proteins are also found in fish with similar functions but varied relative abundances, but the review will focus on studies using mice as the latter have similar otoconia and inner ear properties as humans.

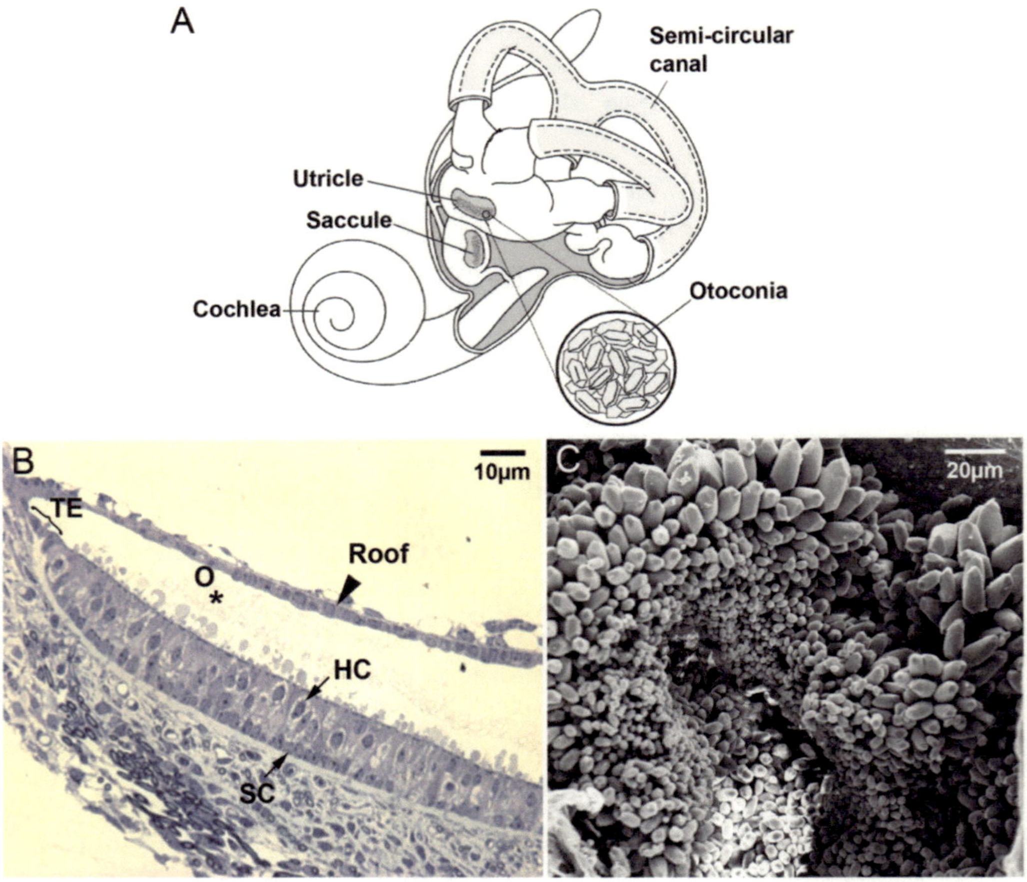

Fig. 1. (**A**) A schematic diagram of the mammalian inner ear. (**B**) A Toluidine blue-stained section of the saccule (P10). (**C**) A scanning electron micrograph of otoconia in the mouse utricle (6.5 months old). HC, hair cells; O, otoconia; SC, supporting cells; TE, transitional epithelium.

2. The roles of otoconial component proteins in crystal formation

Otoconia from higher vertebrates have a barrel-shaped body with triplanar facets at each end (Figure 1C). The core is predominantly organic with a low Ca^{2+} level, and is surrounded by a largely inorganic shell of minute crystallites outlined by the organic matrix (Lim 1984; Lins et al. 2000; Mann et al. 1983; Steyger and Wiederhold 1995; Zhao et al., 2007). Most primitive fishes have apatite otoliths, more advanced fishes have aragonite otoliths, whereas higher levels of vertebrates have calcite otoconia (Carlstrom D 1963; Ross and Pote 1984). Otoliths in lower vertebrates display a daily growth pattern, whereas otoconia in mammals are formed during late embryonic stages, become mature shortly after birth and may undergo maintenance thereafter (Salamat et al. 1980; Thalmann et al. 2001) (Lundberg, unpublished data). Because otoconia/otoliths from animals of different evolutionary levels all have the common $CaCO_3$ component but have various morphologies and crystalline structures and different protein compositions, otoconins (a collective term for otoconial component proteins) must be important for otoconia formation. More importantly, as the mammalian endolymph has an extremely low Ca^{2+} concentration, otoconins may be essential for $CaCO_3$ crystal seeding.

Indeed, recent studies have demonstrated that the shape, size and organization of $CaCO_3$ crystallites in otoconia and otoliths are strictly controlled by an organic matrix (Kang et al. 2008; Murayama et al., 2005; Sollner et al. 2003; Zhao et al. 2007). The organic components of otoconia primarily consist of glycoproteins and proteoglycans (Endo et al. 1991; Ito et al. 1994; Pisam et al. 2002; Pote and Ross 1991; Verpy et al. 1999; Wang et al. 1998; Xu et al. 2010; Zhao et al., 2007). To date, as many as 8 murine otoconins have been identified (Table 1): the predominant otoconial protein, otoconin-90 (Oc90) and other 'minor' otoconins including otolin-1 (aka otolin) (Zhao et al. 2007), fetuin-A (aka countertrypin) (Thalmann et al. 2006; Zhao et al. 2007), osteopontin (aka Spp1) (Sakagami 2000; Takemura et al. 1994; Zhao et al. 2008a), Sparc-like protein 1 (Sc1, aka hevin and Ecm2)(Thalmann et al. 2006; Xu et al. 2010), possibly secreted protein acidic and rich in cysteine (Sparc, aka BM-40 and osteonectin), and dentin matrix protein 1 (DMP1). Those otoconins are expressed in different cells and secreted into the utricular and saccular endolymph. Most of them are highly glycosylated, which confers thermodynamic stability and other properties (see below) on those proteins. They may interact with each other to form the organic scaffold for efficient and orientated deposition of calcium carbonate, and thus determine the size, shape, crystallographic axes and orientation of individual crystallite.

2.1 Otoconin-90 (Oc90) is the essential organizer of the otoconial matrix

Oc90 is the first identified otoconin, and accounts for nearly 90% of the total protein content of otoconia (Pote and Ross 1991; Verpy et al. 1999; Wang et al. 1998). Subsequent studies have revealed that Oc90 is the essential organizer of the otoconial organic matrix by specifically recruiting other matrix components and Ca^{2+} (Yang et al. 2011; Zhao et al. 2007).

Oc90 is structurally similar to secretory phospholipase A2 (sPLA2). Although it likely does not have the catalytic activity of the enzyme due to the substitutions of a few essential residues in the active site (Pote and Ross 1991; Wang et al. 1998), Oc90 possesses the other features of sPLA2. It is a cysteine-rich secretory protein, and has several glycosylation sites and calcium binding capability. The enriched cysteine residues are likely involved in the formation of higher-order protein structures via intra- and inter-molecular disulfide bonds. The intra-molecular disulfide bonds play an important role in protein folding and the stabilization of the tertiary structure, while the disulfide bonds formed between subunits allow dimerization and oligomerization of the protein.

Type	Protein name	Otoconia phenotype of mutant mice	Reference
Constituent proteins	Oc90	Giant otoconia (few to many)	(Zhao et al. 2007)
	Otolin-1	---	---
	Sc1	---	---
	Sparc?	---	---
	KSPG	---	---
	DMP1	---	---
	α-tectorin	Large otoconia but reduced in number	(Legan et al. 2000)
	Osteopontin	Normal otoconia	(Zhao et al. 2008a)
	Fetuin-A	Normal otoconia?	(Xu et al. 2010)
Regulatory proteins	Otopetrin 1	No otoconia	(Hurle et al. 2003)
	Nox3	No otoconia	(Paffenholz et al. 2004)
	Noxo1	No otoconia	(Kiss et al. 2006)
	Noxa1?	---	---
	$p22^{phox}$	No otoconia	(Nakano et al. 2008)
	PMCA2	No otoconia	(Kozel et al. 1998)
	Pendrin	Large otoconia but reduced in number	(Everett et al. 2001)
	TRPVs	---	---
Anchoring proteins	Otogelin	Detached OM	(Simmler et al. 2000a)
	α-tectorin	Large otoconia but reduced in number	(Legan et al. 2000)
	β-tectorin?	---	---
	Otoancorin?	---	---

Table 1. Identified and validated murine otoconial proteins and their importance in otoconia formation by genetic mutation studies. Shaded ones have no measurable impact on bio-crystal formation. ---, no mutant mice available or unknown otoconia/otolith phenotype.

The Ca^{2+} concentrations of the mammalian endolymph are extremely low at ~20 μM (Ferrary et al. 1988; Salt et al. 1989), with a few reporting much higher in the vestibule (Marcus and Wangemann 2009; Salt et al. 1989). This is much lower than what is necessary for the spontaneous formation of calcite crystals, therefore, otoconial proteins are speculated to sequester Ca^{2+}. Indeed, most of the otoconial proteins have structural features for Ca^{2+} binding. Oc90 has 28 (~6%) Glu and 39 (~8%) Asp out of the total 485 amino acids, endowing the molecule with a calculated acidic isoelectric point (pI = 4.5). The measured pI of mature Oc90 is even lower (2.9) due to post-translational modifications such as N-linked glycosylation (Lu et al. 2010). This extreme acidic feature may help Oc90 recruit Ca^{2+} and/or interact with the surface of calcium carbonate crystals to modulate crystal growth. Deletion of Oc90 causes dramatic reduction of matrix-bound Ca^{2+} in the macula of the utricle and saccule (Yang et al. 2011). In the absence of Oc90, the efficiency of crystal formation is reduced by at least 50%, and the organic matrix is greatly reduced, leading to formation of a few giant otoconia with abnormal morphology caused by unordered aggregation of inorganic crystallites (Zhao et al. 2007). A subsequent *in vitro* experiment has also demonstrated that Oc90 can facilitate nucleation, determine the crystal size and morphology in a concentration-dependent manner (Lu et al. 2010). Recent evidence suggests that the formation of otoconia at all in Oc90 null mice may be partially attributed to the compensatory deposition of Sc1 (Xu et al. 2010).

The expression of Oc90 temporally coincides that of otoconia development and growth, also providing evidence for the critical requirement of Oc90 in this unique biomineralization process. Oc90 expression is the earliest among all otolith/otoconia proteins in fish and mice (before embryonic day E9.5 in mice) (Petko et al. 2008; Verpy et al. 1999; Wang et al. 1998), much earlier than the onset of any activities of ion channels/pumps, or the onset of otoconia seeding at around E14.5. Oc90 then recruits other components at the time of their expression to form the organic matrix for calcification (Zhao et al. 2007). When otoconia growth stops at around P7 (postnatal day 7), the expression level of Oc90 significantly decreases in the utricle and saccule (Xu and Lundberg 2012). Although Oc90 has a relatively low abundance in zebrafish otoliths (known as zOtoc1) (Petko et al. 2008), Oc90 morphant fish show more severe phenotypes than morphants for the main otolith matrix protein OMP1 (Murayama et al. 2005; Petko et al. 2008), suggesting that zOc90 (zOtoc1) is essential for the early stages of otolith development (i.e. crystal seeding) whereas OMP regulates crystal growth. Thus, the structure and function of Oc90 is conserved from bony fish to mice (two model systems whose otoconia/otolith are the most studied) regardless of the abundance of the protein in each species.

2.2 Sc1 can partially compensate the function of Oc90

Sc1 was first isolated from a rat brain expression library (Johnston et al. 1990). It is widely expressed in the brain and can be detected from various types of neurons (Lively et al. 2007; McKinnon and Margolskee 1996; Mendis and Brown 1994). As a result, studies of Sc1 have focused on the nervous system. Recently, Thalmann et al. identified Sc1 from mouse otoconia by mass spectrometry (Thalmann et al. 2006). However, Xu et al. (Xu et al. 2010) found that Sc1 was hardly detectable in the wild-type otoconia. Instead, the deposition of Sc1 was drastically increased in otoconia crystals when Oc90 is absent, suggesting a possible role for Sc1 as an alternative process of biomineralization (Xu et al. 2010). *Sc1* knockout mice did not show any obvious phenotypic abnormalities, including vestibular functions (McKinnon et al. 2000)(S. Funk and H. Sage, communication through Thalmann et al. 2006).

Although Sc1 and Oc90 have no significant sequence similarity, the two proteins share analogous structural features. Murine Sc1 is a secreted, acidic and Cys-rich glycoprotein, and belongs to the Sparc family. Its Sparc-like domain consists of a follistatin-like domain followed by an α-helical domain (EC) containing the collagen-binding domain and 2 calcium-binding EF-hands (Maurer et al. 1995). All of these features likely render Sc1 an ideal alternative candidate for otoconia formation in the absence of Oc90. The high abundance of Glu/Asp residues (52 Glu and 87 Asp out of 634 aa) makes the protein highly acidic (pI = 4.2), which, together with the EF-hand motif, provides Sc1 a high affinity for calcium and calcium salts (e.g. calcium carbonate and phosphate). The collagen-binding site in the EC domain can recognize the specific motif of the triple-helical collagen peptide and form a deep 'Phe pocket' upon collagen binding (Hohenester et al. 2008; Sasaki et al. 1998).

The follistatin domain was reported to modulate the process of collagen-binding even though it does not interact with collagen directly (Kaufmann et al. 2004). In addition, the enriched cysteines in the polypeptide backbone of Sc1 may enable the formation of numerous intra- and inter-molecular disulfide bridges, as well as dimerization or even oligomerization of the protein, all of which enable the protein to serve as a rigid and stable framework for inorganic crystal deposition and growth (Chun et al. 2006; Xu et al. 2010).

2.3 Otolin may function similarly to collagen X

Otolin is a secreted glycoprotein present in both otoconial crystals and membranes. The expression level of *otolin* mRNA in the utricle and saccule is much higher than that in the epithelia of non-otolithic inner ear organs (Yang et al. 2011), implicating a potentially critical role of this molecule in otoconia development. In fish, knockdown of otolin led to formation of fused and unstable otoliths (Murayama et al. 2005).

Otolin contains three collagen-like domains in the N-terminal region and a highly conserved globular C1q (gC1q) domain in the C-terminal region, and belongs to the collagen X family and C1q super-family (Deans et al. 2010; Kishore and Reid 1999; Yang et al. 2011). Like collagen X, the N-terminal collagen domains of otolin contain tens of characteristic Gly-X-Y repeats, which can facilitate the formation of collagen triple helix and higher-order structures. Such structural features in otolin may render the protein extremely stable. The C-terminal gC1q domain is more like a target recognition site which may mediate the interaction between otolin and other extracellular proteins. Co-immunoprecipitation experiments demonstrated that Oc90 can interact with both the collagen-like and C1q domains of otolin to form the otoconial matrix framework and to sequester Ca^{2+} for efficient otoconia calcification. Co-expression of Oc90 and otolin in cultured cells leads to significantly increased extracelluar matrix calcification compared with the empty vector, or *Oc90* or *otolin* single transfectants (Yang et al. 2011). Analogously, otolith matrix protein-1 (OMP-1), the main protein in fish otoliths, is required for normal otolith growth and deposition of otolin-1 in the otolith (Murayama et al. 2004; Murayama et al. 2005).

2.4 Keratin sulfate proteoglycan (KSPG) may be critical for otoconia calcification

Proteoglycans are widely distributed at the cell surface and in the extracellular matrix, and are critical for various processes such as cell adhesion, growth, wound healing and fibrosis (Iozzo 1998). A proteoglycan consists of a 'core protein' with covalently attached glycosaminoglycan (GAG) chains. They can interact with other proteoglycans and fibrous matrix proteins, such as collagen, to form a large complex. In addition, proteoglycans have strong negative charges due to the presence of sulfate and uronic acid groups, and can attract positively charged ions, such as Na^{+}, K^{+} and Ca^{2+}. All those features make proteoglycans important players in the extracellular calcification processes. Indeed, both heparan sulfate proteoglycan (HSPG) and chondroitin sulfate proteoglycan (CSPG) are critical for bone and teeth formation. Deletion of those proteins results in various calcification deficiencies (Hassell et al. 2002; Viviano et al. 2005; Xu et al. 1998; Young et al. 2002).

In the inner ear, however, KSPG appears to be the predominant proteoglycan (Xu et al. 2010). KSPG has been detected in chicken and chinchilla otoconia, and shows strong staining in murine otoconia as well (Fermin et al. 1990; Swartz and Santi 1997; Xu et al.

2010). The role of KSPG in otoconia development has not been elucidated yet. It may participate in sequestering and retaining Ca^{2+} for crystal formation because of its strong negative charges. *In vitro* immunoprecipitation results demonstrated that it may interact with Oc90 and otolin to form the matrix framework for the deposition of calcite crystals (Yang et al. 2011).

2.5 Some low abundance otoconins may be dispensable for otoconia formation

Most of the low abundance otoconial proteins play critical roles in bone and/or tooth formation. In contrast, studies by us and other investigators using existing mutant mice have demonstrated that a few of these proteins are dispensable or functionally redundant for otoconia development.

For example, osteopontin, a multifunctional protein initially identified in osteoblasts, is a prominent non-collagen component of the mineralized extracellular matrices of bone and teeth. Osteopontin belongs to the small integrin-binding N-linked glycoprotein (SIBLING) family. As a SIBLING member, osteopontin has an arginine-glycine-aspartate (RGD) motif, which plays an essential role in bone resorption by promoting osteoclast attachment to the bone matrix through cell surface integrins (Oldberg et al. 1986; Rodan and Rodan 1997). Similar to the role of Oc90 in otoconia development, osteopontin acts as an important organizer in bone mineralization. It modulates the bone crystal sizes by inhibiting the hydroxyapatite formation and growth (Boskey et al. 1993; Hunter et al. 1994; Shapses et al. 2003). Osteopontin null mice have altered organization of bone matrix and weakened bone strength, leading to reduced bone fracture toughness (Duvall et al. 2007; Thurner et al. 2010). However, despite its presence in otoconia and vestibular sensory epithelia, osteopontin is dispensable for otoconia formation, and osteopontin knockout mice show normal vestibular morphology and balance function (Zhao et al. 2008a).

Dentin matrix acidic phosphoprotein 1 (DMP1) is another protein that belongs to the SIBLING family. DMP1 was first cloned from dentin and then found in bone. It plays a critical role in apatite crystal seeding and growth in bone and teeth (George et al. 1993; Hirst et al. 1997; MacDougall et al. 1998). DMP1 null mice show severe defects in bone structure. Lv et al. (Lv et al. 2010) recently found that DMP1 null mice developed circling and head shaking behavior resembling vestibular disorders. They attributed these phenotypes to bone defects in the inner ear. However, it should not be excluded that DMP1 deficiency may affect otoconia as the protein is also present in mouse otoconia at a low level (Xu et al. 2010).

Sparc, aka BM-40 or osteonectin, is generally present in tissues undergoing remodeling such as skeletal remodeling and injury repair (Bolander et al. 1988; Hohenester et al. 1997; Sage and Vernon 1994). The protein is a normal component of osteiod, the newly formed bone matrix critical for the initiation of mineralization during bone development (Bianco et al. 1985; Termine et al. 1981). Sparc has a high affinity for both Ca^{2+} and several types of collagen (Bolander et al. 1988; Hohenester et al. 2008; Maurer et al. 1995). These features likely account for the importance of Sparc in bone formation, and possibly in otoconia formation. Indeed, Sparc is also required for otolith formation in fish (Kang et al. 2008). In the wild-type murine otoconia, however, Sparc is present at an extremely low level (Xu et al. 2010) that it may not play a significant role in crystal formation. Instead, the longer form Sc1 is the preferred scaffold protein when Oc90 is absent (Xu et al. 2010).

Fetuin-A, also known as α2-HS-glycoprotein or countertrypin, is a hepatic secreted protein that promotes bone mineralization. It is among the most abundant non-collagen proteins found in bone (Quelch et al. 1984). Several recent studies demonstrated that fetuin-A can bind calcium and phosphate to form a calciprotein particle and prevent the precipitation of these minerals from serum (Heiss et al. 2003; Price et al. 2002), which may explain the role of fetuin-A in bone calcification and its potent inhibition of ectopic mineralization in soft tissues (Schafer et al. 2003; Westenfeld et al. 2007; Westenfeld et al. 2009). However, fetuin-A null mice have normal bone under regular dietary conditions (Jahnen-Dechent et al. 1997). Fetuin-A is present in otoconia crystals (Zhao et al. 2007), but null mice for the protein do not show balance deficits (Jahnen-Dechent, communication in Thalmann et al., 2006), therefore, it is unlikely that the protein has a major impact on otoconia genesis.

Taken together, findings on these low abundance otoconins indicate similarities and differences between bone and otoconia biomineralization.

3. The roles of regulatory proteins in otoconia formation

Otoconia formation depends on both organic and inorganic components that are secreted into the vestibular endolymph. Non-component regulatory proteins affect otoconia development and maintenance likely by several ways: (1) by influencing the secretion (Sollner et al. 2004), structural and functional modification of the component and anchoring proteins (Lundberg, unpublished data), and (2) by spatially and temporally increasing chemical gradients of Ca^{2+}, HCO_3^-, H^+ and possibly other ions/anions to establish an appropriate micro-environmental condition for crystal seeding and growth.

3.1 NADPH oxidase 3 (Nox3) and associated proteins are essential for otoconia formation

The Noxs are a family of enzymes whose primary function is to produce ROS (reactive oxygen species). These proteins participate in a wide range of pathological and physiological processes. To date, seven Nox family members, Nox1-Nox5, Duox1 and Duox2, have been identified in mammals (Bedard and Krause 2007). Noxs serve as the core catalytic components, and their activities are regulated by cytosolic partners such as $p22^{phox}$, Nox organizers (Noxo1, $p47^{phox}$ and $p40^{phox}$), and Nox activators (Noxa1 and $p67^{phox}$).

Among the identified Nox family members, Nox3 is primarily expressed in the inner ear and is essential for otoconia development (Banfi et al. 2004; Cheng et al. 2001; Paffenholz et al. 2004). It interacts with $p22^{phox}$ and Noxo1 to form a functional NADPH oxidase complex, and all three components are required for otoconia development and normal balance in mice (Kiss et al. 2006; Nakano et al. 2007; Nakano et al. 2008; Paffenholz et al. 2004). However, the mechanisms underlying the requirement of Nox-related proteins for otoconia formation are poorly understood. One possible role of Nox3 is to oxidize otoconial proteins, including Oc90, which then undergo conformational changes to trigger crystal nucleation. Indeed, our recent unpublished data show that Nox3 modifies the structures of a few otoconia proteins (Xu et al. 2012).

A novel mechanism proposed by Nakano et al. (Nakano et al. 2008) states that while the Nox3-complex passes electrons from intracellular NADPH to extracellular oxygen, the plasma membrane becomes depolarized. Such depolarization of the apical membrane would elevate endolymphatic Ca^{2+} concentration by preventing cellular Ca^{2+} uptake from endolymph, and by increasing paracellular ion permeability to allow Ca^{2+} influx from perilymph to endolymph. In addition, Nox3-derived superoxide may react with endolymphatic protons and thereby elevate the pH so that $CaCO_3$ can form and be maintained.

3.2 Otopetrin 1 may mobilize Ca^{2+} for $CaCO_3$ formation

Otopetrin (Otop1), a protein with multiple transmembrane domains, is essential for the formation of otoconia/otolith in the inner ear (Hughes et al. 2004; Hurle et al. 2003; Sollner et al., 2004). The protein is conserved in all vertebrates, and its biochemical function was first revealed by studying the phenotypes of two mutants, the *tilted* (*tlt*) and *mergulhador* (*mlh*) mice, which carry single-point mutations in the predicted transmembrane (TM) domains (*tlt*, Ala_{151}→Glu in TM3; *mlh*, Leu_{408}→Gln in TM9) of the *Otop1* gene. Both *tlt* and *mlh* homozygous mutant mice show non-syndromic vestibular disorders caused by the absence of otoconia crystals in the utricle and saccule (Hurle et al. 2003; Zhao et al. 2008b). Those mutations in *Otop1* do not appear to affect other inner ear organs, making *tlt* and *mlh* excellent tools to investigate how Otop1 participates in the development of otoconia and in what aspects the absence of otoconia impacts balance functions.

In fish, expression of *Otop1* is in both hair cells and supporting cells before otolith seeding, but is restricted in hair cells during otolith growth (Hurle et al. 2003; Sollner et al. 2004). In mice, *Otop1* exhibits complementary mRNA expression pattern with Oc90 in the developing otocyst, and high Otop1 protein level is visible in the gelatinous membrane overlying the sensory epithelium, suggesting that it may be integral to the membrane vesicles released into the gelatinous layer (Hurle et al. 2003). However, a more recent study by Kim and colleagues using a different antibody (Kim et al. 2010) demonstrated that Otop1 is expressed in the extrastriolar epithelia of the utricle and saccule, and is specifically localized in the apical end of the supporting cells and a subset of transitional cells. They also found that the *tlt* and *mlh* mutations of Otop1 change the subcelluar localization of the mutant protein, and may underlie its function in otoconia development (Kim et al. 2011).

Both *in vitro* and *ex vivo* studies demonstrated that one of the functions of Otop1 is to modulate intra- and extracellular Ca^{2+} concentrations by specifically inhibiting purinergic receptor P2Y, depleting of endoplasmic reticulum Ca^{2+} stores and mediating influx of extracellular Ca^{2+} (Hughes et al. 2007; Kim et al. 2010). Under normal conditions, the concentration of Ca^{2+} in the mammalian endolymph is much lower than that in the perilymph and other extracellular fluids, and is insufficient to support normal growth of otoconia. Hence, Otop1 may serve as the indispensible Ca^{2+} source that supports otoconia mineralization.

Moreover, Otop1 may also regulate the secretion of components required for otoconia formation. In zebrafish, Otop1 was shown to affect the secretion of *starmaker*, a protein essential for otolith formation, in the sensory epithelia (Sollner et al. 2004).

3.3 PMCA2 is a critical source of Ca^{2+} for $CaCO_3$ formation

Calmodulin-sensitive plasma membrane Ca^{2+}-ATPases (PMCAs) are vital regulators of otoconia formation by extruding Ca^{2+} from hair cells and thereby maintaining the appropriate Ca^{2+} concentration near the plasma membrane. There are four isoforms of mammalian PMCA (PMCA1-4) encoded by four distinct genes and each of them undergoes alternative exon splicing in two regions (Keeton et al. 1993). All four PMCAs are expressed in the mammalian cochlea and extrude Ca^{2+} from hair cell stereocilia, whereas PMCA2a, a protein encoded by *Atp2b2* gene, is the only PMCA isoform present in vestibular hair bundles (Crouch and Schulte 1996; Dumont et al. 2001; Furuta et al. 1998; Yamoah et al. 1998). Null mutation in *Atp2b2* results in the absence of otoconia and subsequent balance deficits (Kozel et al. 1998), underpinning the importance of PMCA2 in otoconial genesis.

3.4 Pendrin regulates endolymph pH, composition and volume

Pendrin, encoded by *Slc26a4*, is an anion transporter which mediates the exchange of Cl^-, I^-, OH^-, HCO_3^-, or formate, across a variety of epithelia (Scott et al. 1999; Scott and Karniski 2000). In the inner ear, pendrin is primarily expressed in the endolymphatic duct and sac, the transitional epithelia adjacent to the macula of the utricle and saccule, and the external sulcus of the cochlea (Everett et al. 1999). Pendrin is critical for maintaining the appropriate anionic and ionic composition and volume of the endolymphatic fluid, presumably due to HCO_3^- secretion. Mutations in human *SLC26A4* are responsible for Pendred syndrome, a genetic disorder which causes early hearing loss in children (Dai et al. 2009; Luxon et al. 2003). Studies using an *Slc26a4* knockout mouse model have revealed that pendrin dysfunction can cause an enlargement and acidification of inner ear membrane labyrinth and thyroid at embryonic stages, leading to deafness, balance disorders and goiter similar to the symptoms of human Pendred syndrome (Everett et al. 2001; Kim and Wangemann 2010; Kim and Wangemann 2011). The mice have much lower endolymphatic pH, resulting in the formation of giant crystals with reduced numbers in both the utricle and saccule (Everett et al. 2001; Nakaya et al. 2007). Recently, Dror et al. have also demonstrated that a recessive missense mutation within the highly conserved region of *slc26a4* results in a mutant pendrin protein with impaired transport activity. This mutant mouse has severely abnormal mineral composition, size and shape of otoconia, i.e., giant $CaCO_3$ crystals in the utricle at all ages, giant CaOx crystals in the saccule of older adults, and ectopic giant stones in the crista (Dror et al. 2010). Therefore, pendrin participates in otoconia formation through providing HCO_3^-, which is essential for forming $CaCO_3$ crystals and for buffering the endolymphatic pH. Pendrin can also buffer pH through other anions such as formate.

3.5 Carbonic anhydrase (CA) provides HCO_3^- and maintains appropriate pH for otoconia formation and maintenance

CA catalyzes the hydration of CO_2 to yield HCO_3^- and related species, and is thus thought to be important for otoconia formation by producing HCO_3^- and keeping appropriate endolymph pH. CA is widely present in the sensory and non-sensory epithelia of the inner ear (Lim et al. 1983; Pedrozo et al. 1997), especially the developing endolymphatic sac of mammalian embryos contain high levels of CA. Administration of acetazolamide, a CA inhibitor, in the latter tissue can decrease the luminal pH and HCO_3^- concentration (Kido et al. 1991; Tsujikawa et al. 1993). Injection of acetazolamide into the yolk sac of developing chick embryos alters and inhibits normal otoconial morphogenesis (Kido et al. 1991). Activation/deactivation of macular CA under different gravity is associated with changes in otolith sizes in fish (Anken et al. 2004). Immunohistochemstry shows that CAII is co-expressed with pendrin in the same cells in the endolymphatic sac, suggesting that those two proteins may cooperate in maintaining the normal function of the endolymphatic sac (Dou et al. 2004), which is an important tissue for endolymph production.

In addition to CA, HCO_3^--ATPase and Cl^-/HCO_3^--exchangers are involved in the transepithelial transport of bicarbonate ions to the endolymph, and affect carbon incorporation into otoliths (Tohse and Mugiya 2001).

3.6 Transient receptor potential vanilloids (TRPVs) may also regulate endolymph homeostasis

Studies suggest that TRPVs may also play an important part in fluid homeostasis of the inner ear. All TRPVs (TRPV1-6) are expressed in vestibular and cochlear sensory epithelia (Ishibashi et al. 2008; Takumida et al. 2009). In addition, TRPV4 is also present in the endolymphatic sac and presumably acts as an osmoreceptor in cell and fluid volume regulation (Kumagami et al. 2009). Both TRPV5 and TRPV6 are found in vestibular semi-circular canal ducts (Yamauchi et al. 2010). In pendrin-deficient mice, the acidic vestibular endolymphatic pH is thought to inhibit the acid-sensitive TRPV5/6 calcium channels and lead to a significantly higher Ca^{2+} concentration in the endolymph, which may be another factor causing the formation of abnormal otoconia crystals (Nakaya et al. 2007). However, direct evidence has yet to be presented on whether TRPV-deficiency will lead to otoconia abnormalities.

4. The roles of anchoring proteins in the pathogenesis of otoconia-related imbalance and dizziness/vertigo

The inner ear acellular membranes, namely the otoconial membranes in the utricule and saccule, the cupula in the ampulla, and the tectorial membrane in the cochlea, cover their corresponding sensory epithelia, have contact with the stereocilia of hair cells and thus play crutial role in mechanotransduction. In the utricle and saccule, otoconia crystals are attached to and partially embedded in a honeycomb layer above a fibrous meshwork, which are collectively called otoconial membranes, and are responsible for the site-specific anchoring of otoconia. Disruption of the otoconial membrane structure may cause the detachment and dislocation of otoconia and thus vestibular disorders.

The acellular structures of the inner ear consist of collagenous and non-collagenous glycoproteins and proteoglycans. Several types of collagen, including type II, IV, V and IX, have been identified in the mammalian tectorial membrane (Richardson et al. 1987; Slepecky et al. 1992). In the otoconial membranes, however, otolin is likely the main collagenous component. As to the noncollagenous constituents, three glycoproteins, otogelin, α-tectorin and β-tectorin, have been identified in the inner ear acellular membranes in mice to date (Cohen-Salmon et al. 1997; Legan et al. 1997). The proteoglycan in mouse otoconia is keratin sulfate proteoglycan (KSPG) (Xu et al. 2010).

Otogelin is a glycoprotein that is present and restricted to all acellular membranes of the inner ear (Cohen-Salmon et al. 1997). At early embryonic stages, otogelin is produced by the supporting cells of the sensory epithelia of the developing vestibule and cochlea, and presents a complementary distribution pattern with Myosin VIIA, a marker of hair cells and precursors (El-Amraoui et al. 2001). At adult stages, otogelin is still expressed in the vestibular supporting cells, but become undetectable in the cochlear cells. Otogelin may be required for the attachment of the otoconial membranes and consequently site-specific anchoring of otoconia crystals. Dysfunction of otogelin in either the *Otog* knockout mice or the twister mutant mice leads to severe vestibular deficits, which is postulated to be caused by displaced otoconial membranes in the utricle and saccule (Simmler et al. 2000a; Simmler et al. 2000b).

α-tectorin and β-tectorin, named with reference to their localization, are major non-collagenous glycoproteins of the mammalian tectorial membrane (Legan et al. 1997). In addition, these two proteins are abundant constituents of the otoconial membranes, but are not present in the cupula (Goodyear and Richardson 2002; Xu et al. 2010). In the mouse vestibule, α-tectorin is mainly expressed between E12.5 and P15 in the transitional zone, as well as in a region that is producing the accessory membranes of the utricle and saccule, but absent in the ampullae of semicircular canals (Rau et al. 1999). Mice with targeted deletion of α-tectorin display reduced otoconial membranes and a few scattered giant otoconia (Legan et al. 2000).

β-tectorin has a spatial and temporal expression pattern distinct from that of α-tectorin in the vestibule. It is expressed in the striolar region of the utricule and saccule from E14.5 until at least P150 (Legan et al. 1997; Rau et al. 1999), suggesting that the striolar and extrastriolar region of the otoconial membranes may have different composition. *Tectb* null mice show structural disruption of the tectorial membrane and hearing loss at low frequencies (Russell et al. 2007). However, no vestibular defects have been reported.

Interestingly, both otogelin and α-tectorin possess several von Willebrand factor type D (VWFD) domains containing the multimerization consensus site CGLC (Mayadas and Wagner 1992). This structural feature is probably essential for the multimer assembly of those proteins to form filament and higher order structures.

Otoancorin is a glycosylphosphatidylinositol (GPI)-anchored protein specific to the interface between the sensory epithelia and their overlying acellular membranes of the inner ear (Zwaenepoel et al. 2002). In the vestibule, otoancorin is expressed on the apical surface of the supporting cells in the utricle, saccule and crista. Although the function of otoancorin has not been elucidated, the C-terminal GPI anchor motif of this protein likely facilitates the otoancorin-cell surface adhesion. It is proposed that otoancorin may interact with the other components of the otoconial membranes, such as otogelin and tectorins, and with the epithelial surface, thus mediating the attachment of otoconial membranes to the underlying sensory epithelia (Zwaenepoel et al. 2002).

5. Summary and future direction

Like other biominerals such as bone and teeth, otoconia primarily differ from their non-biological counterparts by their protein-mediated nucleation, growth and maintenance processes. With only $CaCO_3$ crystallites and less than a dozen glycoprotein/proteoglycan components, otoconia are seemingly simple biological structures compared to other tissues. Yet, the processes governing otoconia formation are multiple and involve many more molecules and much complicated cellular and extracellular events including matrix assembly, endolymph homeostasis and proper function of ion channels/pumps. Expression of the involved genes is well orchestrated temporally and spatially, and the functions of their proteins are finely coordinated for optimal crystal formation. Some of these proteins also play vital roles in normal cellular activities (e.g. hair cell stimulation) and other vestibular function. Some other proteins (e.g. otolin, tectorins and otoancorin) still need to be further investigated of their functions. Animal models with targeted disruption of otolin and otoancorin are not yet available, and animal models with double mutant genes (e.g. Oc90 and Sc1) have not been studied but can yield more information on the precise role of the organic matrix in $CaCO_3$ nucleation and growth. Additional studies are needed to further uncover the mechanisms underlying the spatial specific formation of otoconia. The high prevalence and debilitating nature of otoconia-related dizziness/vertigo and balance disorders necessitate these types of studies as they are the foundation required to uncover the molecular etiology.

6. Acknowledgements

The work was supported by grants from the National Institute on Deafness and Other Communication Disorders (R01 DC008603 and DC008603-S1 to Y.W.L.).

7. References

Anken RH, Beier M, Rahmann H. Hypergravity decreases carbonic anhydrase-reactivity in inner ear maculae of fish. J.Exp.Zoolog.A Comp Exp.Biol. 301:815-819, 2004.

Anniko M, Wenngren BI, Wroblewski R. Aberrant elemental composition of otoconia in the dancer mouse mutant with a semidominant gene causing a morphogenetic type of inner ear defect. Acta Otolaryngol. 106:208-212, 1988.

Banfi B, Malgrange B, Knisz J, Steger K, Dubois-Dauphin M, Krause KH. NOX3, a superoxide-generating NADPH oxidase of the inner ear. J.Biol.Chem. 279:46065-46072, 2004.

Bedard K and Krause KH. The NOX family of ROS-generating NADPH oxidases: physiology and pathophysiology. Physiol Rev. 87:245-313, 2007.

Bianco P, Hayashi Y, Silvestrini G, Termine JD, Bonucci E. Osteonectin and Gla-protein in calf bone: ultrastructural immunohistochemical localization using the Protein A-gold method. Calcif.Tissue Int. 37:684-686, 1985.

Bolander ME, Young MF, Fisher LW, Yamada Y, Termine JD. Osteonectin cDNA sequence reveals potential binding regions for calcium and hydroxyapatite and shows homologies with both a basement membrane protein (SPARC) and a serine proteinase inhibitor (ovomucoid). Proc.Natl.Acad.Sci.U.S.A 85:2919-2923, 1988.

Boskey AL, Maresca M, Ullrich W, Doty SB, Butler WT, Prince CW. Osteopontin-hydroxyapatite interactions in vitro: inhibition of hydroxyapatite formation and growth in a gelatin-gel. Bone Miner. 22:147-159, 1993.

Carlstrom D. Crystallographic study of vertebrate otoliths. Biological Bulletin 125:441-463, 1963.

Cheng G, Cao Z, Xu X, van Meir EG, Lambeth JD. Homologs of gp91phox: cloning and tissue expression of Nox3, Nox4, and Nox5. Gene 269:131-140, 2001.

Chun YH, Yamakoshi Y, Kim JW, Iwata T, Hu JC, Simmer JP. Porcine SPARC: isolation from dentin, cDNA sequence, and computer model. Eur.J.Oral Sci. 114 Suppl 1:78-85, 2006.

Cohen-Salmon M, El-Amraoui A, Leibovici M, Petit C. Otogelin: a glycoprotein specific to the acellular membranes of the inner ear. Proc.Natl.Acad.Sci.U.S.A 94:14450-14455, 1997.

Crouch JJ and Schulte BA. Identification and cloning of site C splice variants of plasma membrane Ca-ATPase in the gerbil cochlea. Hear.Res. 101:55-61, 1996.

Dai P, Stewart AK, Chebib F, Hsu A, Rozenfeld J, Huang D, Kang D, Lip V, Fang H, Shao H, Liu X, Yu F, Yuan H, Kenna M, Miller DT, Shen Y, Yang W, Zelikovic I, Platt OS, Han D, Alper SL, Wu BL. Distinct and novel SLC26A4/Pendrin mutations in Chinese and U.S. patients with nonsyndromic hearing loss. Physiol Genomics 38:281-290, 2009.

Deans MR, Peterson JM, Wong GW. Mammalian Otolin: a multimeric glycoprotein specific to the inner ear that interacts with otoconial matrix protein Otoconin-90 and Cerebellin-1. PLoS.ONE. 5:e12765-2010.

Dou H, Xu J, Wang Z, Smith AN, Soleimani M, Karet FE, Greinwald JH, Jr., Choo D. Co-expression of pendrin, vacuolar H+-ATPase alpha4-subunit and carbonic anhydrase II in epithelial cells of the murine endolymphatic sac. J.Histochem.Cytochem. 52:1377-1384, 2004.

Dror AA, Politi Y, Shahin H, Lenz DR, Dossena S, Nofziger C, Fuchs H, Hrabe de AM, Paulmichl M, Weiner S, Avraham KB. Calcium oxalate stone formation in the inner ear as a result of an Slc26a4 mutation. J.Biol.Chem. 285:21724-21735, 2010.

Dumont RA, Lins U, Filoteo AG, Penniston JT, Kachar B, Gillespie PG. Plasma membrane Ca2+-ATPase isoform 2a is the PMCA of hair bundles. J.Neurosci. 21:5066-5078, 2001.

Duvall CL, Taylor WR, Weiss D, Wojtowicz AM, Guldberg RE. Impaired angiogenesis, early callus formation, and late stage remodeling in fracture healing of osteopontin-deficient mice. J.Bone Miner.Res. 22:286-297, 2007.

El-Amraoui A, Cohen-Salmon M, Petit C, Simmler MC. Spatiotemporal expression of otogelin in the developing and adult mouse inner ear. Hear.Res. 158:151-159, 2001.

Endo S, Sekitani T, Yamashita H, Kido T, Masumitsu Y, Ogata M, Miura M. Glycoconjugates in the otolithic organ of the developing chick embryo. Acta Otolaryngol.Suppl 481:116-120, 1991.

Everett LA, Belyantseva IA, Noben-Trauth K, Cantos R, Chen A, Thakkar SI, Hoogstraten-Miller SL, Kachar B, Wu DK, Green ED. Targeted disruption of mouse Pds provides insight about the inner-ear defects encountered in Pendred syndrome. Hum.Mol.Genet. 10:153-161, 2001.

Everett LA, Morsli H, Wu DK, Green ED. Expression pattern of the mouse ortholog of the Pendred's syndrome gene (Pds) suggests a key role for pendrin in the inner ear. Proc.Natl.Acad.Sci.U.S.A 96:9727-9732, 1999.

Fermin CD, Lovett AE, Igarashi M, Dunner K, Jr. Immunohistochemistry and histochemistry of the inner ear gelatinous membranes and statoconia of the chick (Gallus domesticus). Acta Anat.(Basel) 138:75-83, 1990.

Ferrary E, Tran Ba HP, Roinel N, Bernard C, Amiel C. Calcium and the inner ear fluids. Acta Otolaryngol.Suppl 460:13-17, 1988.

Furuta H, Luo L, Hepler K, Ryan AF. Evidence for differential regulation of calcium by outer versus inner hair cells: plasma membrane Ca-ATPase gene expression. Hear.Res. 123:10-26, 1998.

George A, Sabsay B, Simonian PA, Veis A. Characterization of a novel dentin matrix acidic phosphoprotein. Implications for induction of biomineralization. J.Biol.Chem. 268:12624-12630, 1993.

Goodyear RJ and Richardson GP. Extracellular matrices associated with the apical surfaces of sensory epithelia in the inner ear: molecular and structural diversity. J.Neurobiol. 53:212-227, 2002.

Hassell J, Yamada Y, rikawa-Hirasawa E. Role of perlecan in skeletal development and diseases. Glycoconj.J. 19:263-267, 2002.

Heiss A, DuChesne A, Denecke B, Grotzinger J, Yamamoto K, Renne T, Jahnen-Dechent W. Structural basis of calcification inhibition by alpha 2-HS glycoprotein/fetuin-A. Formation of colloidal calciprotein particles. J.Biol.Chem. 278:13333-13341, 2003.

Hirst KL, Ibaraki-O'Connor K, Young MF, Dixon MJ. Cloning and expression analysis of the bovine dentin matrix acidic phosphoprotein gene. J.Dent.Res. 76:754-760, 1997.

Hohenester E, Maurer P, Timpl R. Crystal structure of a pair of follistatin-like and EF-hand calcium-binding domains in BM-40. EMBO J. 16:3778-3786, 1997.

Hohenester E, Sasaki T, Giudici C, Farndale RW, Bachinger HP. Structural basis of sequence-specific collagen recognition by SPARC. Proc.Natl.Acad.Sci.U.S.A 105:18273-18277, 2008.

Hughes I, Blasiole B, Huss D, Warchol ME, Rath NP, Hurle B, Ignatova E, Dickman JD, Thalmann R, Levenson R, Ornitz DM. Otopetrin 1 is required for otolith formation in the zebrafish Danio rerio. Dev.Biol. 276:391-402, 2004.

Hughes I, Saito M, Schlesinger PH, Ornitz DM. Otopetrin 1 activation by purinergic nucleotides regulates intracellular calcium. Proc.Natl.Acad.Sci.U.S.A 104:12023-12028, 2007.

Hunter GK, Kyle CL, Goldberg HA. Modulation of crystal formation by bone phosphoproteins: structural specificity of the osteopontin-mediated inhibition of hydroxyapatite formation. Biochem.J. 300 (Pt 3):723-728, 1994.

Hurle B, Ignatova E, Massironi SM, Mashimo T, Rios X, Thalmann I, Thalmann R, Ornitz DM. Non-syndromic vestibular disorder with otoconial agenesis in tilted/mergulhador mice caused by mutations in otopetrin 1. Hum.Mol.Genet. 12:777-789, 2003.

Iozzo RV. Matrix proteoglycans: from molecular design to cellular function. Annu.Rev.Biochem. 67:609-652, 1998.

Ishibashi T, Takumida M, Akagi N, Hirakawa K, Anniko M. Expression of transient receptor potential vanilloid (TRPV) 1, 2, 3, and 4 in mouse inner ear. Acta Otolaryngol. 128:1286-1293, 2008.

Ito M, Spicer SS, Schulte BA. Histochemical detection of glycogen and glycoconjugates in the inner ear with modified concanavalin A-horseradish peroxidase procedures. Histochem.J. 26:437-446, 1994.

Jahnen-Dechent W, Schinke T, Trindl A, Muller-Esterl W, Sablitzky F, Kaiser S, Blessing M. Cloning and targeted deletion of the mouse fetuin gene. J.Biol.Chem. 272:31496-31503, 1997.

Johnston IG, Paladino T, Gurd JW, Brown IR. Molecular cloning of SC1: a putative brain extracellular matrix glycoprotein showing partial similarity to osteonectin/BM40/SPARC. Neuron 4:165-176, 1990.

Jones SM, Erway LC, Bergstrom RA, Schimenti JC, Jones TA. Vestibular responses to linear acceleration are absent in otoconia-deficient C57BL/6JEi-het mice. Hear.Res. 135:56-60, 1999.

Jones SM, Erway LC, Johnson KR, Yu H, Jones TA. Gravity receptor function in mice with graded otoconial deficiencies. Hear.Res. 191:34-40, 2004.

Kang YJ, Stevenson AK, Yau PM, Kollmar R. Sparc protein is required for normal growth of zebrafish otoliths. J.Assoc.Res.Otolaryngol. 9:436-451, 2008.

Kaufmann B, Muller S, Hanisch FG, Hartmann U, Paulsson M, Maurer P, Zaucke F. Structural variability of BM-40/SPARC/osteonectin glycosylation: implications for collagen affinity. Glycobiology 14:609-619, 2004.

Keeton TP, Burk SE, Shull GE. Alternative splicing of exons encoding the calmodulin-binding domains and C termini of plasma membrane Ca(2+)-ATPase isoforms 1, 2, 3, and 4. J.Biol.Chem. 268:2740-2748, 1993.

Kido T, Sekitani T, Yamashita H, Endo S, Masumitsu Y, Shimogori H. Effects of carbonic anhydrase inhibitor on the otolithic organs of developing chick embryos. Am.J.Otolaryngol. 12:191-195, 1991.

Kim E, Hyrc KL, Speck J, Lundberg YW, Salles FT, Kachar B, Goldberg MP, Warchol ME, Ornitz DM. Regulation of cellular calcium in vestibular supporting cells by Otopetrin 1. J.Neurophysiol.2010.

Kim E, Hyrc KL, Speck J, Salles FT, Lundberg YW, Goldberg MP, Kachar B, Warchol ME, Ornitz DM. Missense mutations in Otopetrin 1 affect subcellular localization and inhibition of purinergic signaling in vestibular supporting cells. Mol.Cell Neurosci. 46:655-661, 2011.

Kim HM and Wangemann P. Failure of fluid absorption in the endolymphatic sac initiates cochlear enlargement that leads to deafness in mice lacking pendrin expression. PLoS.ONE. 5:e14041-2010.

Kim HM and Wangemann P. Epithelial cell stretching and luminal acidification lead to a retarded development of stria vascularis and deafness in mice lacking pendrin. PLoS.ONE. 6:e17949-2011.

Kishore U and Reid KB. Modular organization of proteins containing C1q-like globular domain. Immunopharmacology 42:15-21, 1999.

Kiss PJ, Knisz J, Zhang Y, Baltrusaitis J, Sigmund CD, Thalmann R, Smith RJ, Verpy E, Banfi B. Inactivation of NADPH oxidase organizer 1 Results in Severe Imbalance. Curr.Biol. 16:208-213, 2006.

Kozel PJ, Friedman RA, Erway LC, Yamoah EN, Liu LH, Riddle T, Duffy JJ, Doetschman T, Miller ML, Cardell EL, Shull GE. Balance and hearing deficits in mice with a null mutation in the gene encoding plasma membrane Ca2+-ATPase isoform 2. J.Biol.Chem. 273:18693-18696, 1998.

Kumagami H, Terakado M, Sainoo Y, Baba A, Fujiyama D, Fukuda T, Takasaki K, Takahashi H. Expression of the osmotically responsive cationic channel TRPV4 in the endolymphatic sac. Audiol.Neurootol. 14:190-197, 2009.

Legan PK, Lukashkina VA, Goodyear RJ, Kossi M, Russell IJ, Richardson GP. A targeted deletion in alpha-tectorin reveals that the tectorial membrane is required for the gain and timing of cochlear feedback. Neuron 28:273-285, 2000.

Legan PK, Rau A, Keen JN, Richardson GP. The mouse tectorins. Modular matrix proteins of the inner ear homologous to components of the sperm-egg adhesion system. J.Biol.Chem. 272:8791-8801, 1997.

Lim DJ. Otoconia in health and disease. A review. Ann.Otol.Rhinol.Laryngol.Suppl 112:17-24, 1984.

Lim DJ, Karabinas C, Trune DR. Histochemical localization of carbonic anhydrase in the inner ear. Am.J.Otolaryngol. 4:33-42, 1983.

Lins U, Farina M, Kurc M, Riordan G, Thalmann R, Thalmann I, Kachar B. The otoconia of the guinea pig utricle: internal structure, surface exposure, and interactions with the filament matrix. J.Struct.Biol. 131:67-78, 2000.

Lively S, Ringuette MJ, Brown IR. Localization of the extracellular matrix protein SC1 to synapses in the adult rat brain. Neurochem.Res. 32:65-71, 2007.

Lu W, Zhou D, Freeman JJ, Thalmann I, Ornitz DM, Thalmann R. In vitro effects of recombinant otoconin 90 upon calcite crystal growth. Significance of tertiary structure. Hear.Res. 268:172-183, 2010.

Luxon LM, Cohen M, Coffey RA, Phelps PD, Britton KE, Jan H, Trembath RC, Reardon W. Neuro-otological findings in Pendred syndrome. Int.J.Audiol. 42:82-88, 2003.

Lv K, Huang H, Lu Y, Qin C, Li Z, Feng JQ. Circling behavior developed in Dmp1 null mice is due to bone defects in the vestibular apparatus. Int.J.Biol.Sci. 6:537-545, 2010.

MacDougall M, Gu TT, Luan X, Simmons D, Chen J. Identification of a novel isoform of mouse dentin matrix protein 1: spatial expression in mineralized tissues. J.Bone Miner.Res. 13:422-431, 1998.

Mann S, Parker SB, Ross MD, Skarnulis AJ, Williams RJ. The ultrastructure of the calcium carbonate balance organs of the inner ear: an ultra-high resolution electron microscopy study. Proc.R.Soc.Lond B Biol.Sci. 218:415-424, 1983.

Marcus DC and Wangemann P. Cochlear and Vestibular Function and Dysfunction. In *Physiology and Pathology of Chloride Transporters and Channels in the Nervous System--From molecules to diseases.* Edited by Alvarez-Leefmans FJ, Delpire E. Elsevier; 2009:421-433.

Maurer P, Hohenadl C, Hohenester E, Gohring W, Timpl R, Engel J. The C-terminal portion of BM-40 (SPARC/osteonectin) is an autonomously folding and crystallisable domain that binds calcium and collagen IV. J.Mol.Biol. 253:347-357, 1995.

Mayadas TN and Wagner DD. Vicinal cysteines in the prosequence play a role in von Willebrand factor multimer assembly. Proc.Natl.Acad.Sci.U.S.A 89:3531-3535, 1992.

McKinnon PJ and Margolskee RF. SC1: a marker for astrocytes in the adult rodent brain is upregulated during reactive astrocytosis. Brain Res. 709:27-36, 1996.

McKinnon PJ, McLaughlin SK, Kapsetaki M, Margolskee RF. Extracellular matrix-associated protein Sc1 is not essential for mouse development. Mol.Cell Biol. 20:656-660, 2000.

Mendis DB and Brown IR. Expression of the gene encoding the extracellular matrix glycoprotein SPARC in the developing and adult mouse brain. Brain Res.Mol.Brain Res. 24:11-19, 1994.

Murayama E, Herbomel P, Kawakami A, Takeda H, Nagasawa H. Otolith matrix proteins OMP-1 and Otolin-1 are necessary for normal otolith growth and their correct anchoring onto the sensory maculae. Mech.Dev. 122:791-803, 2005.

Murayama E, Takagi Y, Nagasawa H. Immunohistochemical localization of two otolith matrix proteins in the otolith and inner ear of the rainbow trout, Oncorhynchus mykiss: comparative aspects between the adult inner ear and embryonic otocysts. Histochem.Cell Biol. 121:155-166, 2004.

Nakano Y, Banfi B, Jesaitis AJ, Dinauer MC, Allen LA, Nauseef WM. Critical roles for p22phox in the structural maturation and subcellular targeting of Nox3. Biochem.J. 403:97-108, 2007.

Nakano Y, Longo-Guess CM, Bergstrom DE, Nauseef WM, Jones SM, Banfi B. Mutation of the Cyba gene encoding p22phox causes vestibular and immune defects in mice. J.Clin.Invest 118:1176-1185, 2008.

Nakaya K, Harbidge DG, Wangemann P, Schultz BD, Green ED, Wall SM, Marcus DC. Lack of pendrin HCO3- transport elevates vestibular endolymphatic [Ca2+] by inhibition of acid-sensitive TRPV5 and TRPV6 channels. Am.J.Physiol Renal Physiol 292:F1314-F1321, 2007.

Oldberg A, Franzen A, Heinegard D. Cloning and sequence analysis of rat bone sialoprotein (osteopontin) cDNA reveals an Arg-Gly-Asp cell-binding sequence. Proc.Natl.Acad.Sci.U.S.A 83:8819-8823, 1986.

Paffenholz R, Bergstrom RA, Pasutto F, Wabnitz P, Munroe RJ, Jagla W, Heinzmann U, Marquardt A, Bareiss A, Laufs J, Russ A, Stumm G, Schimenti JC, Bergstrom DE. Vestibular defects in head-tilt mice result from mutations in Nox3, encoding an NADPH oxidase. Genes Dev. 18:486-491, 2004.

Pedrozo HA, Schwartz Z, Dean DD, Harrison JL, Campbell JW, Wiederhold ML, Boyan BD. Evidence for the involvement of carbonic anhydrase and urease in calcium carbonate formation in the gravity-sensing organ of Aplysia californica. Calcif.Tissue Int. 61:247-255, 1997.

Petko JA, Millimaki BB, Canfield VA, Riley BB, Levenson R. Otoc1: a novel otoconin-90 ortholog required for otolith mineralization in zebrafish. Dev.Neurobiol. 68:209-222, 2008.

Pisam M, Jammet C, Laurent D. First steps of otolith formation of the zebrafish: role of glycogen? Cell Tissue Res. 310:163-168, 2002.

Pote KG and Ross MD. Each otoconia polymorph has a protein unique to that polymorph. Comp Biochem.Physiol B 98:287-295, 1991.

Price PA, Thomas GR, Pardini AW, Figueira WF, Caputo JM, Williamson MK. Discovery of a high molecular weight complex of calcium, phosphate, fetuin, and matrix gamma-carboxyglutamic acid protein in the serum of etidronate-treated rats. J.Biol.Chem. 277:3926-3934, 2002.

Quelch KJ, Cole WG, Melick RA. Noncollagenous proteins in normal and pathological human bone. Calcif.Tissue Int. 36:545-549, 1984.

Rau A, Legan PK, Richardson GP. Tectorin mRNA expression is spatially and temporally restricted during mouse inner ear development. J.Comp Neurol. 405:271-280, 1999.

Richardson GP, Russell IJ, Duance VC, Bailey AJ. Polypeptide composition of the mammalian tectorial membrane. Hear.Res. 25:45-60, 1987.

Rodan SB and Rodan GA. Integrin function in osteoclasts. J.Endocrinol. 154 Suppl:S47-S56, 1997.

Ross MD and Pote KG. Some properties of otoconia. Philos.Trans.R.Soc.Lond B Biol.Sci. 304:445-452, 1984.

Russell IJ, Legan PK, Lukashkina VA, Lukashkin AN, Goodyear RJ, Richardson GP. Sharpened cochlear tuning in a mouse with a genetically modified tectorial membrane. Nat.Neurosci. 10:215-223, 2007.

Sage EH and Vernon RB. Regulation of angiogenesis by extracellular matrix: the growth and the glue. J.Hypertens.Suppl 12:S145-S152, 1994.

Sakagami M. Role of osteopontin in the rodent inner ear as revealed by in situ hybridization. Med.Electron Microsc. 33:3-10, 2000.

Salamat MS, Ross MD, Peacor DR. Otoconial formation in the fetal rat. Ann.Otol.Rhinol.Laryngol. 89:229-238, 1980.

Salt AN, Inamura N, Thalmann R, Vora A. Calcium gradients in inner ear endolymph. Am.J.Otolaryngol. 10:371-375, 1989.

Salvinelli F, Firrisi L, Casale M, Trivelli M, D'Ascanio L, Lamanna F, Greco F, Costantino S. Benign paroxysmal positional vertigo: diagnosis and treatment. Clin.Ter. 155:395-400, 2004.

Sasaki T, Hohenester E, Gohring W, Timpl R. Crystal structure and mapping by site-directed mutagenesis of the collagen-binding epitope of an activated form of BM-40/SPARC/osteonectin. EMBO J. 17:1625-1634, 1998.

Schafer C, Heiss A, Schwarz A, Westenfeld R, Ketteler M, Floege J, Muller-Esterl W, Schinke T, Jahnen-Dechent W. The serum protein alpha 2-Heremans-Schmid glycoprotein/fetuin-A is a systemically acting inhibitor of ectopic calcification. J.Clin.Invest 112:357-366, 2003.

Schuknecht HF. Cupulolithiasis. Arch.Otolaryngol. 90:765-778, 1969.

Schuknecht HF. Positional vertigo: clinical and experimental observations. Trans.Am.Acad.Ophthalmol.Otolaryngol. 66:319-332, 1962.

Scott DA and Karniski LP. Human pendrin expressed in Xenopus laevis oocytes mediates chloride/formate exchange. Am.J.Physiol Cell Physiol 278:C207-C211, 2000.

Scott DA, Wang R, Kreman TM, Sheffield VC, Karniski LP. The Pendred syndrome gene encodes a chloride-iodide transport protein. Nat.Genet. 21:440-443, 1999.

Shapses SA, Cifuentes M, Spevak L, Chowdhury H, Brittingham J, Boskey AL, Denhardt DT. Osteopontin facilitates bone resorption, decreasing bone mineral crystallinity and content during calcium deficiency. Calcif.Tissue Int. 73:86-92, 2003.

Simmler MC, Cohen-Salmon M, El-Amraoui A, Guillaud L, Benichou JC, Petit C, Panthier JJ. Targeted disruption of otog results in deafness and severe imbalance. Nat.Genet. 24:139-143, 2000a.

Simmler MC, Zwaenepoel I, Verpy E, Guillaud L, Elbaz C, Petit C, Panthier JJ. Twister mutant mice are defective for otogelin, a component specific to inner ear acellular membranes. Mamm.Genome 11:960-966, 2000b.

Slepecky NB, Savage JE, Yoo TJ. Localization of type II, IX and V collagen in the inner ear. Acta Otolaryngol. 112:611-617, 1992.

Sollner C, Burghammer M, Busch-Nentwich E, Berger J, Schwarz H, Riekel C, Nicolson T. Control of crystal size and lattice formation by starmaker in otolith biomineralization. Science 302:282-286, 2003.

Sollner C, Schwarz H, Geisler R, Nicolson T. Mutated otopetrin 1 affects the genesis of otoliths and the localization of Starmaker in zebrafish. Dev.Genes Evol. 214:582-590, 2004.

Squires TM, Weidman MS, Hain TC, Stone HA. A mathematical model for top-shelf vertigo: the role of sedimenting otoconia in BPPV. J.Biomech. 37:1137-1146, 2004.

Steyger PS and Wiederhold ML. Visualization of newt aragonitic otoconial matrices using transmission electron microscopy. Hear.Res. 92:184-191, 1995.

Swartz DJ and Santi PA. Immunohistochemical localization of keratan sulfate in the chinchilla inner ear. Hear.Res. 109:92-101, 1997.

Takemura T, Sakagami M, Nakase T, Kubo T, Kitamura Y, Nomura S. Localization of osteopontin in the otoconial organs of adult rats. Hear.Res. 79:99-104, 1994.

Takumida M, Ishibashi T, Hamamoto T, Hirakawa K, Anniko M. Age-dependent changes in the expression of klotho protein, TRPV5 and TRPV6 in mouse inner ear. Acta Otolaryngol. 129:1340-1350, 2009.

Termine JD, Kleinman HK, Whitson SW, Conn KM, McGarvey ML, Martin GR. Osteonectin, a bone-specific protein linking mineral to collagen. Cell 26:99-105, 1981.

Thalmann I, Hughes I, Tong BD, Ornitz DM, Thalmann R. Microscale analysis of proteins in inner ear tissues and fluids with emphasis on endolymphatic sac, otoconia, and organ of Corti. Electrophoresis 27:1598-1608, 2006.

Thalmann R, Ignatova E, Kachar B, Ornitz DM, Thalmann I. Development and maintenance of otoconia: biochemical considerations. Ann.N.Y.Acad.Sci. 942:162-178, 2001.

Thurner PJ, Chen CG, Ionova-Martin S, Sun L, Harman A, Porter A, Ager JW, III, Ritchie RO, Alliston T. Osteopontin deficiency increases bone fragility but preserves bone mass. Bone 46:1564-1573, 2010.

Tohse H and Mugiya Y. Effects of enzyme and anion transport inhibitors on in vitro incorporation of inorganic carbon and calcium into endolymph and otoliths in salmon Oncorhynchus masou. Comp Biochem.Physiol A Mol.Integr.Physiol 128:177-184, 2001.

Trune DR and Lim DJ. The behavior and vestibular nuclear morphology of otoconia-deficient pallid mutant mice. J.Neurogenet. 1:53-69, 1983.

Tsujikawa S, Yamashita T, Tomoda K, Iwai H, Kumazawa H, Cho H, Kumazawa T. Effects of acetazolamide on acid-base balance in the endolymphatic sac of the guinea pig. Acta Otolaryngol.Suppl 500:50-53, 1993.

Verpy E, Leibovici M, Petit C. Characterization of otoconin-95, the major protein of murine otoconia, provides insights into the formation of these inner ear biominerals. Proc.Natl.Acad.Sci.U.S.A 96:529-534, 1999.

Viviano BL, Silverstein L, Pflederer C, Paine-Saunders S, Mills K, Saunders S. Altered hematopoiesis in glypican-3-deficient mice results in decreased osteoclast differentiation and a delay in endochondral ossification. Dev.Biol. 282:152-162, 2005.

Wang Y, Kowalski PE, Thalmann I, Ornitz DM, Mager DL, Thalmann R. Otoconin-90, the mammalian otoconial matrix protein, contains two domains of homology to secretory phospholipase A2. Proc.Natl.Acad.Sci.U.S.A 95:15345-15350, 1998.

Westenfeld R, Schafer C, Kruger T, Haarmann C, Schurgers LJ, Reutelingsperger C, Ivanovski O, Drueke T, Massy ZA, Ketteler M, Floege J, Jahnen-Dechent W. Fetuin-A protects against atherosclerotic calcification in CKD. J.Am.Soc.Nephrol. 20:1264-1274, 2009.

Westenfeld R, Schafer C, Smeets R, Brandenburg VM, Floege J, Ketteler M, Jahnen-Dechent W. Fetuin-A (AHSG) prevents extraosseous calcification induced by uraemia and phosphate challenge in mice. Nephrol.Dial.Transplant. 22:1537-1546, 2007.

Xu T, Bianco P, Fisher LW, Longenecker G, Smith E, Goldstein S, Bonadio J, Boskey A, Heegaard AM, Sommer B, Satomura K, Dominguez P, Zhao C, Kulkarni AB, Robey PG, Young MF. Targeted disruption of the biglycan gene leads to an osteoporosis-like phenotype in mice. Nat.Genet. 20:78-82, 1998.

Xu Y, Zhang H, Yang H, Zhao X., Lovas S, Lundberg YW. Expression, functional and structural analysis of proteins critical for otoconia development. Dev.Dyn. 239:2659-2673, 2010.

Xu Y and Lundberg Y.W. Temporally and spatially regulated expression of otoconial genes. 35th Association for Research in Otolaryngology MidWinter Meeting #282,2012.

Xu Y, Yang L, Jones S.M., Zhao X., Zhang Y, Lundberg Y.W. Functional cooperation of two otoconial proteins Oc90 and Nox3. 35th Association for Research in Otolaryngology MidWinter Meeting #281:2012.

Yamauchi D, Nakaya K, Raveendran NN, Harbidge DG, Singh R, Wangemann P, Marcus DC. Expression of epithelial calcium transport system in rat cochlea and vestibular labyrinth. BMC.Physiol 10:1-2010.

Yamoah EN, Lumpkin EA, Dumont RA, Smith PJ, Hudspeth AJ, Gillespie PG. Plasma membrane Ca2+-ATPase extrudes Ca2+ from hair cell stereocilia. J.Neurosci. 18:610-624, 1998.

Yang H, Zhao X, Xu Y, Wang L, He Q, Lundberg YW. Matrix recruitment and calcium sequestration for spatial specific otoconia development. PLoS.ONE. 6:e20498-2011.

Young MF, Bi Y, Ameye L, Chen XD. Biglycan knockout mice: new models for musculoskeletal diseases. Glycoconj.J. 19:257-262, 2002.

Zhao X, Jones SM, Thoreson WB, Lundberg YW. Osteopontin is not critical for otoconia formation or balance function. J.Assoc.Res.Otolaryngol. 9:191-201, 2008a.

Zhao X, Jones SM, Yamoah EN, Lundberg YW. Otoconin-90 deletion leads to imbalance but normal hearing: a comparison with other otoconia mutants. Neuroscience 153:289-299, 2008b.

Zhao X, Yang H, Yamoah EN, Lundberg YW. Gene targeting reveals the role of Oc90 as the essential organizer of the otoconial organic matrix. Dev.Biol. 304:508-524, 2007.

Zwaenepoel I, Mustapha M, Leibovici M, Verpy E, Goodyear R, Liu XZ, Nouaille S, Nance WE, Kanaan M, Avraham KB, Tekaia F, Loiselet J, Lathrop M, Richardson G, Petit C. Otoancorin, an inner ear protein restricted to the interface between the apical surface of sensory epithelia and their overlying acellular gels, is defective in autosomal recessive deafness DFNB22. Proc.Natl.Acad.Sci.U.S.A 99:6240-6245, 2002.

Section 2

Rhinology

2

Epistaxis

Jin Hee Cho and Young Ha Kim
College of Medicine, The Catholic University of Korea
South Korea

1. Introduction

Epistaxis occur due to trauma, disorders in mucosa or vessels, or coagulopathy. It is a very common disease, as 10% of all population experience severe epistaxis, about 30% of children aged 0~5, 56% of children aged 6~10 and 64% of children aged 11~15 are reported to experience one or more episode of epistaxis. (Cho, 2009)

Although most cases of epistaxis are mild, that can be self-managed, life-threatening condition can be also possible. When encounter patient with severe epistaxis, it is important to find the bleeding focus and to analyse the causes of epistaxis fast and accurately, to treat the patient promptly to avoid complications such as hypotension, hypoxia, anemia, aspiration or death.

2. Anatomy

Nasal bleeding can conveniently be divided into anterior and posterior epistaxis. Anterior bleeds come out the front of the nose, whereas posterior bleeds run down the back of the nose into the pharynx. Roughly 90% of cases of epistaxis can be classified as anterior. The common sites of anterior bleeding include the anterior aspect of the nasal septum, anterior edge of the inferior turbinate and the anterior ethmoid sinus. Among them, the anterior aspect of the nasal septum is the single most common site, where sometimes referred to as Kisselbach's plexus (Little's area). Kisselbach's plexus contains a rich capillary blood supply that is at the confluence of four different arterial blood supplies, which are sphenopalatine artery, greater palatine artery, superior labial artery, and anterior ethmoid artery (Figure 1).

Posterior epistaxis typically arises from vessels on the posterior septum, on the floor of the nose in the posterior choana, or from the back of the middle or inferior turbinate. The area at the back of the inferior turbinate is specified as Woodruff's plexus (Figure 2). Recently, it is known that the Woodruff plexus is a venous plexus located at the back of the inferior meatus, not an arterial plexus.

3. Causes of epistaxis

The causes of the epistaxis cannot be found in 80 to 90% of patients. It is easy to injure nasal mucosa and generate epistaxis, as it is rich with blood vessels just underneath mucosa. A number of factors and conditions contribute to the development, severity and recurrence of epistaxis. (Table 1)

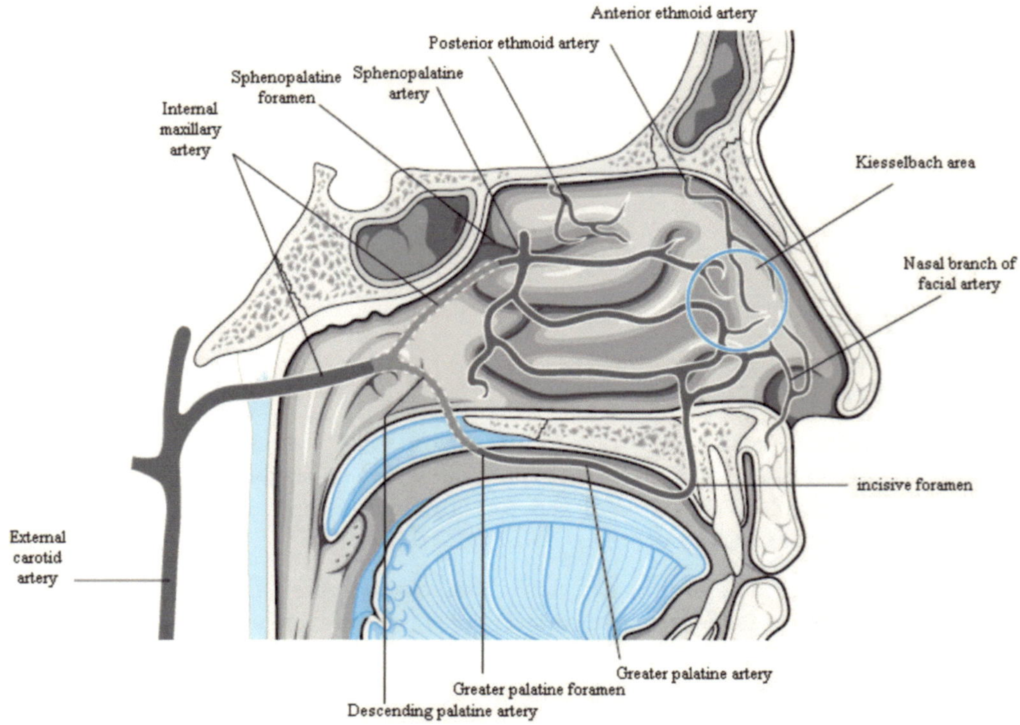

Fig. 1. Blood supply of nasal septum showing Kiesselbach area. (Cho, 2009)

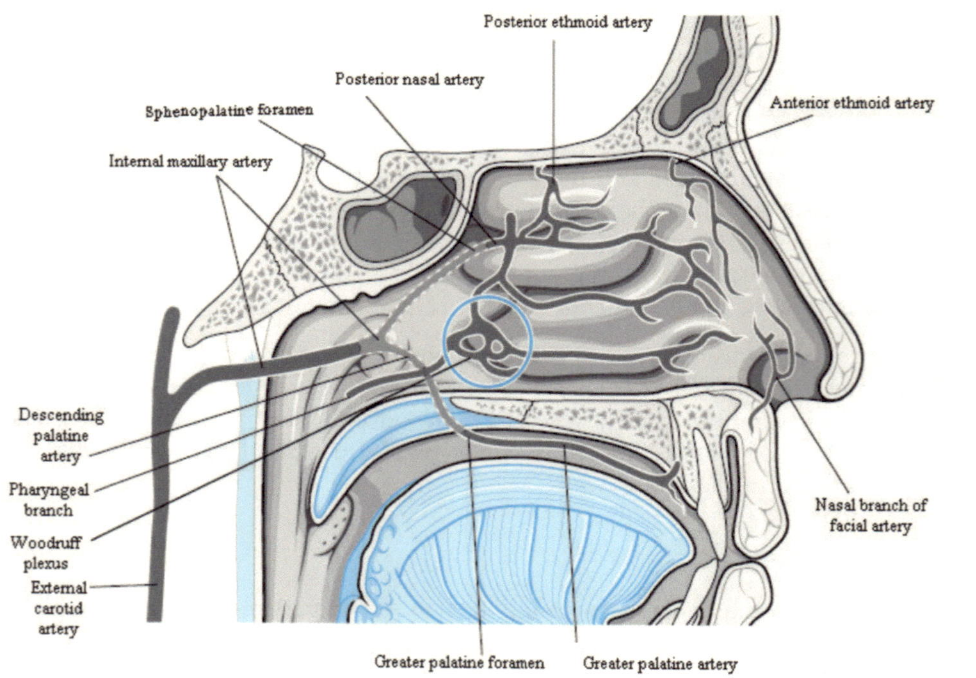

Fig. 2. Blood supply of lateral nasal wall showing Woodruff area. (Cho, 2009)

Local causes
Trauma
Digital
Nose blowing
Blunt
Penetrating
Iatrogenic
Chronic irritation
Mucosal dehydration
Deviated septum
Arid environment
Inflammation
Rhinitis
Sinusitis
Autoimmune disorders
Environmental irritants
Tumors
Benign
Inverted papilloma
Juvenile nasopharyngeal angiofibroma
Malignant
Nasopharyngeal carcinoma
Esthesioneuroblastoma
Systemic causes
Age
Hypertension
Cogulopathy
Hemophilia
Thrombocytopenia
Renal failure
Cancer chemotherapy
Medication-related
Aspirin
Coumadin
Heparin
Hereditary Hemorrhagic Telangiectasia

Table 1. Causes of Epistaxis.

3.1 Local causes

3.1.1 Trauma

Especially in children or patients with mental problem, finger manipulation of the nose is an almost ubiquitous behavior. Continuous mechanical trauma to the nasal mucosa can lead to mucosal abrasion and, eventually, ulceration. This initially leads to a small amount of blood that merely coats the ulceration, leading to a fibrous clot that dries into scab formation.

Removal of the scab causes further injury to the mucosa, which can result in more significant bleeding.

It is possible to cause rupture of superficial vessels of the mucosa by violent nose blowing. Nose blowing is an especially prominent source of trauma in patients who have undergone recent surgery on the nose or sinuses or who have preexisting bleeding sites.

The trauma may be in the form of blunt trauma to the nose or sinuses as a result of traffic accident or during sports, resulting in fracture of the septum, lateral wall, or one of the sinuses. The fracture leads to disruption of the mucosal lining, tearing of blood vessels, and bleeding.

Chronic irritation of nasal mucosa can also cause epistaxis. For example, nasal abuse of cocaine, nasal smoke or misuse of nasal spray can cause nasal irritation and dehydration which can lead to epistaxis or even septal perforation.

3.1.2 Dehydration

Drying of the nasal mucosa is one of the common factors contributing to epistaxis. The possibility of epistaxis increases when the nasal humidifying function falls as the nasal secretion decreases, or when nasal mucosa expose to the cold, dry environmental air as a seasonal factor. Also, when the septum is significantly deviated, or when nasal airway is altered as a result of surgery, there can be an abnormally high airflow that are no longer able to humidify the air adequately and as a result, epistaxis can occur.

Number of epistaxis patients who visit emergency department increases as temperature and humidity decrease. Also, the number of patients who admit to hospital increases in winter. Comparing in-patients number with air temperature, admission increases 30% in days with average temperature under 5°C than days with average temperature over 5°C. (Viducich et al., 1995)

3.1.3 Inflammation

Inflammatory conditions such as acute upper respiratory infection, allergic rhinitis, sinusitis and nasal foreign bodies can often lead to nasal bleeding. Nasal decongestant or intranasal steroid spray also can cause nasal dryness and epistaxis. Any factors that cause nasal inflammation can make the mucosa more fragile and make patients to blow the nose more frequently, weak vessels can be damaged easily. Nasal granulomatous diseases such as Wegener's granulomatosis, sarcoidosis, nasal tuberculosis and nasal syphilis lead to mucosal ulceration or extreme inflammation that may predispose the patient to crusting, abrasion, and eventually, bleeding.

3.1.4 Tumors and aneurysms

Juvenile nasopharyngeal angiofibroma classically presents as recurrent epistaxis in adolescents or young adult men, malignant tumors such as malignant melanoma and squamous cell carcinoma present as unilateral nasal stuffiness with epistaxis in adults. Intracavernous aneurysm of internal carotid artery after trauma can cause severe epistaxis. This posttraumatic aneurysm occurs about 7 weeks after trauma, and mortality rate reaches 50%.

3.2 Systemic causes

3.2.1 Age

In elderly, changes in vessel wall, especially in arterial wall fibrosis, are related with epistaxis. In children, previously mentioned mechanical trauma, nasal foreign body and nasal mucosal inflammation are the causes of epistaxis.

3.2.2 Hypertension

Hypertension and epistaxis commonly occur simultaneously among adults of general population. It is uncertain whether the hypertension is an etiologic factor in all of these patients. It is known that hypertension in epistaxis patients is caused by anxiety. However, one study that analyzed 200 epistaxis patients reported that 75% showed elevated blood pressure during nose bleeding and 30% was severe hypertension patients. (Herkner et al., 2000)

Elevated blood pressure can contribute to epistaxis in two different ways. First, the high pressure causes chronic damage of a blood vessel wall in the nasal or sinus mucosa. Second, 20% of epistaxis patients experience elevated blood pressure because the natural response to seeing blood from one's nose is to get agitated, which can directly lead to elevation of the blood pressure. Practically, active bleeding patients in emergency department were related to hypertension and patients without active nasal bleeding had less related to hypertension.

3.2.3 Coagulopathy

Coagulopathy leads to unwanted bleeding due to the absence or inactivity of one of the clotting factors. These conditions are rare, but affected patients tend to have severe nosebleeds from an early age. There are also patients with inherent disorders of platelet function. Conditions such as hemophilia, von Willebrand disease, thrombocytopenia, AIDS or liver disease can often cause epistaxis. And among them, von Willebrand disease is most common.

Patients with chronic renal failure commonly have problems with epistaxis. This is due to the two-prolonged problem of regularly receiving heparin during dialysis and having poor clotting secondary to the renal failure. In these patients, epistaxis tends to occur either while the patient is undergoing dialysis or shortly after the dialysis. Patients with septic shock develop a condition of poor clotting that may progress to disseminated intravascular coagulation (DIC). This starts out as uncontrolled clotting of the blood within the vascular system and progresses to a coagulopathy secondary to consumption of all available clotting factors.

Finally, there are patients who acquire clotting deficiencies as a result of cancer therapy. This may occur secondary to high-dose chemotherapy, leading to transient decrease in the platelet count. Alternatively, the coagulopathy may be caused by depletion of bone marrow reserves of platelets due to bone marrow transplant. In both of these cases, thrombocytopenia becomes a clinical reality and epistaxis may result.

3.2.4 Medications

There are several medications that interfere normal blood clotting process, for example, warfarin, heparin and nonsteroid anti-inflammatory drugs(NSAIDs). Most commonly used medication is NSAIDs, including aspirin. Aspirin, by inhibiting the enzyme cyclooxygenase, interferes with platelet function. This results in significant increases in bleeding time, but should not increase the incidence of nosebleeds. Millions of patients are currently taking a regular dose of aspirin, as prescribed by their doctors, for prevention of stroke, heart attack, and clotting in prosthetic arteries. For this reason, aspirin use is becoming an increasingly important risk factor for epistaxis in adults.

3.2.5 Hereditary hemorrhagic telangiectasia

Hereditary hemorrhagic telangiectasia (HHT), also known as *Rendu-Osler-Weber disease,* is a rare systemic fibrovascular dysplasia with autosomal dominant inheritance. Multiple telangiectasic vascular malformations can be seen on the skin and in the mucosa of the digestive tract and respiratory airways. 20% of patients have family history and the incidence is 1~2 per 100,000. Several elevated small cherry red spots in lip and oral cavity mucosa can be seen and they become pale when pressed. Dilatation of arterioles under basement membrane is referred to as telangiectasia, and these arterioles can easily be damaged as they do not have elastic tissue under endothelial layer. If the patient is diagnosed of HHT, arteriovenous malformation should be checked in other organs. Other manifestations of the disease occur in the internal organs such as the lungs, liver, or the central nervous system. It is estimated that at least 30% of HHT patients have pulmonary, 30% hepatic, and 10–20% cerebral involvement. (Guttmacher et al., 1995)

Diagnosis is made according to the Curaçao Criteria: telangiectasia on the face, hands and in oral cavity, recurrent epistaxis, arteriovenous malformations with visceral involvement, family history. Diagnosis is confirmed upon the presence of at least three of these manifestations. HHT is an uncommon cause of epistaxis, but an important cause owing to the severity of the condition and the special measures required for treatment. In any patient with recurrent epistaxis, a careful examination of the mucosal surfaces in the nose should be performed to rule out HHT lesions. The presence of three or more suggestive vascular lesions should alert the physician to the possibility that the patient may have HHT. (Fuchizaki et al., 2003)

4. Diagnosis

When the patient with epistaxis initially presents for treatment, it is important to perform a systematic evaluation. One may be tempted to proceed directly to managing the patient's symptoms without performing a careful history and physical examination. Indeed, in cases of heavy bleeding, this may be necessary. For most patients, nose with Neo-Synephrine-soaked cotton pledgets, should control the bleeding sufficiently to allow the physician to perform a proper evaluation before initiating definitive treatment.

4.1 History

During the initial inquiry, it is important to investigate the duration of bleeding, frequency of bleeding, and amount of bleeding. If not in an emergency situation, it is also important to determine the side of the bleeding and its primary site of origin and flow: out the front of the nose, down the back of the nose or a combination of the two. It may be possible during history taking to elicit information that will provide clues to the underlying cause of the bleeding, such as trauma, surgery, history of coagulopathy or medication history.

4.2 Physical examination

After stabilize the patient, the initial examination of the nose should be performed to find the origin site by anterior rhinoscopy after removal of the blood clot and minimize the edema using decongestant, using adequate light source to visualize whole nasal cavity. If the bleeding has stopped after the removal of clots, additional immediate treatment is not needed. Packing of the nasal cavity without evidence of continuous bleeding can damage the nasal mucosa and cause epistaxis rather than stopping it. The most likely finding is a superficial vessel that has eroded on anterior nasal septum, or medial portion of the turbinate in patients with no specific cause, so special cautions are needed in those parts of the nose.

4.3 Endoscopy

In cases of either acute or recurrent epistaxis without an obvious bleeding source on anterior rhinoscopy, an endoscopic examination is indicated to attempt to identify the site. This is usually performed bilaterally and with thorough decongestion and topical anesthesia. Either a flexible or rigid endoscope can be used. The flexible scope is perhaps easier to use and less uncomfortable. However, the rigid scopes have superior optics, with better image resolution and are easy to use instruments.

4.4 Radiologic evaluation

Routine radiologic studies have little role in the initial diagnosis of epistaxis. However, in patients with recurrent epistaxis without a known source or cause, imaging studies have important role in diagnosis. The imaging study of choice for initial evaluation of most nasal or sinus pathologic conditions, including epistaxis, is the CT scan and tumors that cause epistaxis are often found.

5. Management

It is important to evaluate epistaxis patients thoroughly because the method of controlling epistaxis depends largely on the specifics of an individual case, with an entire menu of options available. (Table 2)

Anterior flexion of head can prevent nausea or airway obstruction, as blood does not flow back to pharynx. It is important to keep the blood pressure low and keep the airway clean. Also, fluid replacement can be considered according to the amount of blood loss. Systemic diseases can cause multiple bleeding sites or frequent recurrent epistaxis so blood testing should be performed in patients with those findings. Patients with posterior epistaxis, coagulopathy, coronary artery disease, uncontrolled hypertension, severe anemia or old age should be considered to treat as in-patient basis.

5.1 Medical treatment

On the first visit of a patient with minimal or moderate history of nasal bleeding, an empiric trial of medical therapy is advised. This includes several measures designed to increase humidification of the mucosa to allow the bleeding site to heal. This approach is based on the assumption that dryness is one of the most important factors causing epistaxis. The

Medical Management
Nasal packing Traditional anterior pack Nasal sponges Gelfoam Traditional posterior pack Nasal balloon
Cautery Silver nitrate Endoscopic electrocautery Laser cautery
Embolization
Arterial ligation Transantral ligation of the internal maxillary artery External ligation of the ethmoid arteries Endoscopic ligation of the sphenopalatine artery
Surgery Septoplasty Septal dermoplasty

Table 2. Management options of epistaxis.

recommendations include applying an ointment to the anterior nose each morning and night. In between ointment applications, nasal saline is sprayed into the nose every 2 to 3 hours. In addition, every effort should be made to humidify the air of the home environment. This usually requires using a room air humidifier in the bedroom every night. Maximum effect is achieved by running the humidifier on full with the doors and windows to the room closed.

Also, medical conditions that contribute to epistaxis should be controlled. For example, in patients with hypertension, medication should be administered to lower the blood pressure to within normal range. For patients with coagulopathy, every attempt should be made to normalize clotting function. This may require discontinuing Coumadin or aspirin therapy. For patients with acute and life-threatening bleeding, platelet or plasma transfusions may be administered to reverse the bleeding disorder.

Patients with epistaxis should also minimize their activity while the nose is healing. Exercise should be deferred until the bleeding has stopped for at least 1 week. Bed rest is generally not necessary, nor is staying home from work or school. However, patients should be aware of their level of activity and take steps to avoid any activities that would elevate the blood pressure. Nose blowing should be minimized, and patients should be instructed to blow gently. Patients should also be instructed to avoid rubbing and picking at the nose. Finally, adjunctive therapy, including stool softeners and antitussives, should be considered in selected patients.

If initial attempts to control epistaxis with these conservative medical therapies fail, a more comprehensive approach to the problem should be initiated. This may include specific investigations to evaluate the haemoglobin, platelet levels and coagulation function. An endoscopic examination, if not already performed, should also be considered. This subset of patients might also benefit from a CT scan to rule out the possibility of an occult tumor.

Second-line therapy is then indicated, including nasal packing, cauterization, and vessel ligation.

5.2 General treatment

5.2.1 General treatment for anterior epistaxis

If the bleeding site is identified, it is recommended to use pledgets impregnated with decongestant containing bosmin or phenylephrine solution. Compress both nasal dorsum directly for at least 5 minutes after packing the nasal cavity with gauzes impregnated with decongestant and anesthetic agent.

In cases with coagulopathy, packing with pledget can damage the mucosa so hemostatic agents such as Avitene, Surgicel or gelfoam can be used. Electric cautery should be performed carefully because it can damage surrounding normal tissue. Also, physician should keep in mind that electric cautery on bilateral septum can lead to septal perforation.

In case epistaxis continues with former treatments, nasal packing using gauze with Vaseline and antibiotics, from posterior to anterior and from inferior to superior, should be done. Using bayonet forceps, grasp the packing about 10 cm from one end and place into the back of the nose. Loops of the packing are then placed one on top of another, gently but firmly pressing the loop onto the floor of the nose as each is placed. In this way, the pack is built up sequentially. The final pack should tightly fill the nasal cavity. (Figure 3)

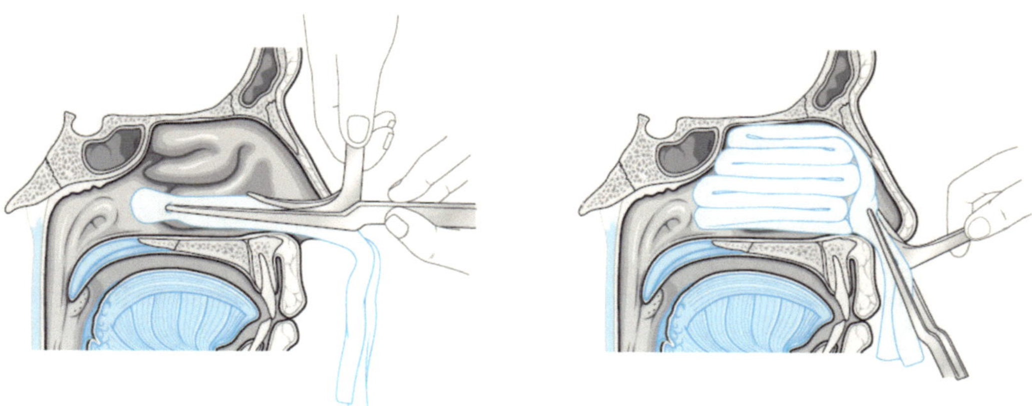

Fig. 3. Placement of traditional or standard anterior nasal packing. A. The gauze is grasped 10cm from one end and placed into the posterior choanae. B. The gauze is layered one length at a time to build up the pack. (Cho, 2009)

Instead of gauze, compressed sponge (Merocel) can be used. The pack is introduced in a dehydrated state and is expanded by either instilling saline or by absorbing blood from the patient. As the material expands, it fills the nasal or sinus cavity, helping to stop the bleeding in two ways: by applying pressure against the mucosa and by providing a surface against which the blood can clot.

The packs are maintained for a period of 2 to 5 days depending on the circumstances. The patient can be sent home with an anterior pack in the nose. It is recommended to coat sponge with antistaphyloccocal ointment to prevent toxic shock syndrome, which is a side effect of prolonged packing. It is advisable to prescribe antistaphylococcal antibiotics for the duration of time the pack is in place for same reason. The patient should be advised to restrict activity. Absolute bed rest is not necessary, but the patient should avoid strenuous activity and should not attempt to maintain normal activity levels.

5.2.2 General treatment for posterior epistaxis

If posterior epistaxis does not stop with anterior packing, balloon insertion or posterior packing should be done. Posterior epistaxis is typically heavy and cannot be controlled with an anterior pack or by anterior compression of the nose. Posterior packing is the traditional first-line therapy for posterior epistaxis. However, with the many options available today, many otolaryngologists prefer not to use the traditional posterior pack.

The benefits of the posterior pack are that, if properly placed, this method almost always results in control of the bleeding. Also, it can be created with minimal supplies available in all emergency rooms and on all nursing units. However, there are significant disadvantages to this method. The most important is that it is very uncomfortable to place as well as to maintain for any length of time. And these packs tend to cause significant injury to the nasal mucosa. Ulcerations are common and abrasions are universal. Finally, there is a significant risk for development of hypoxia with this pack. Nasal pulmonary reflex is suspected to be the cause of unexplained hypoxia, but it is still controversial.

Several methods can be used for posterior packing. First is the foley catheter technique. With the foley catheter technique, catheter is placed through each side of the nose, grasped in the pharynx, and brought out through the mouth. Inflate the balloon with 3~4 ml of water or air and then withdraw through the nose pulling the balloon into the nasopharynx. The size of the posterior pack should be enough to fill up the posterior choana. A full anterior pack is placed in front of the posterior pack and is then fixed with umbilical clamp over the anterior nasal spine. It is important to put a soft dressing to prevent necrosis on columella.

Second method is a gauze sponge method. A gauze sponge can be rolled, tied up and is moistened with antibiotics ointment and iodine solution before use. Before placing a traditional posterior nasal pack, the patient should be well decongested and anesthetized on nasal cavity and pharynx. The gauze is tied with 2-0 silk to make two strings on one side and with 3-0 silk to make a string on the other side, and use 3-0 silk string when removing the posterior pack. The nelaton catheter is placed through nose, visualized in pharynx and brought out through the mouth. One 2-0 silk string tied to the pack is tied to the catheter and pull the catheter and 2-0 silk string from anterior nostril and place the posterior pack in posterior choana with finger tip at the same time. A full anterior pack is placed in front of the posterior pack and the 2-0 silk string through the nose is pulled tight to add the desired pressure and is the tied around the gauze bolster over the anterior nasal spine to protect the columella from pressure necrosis. (Figure 4) The anterior pack is partially removed start from the third day and the posterior pack is removed via oral cavity on fifth day.

After placing the posterior pack, the patient should be observed in a monitored bed with saturation monitoring. For the entire time that the posterior pack is in place, humidified oxygen should be administered to prevent drying of the pharynx. Intravenous antibiotics are prescribed to prevent sinus infection and to prevent toxic shock syndrome. The pack is normally kept in place for 3 to 5 days and then gradually deflated.

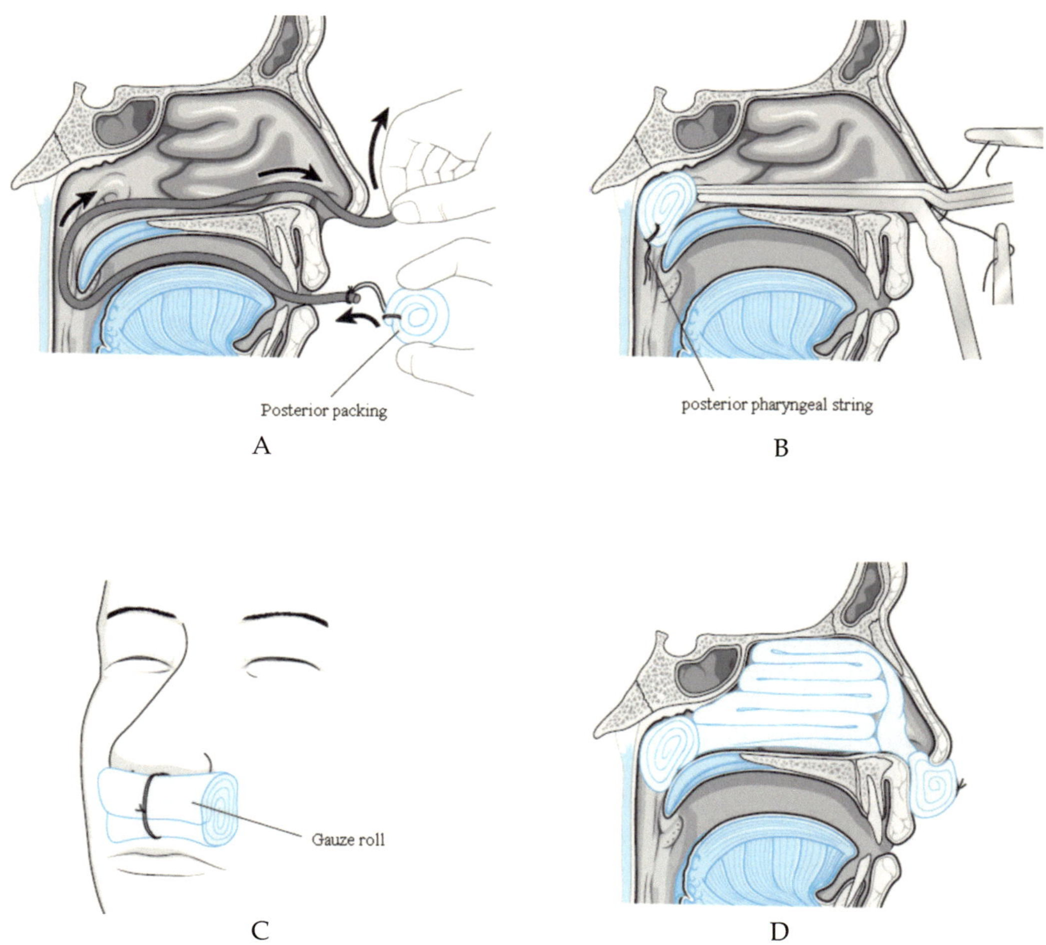

Fig. 4. A Gauze sponge posterior packing method. A. Insertion of a nelaton catheter into nasal cavity. Pull the catheter from oropharynx to take out the tip through oral cavity. Tie the two 2-0 silk with nelaton tip. B. Pull the nelaton catheter from nasal cavity to place the posterior pack in posterior choana. Hold the 2-0 silk which were tied to nelaton on nostril and do the anterior packing. C. Place a gauze roll in front of nostril and tie up the 2-0 silk on the gauze roll. D. Sagittal picture with anterior and posterior nasal packing in situ. (Cho, 2009)

5.3 Cautery

Cauterization is an effective and simple way of controlling epistaxis. There are currently two methods of applying cautery in the nose. The first is the use of chemical agent, such as silver nitrate and is primarily applicable to anterior epistaxis. The second is electrocautery, which can be used throughout the nose.

5.3.1 Chemical cautery

Usually silver nitrate is used for chemical cautery. The most convenient and usual method of delivery is via a silver nitrate applicator stick. When touched to the mucosa, this causes a chemical burn that coagulates the tissue. This method should be applied to selected cases of epistaxis from the small superficial vessels. The best indication for use of silver nitrate is for active bleeding from an anterior nasoseptal vessel. The depth of coagulation is both an advantage and a limitation of this technique. The advantage is that there is minimal tissue damage and, therefore, minimal discomfort and rapid healing. The limitation is that only superficial, small vessels can be coagulated.

For chemical cauterization, the nose is first decongested and anesthetized with topical anesthesia. For actively bleeding vessels, one or two sticks are pressed against the vessel and slowly rolled to release the chemical. A piece of moistened cotton is then pressed over the area, pushing the sticks onto the vessel. After 15 to 30 seconds, the cotton and sticks are removed and the area of the cautery should be reinforced with Gelfoam or other suitable packing.

5.3.2 Endoscopic cautery

Endoscopic cauterization is rising as a valuable management tool for intractable epistaxis. Posterior endoscopic cauterization can replace arterial ligation method in many cases. Endoscopic cautery is indicated for controlling posterior epistaxis and epistaxis that stems from the septum and lateral wall, both of which lie beyond the reach of a silver nitrate stick. This procedure is very effective if the exact location of the bleeding vessel is known or the bleeding is active at the time of the procedure. The result of endoscopic cautery is largely dependent upon the experience on sinus endoscopy of the surgeon. To cauterize the bleeding on lateral wall of nasal cavity, a greater palatine block is needed to minimize the pain. In case of severe posterior epistaxis, cauterization in operating room under general anesthesia is recommended for safety.

The nose is examined using a 0-degree or 30-degree to find the bleeding focus. When doing this, use of decongestant should be avoided, as the agent can stop bleeding temporarily. If the bleeding focus is not found, it is helpful to irritate suspicious site of bleeding with suction tip. Mucosal ulceration, mucosal injury, fresh blood clot or prominent blood capillaries are common findings to suspect recent bleeding. Cautery is performed on the bleeding focus using a suction cautery unit with the power of 15 to 20 watt. If a suction cautery is not equipped, monopolar cautery is used after cover all raw surface of suction except tip with insulating tape. Although nasal packing is usually not necessary, decision is made by the surgeon after consideration of the amount of bleeding and the status of patients.

Endoscopic cautery is widely used as an effective treatment method for epistaxis, as success rate is up to 89% and also, this method can reduce the rate of nasal packing and admission.

5.4 Arterial ligation

At the era before internal maxillary artery ligation via transantral approach was introduced, external carotid artery ligation was commonly used to treat intractable epistaxis. Although transantral approach for internal maxillary artery ligation attained less morbidity than external carotid artery ligation, it still has had weak points. Transantral approach showed high failure rate as it cannot identify the divergences of internal maxillary artery and had several complication that cannot be bypassed, such as infraorbital nerve paresthesia, oroantraol fistula, teeth injury, sinusitis or rarely blindness.

5.4.1 Transantral ligation of the internal maxillary artery

This procedure is the traditional procedure of choice for controlling posterior epistaxis. When comparing this procedure traditional posterior packing for posterior epistaxis in terms of cost-effectiveness and length of hospitalization, surgical procedure was superior to the packing. Nevertheless, most patients would prefer not to have a surgical procedure, and the morbidity of the transantral procedure is significant.

Under general anesthesia, the sublabial incison is made with a No. 15 scalpel through the mucosa. The incision is located 5mm above the gingivolabial sulcus and extends from the midline to the first molar. The periosteum is incised and a subperiosteal elevation is performed over the anterior wall of the maxillary sinus. The maxillary sinus is entered over the canine fossa using a 4mm osteotome and mallet. The opening is enlarged with a Kerrison rongeur. The opening should be maximized by removing the anterior wall medially to the medial buttress, laterally to the lateral wall, inferiorly to the floor of the sinus, and superiorly to the infraorbital nerve. Then, maxillary posterior wall is drilled or removed with chisel. The initial bone removal of the posterior wall should start 1 to 2 cm below the floor of the orbit. A 4mm osteotome can be used in a controlled fashion with very light taps to fracture the thin bone of this area. Incision is made on periosteum after cauterization with a bayonet type bipolar forceps in a cruciate fashion. vessels in pterygopalatine fossa is divided and proximal vessel and distal vessels, such as sphenopalatine artery and descending palatine artery, are double ligated using hemoclips. The anatomy of the vessel is somewhat variable. However, there are several branches that can usually be identified, including the descending palatine, the superior alveolar, the infraorbital, and the sphenopalatine. Nasal packing materials are removed after the procedure and the nose is suctioned. Sinus packing with strip gauze is performed and the sublabial incision is then closed using interrupted 3-0 Vicryl suture.

This method has a high probability of failure because of anatomic variation in arterial positions. Recurrent bleeding is possible but unusual after this operation. The primary cause of rebleeding is misdiagnosis of the source of bleeding, the other cause is failure to ligate the appropriate vessels. The problem in the case of rebleeding is that it is difficult to distinguish between these two possibilities based on examination or history. In the case of rebleeding after transantral ligation of the sphenopalatine vessel, the recommended management is to perform an arteriogram. This will reliably distinguish between these situations, and also affords the option of embolization if amenable.

5.4.2 External ligation of the ethmoid artery

Epistaxis from anterior ethmoid artery is rare, however, trauma patients with fractures through the skull base that avulse or lacerate the anterior ethmoid artery can occur. Anterior ethmoid artery ligation via external approach is usually used in cases of epistaxis after facial trauma. Also, following endoscopic sinus surgery, some patients may develop heavy bleeding from the anterior or posterior ethmoid arteries that may not respond to packing. These can be treated with endoscopic cautery in most of cases. In certain cases, it may be preferable to ligate the vessel. Finally, patients with HHT may require vessel ligation to minimize the frequency or severity of epistaxis.

Under general anesthesia, operation starts with incision. In most cases, the nose is packed and there may be a posterior pack or nasal balloon. If possible, it is best to leave this in place until after the procedure is finished. Lynch incision is made on epistaxis side and the subcutaneous tissue is divided down through the periosteum to the bone. The angular artery will be encountered in the inferior aspect of the wound and should be controlled with either ligation or bipolar cautery. The soft tissues are retracted and the eye is elevated from the orbital bone with a Freer elevator. Lacrimal fossa and frontoethmoidal suture line can be identified. While advancing posteriorly along the frontoethmoid suture line, anterior ethmoid artery is found 20 to 24 mm posterior to the anterior lacrimal crest and this should be double ligated or cauterized. The preferred technique is to use bipolar cautery, as the clips tend to fall off and can lead to orbital hematoma. It is important to make sure that the full diameter of the artery is cauterized. Once the artery is fully cauterized or clipped, Jameson scissors are used to transect the artery in the middle, making sure that there is room to cauterize each stump if necessary. The dissection is then carried posteriorly for another 10 to 12mm until reaching the posterior ethmoid artery. Posterior ethmoid artery goes close to optic nerve and is not a major vessel that causes epistaxis, so ligation is usually not considered. After the arteries are divided, the wound is closed. Hemostasis should be achieved using bipolar cautery on the orbital tissues and monopolar cautery on the subcutaneous tissues.

All patients should be observed at least overnight after this surgery for two significant concerns: orbital hematoma and rebleeding. Orbital edema and ecchymosis are expected. However, there should not be any chemosis, true proptosis, or limitation of extraocular movements. Any of these signs suggests orbital hematoma and should be managed immediately according to the management protocol for orbital hematoma.

5.4.3 Endoscopic ligation of sphenopalatine artery

Endoscopic ligation of the internal maxillary artery is the newest addition to the surgical arsenal of the rhinologist for posterior epistaxis that can lower the complication of transantral approach and pterygomaxillary fossa dissection, and can prevent the collateral vessel formation as the most distal part of the artery is ligated, compared to other methods.

General anesthesia is achieved with orotracheal intubation. Before the nasal pack is removed, a transpalatal injection of the greater palatine foramen is performed using local anesthetic agent to minimize the bleeding after removal of the posterior pack. After removal of posterior pack, using 0 degree endoscope, thorough suction in the nasal cavity is performed for visualization. The posterior attachment of the middle turbinate is identified and an incision is made in the mucosa about 1 cm anterior to this point, extending from the inferior turbinate to the ethmoid sinus. The mucoperiosteal flap is elevated posterosuperiorly then surgeon can identify bundle of vessels and nerves originated from sphenopalatine foramen. The vessels are then carefully dissected with Freer elevator to identify sphenopalatine artery and ligation of the artery with surgical clip is performed. The mucoperiosteal flap is then repositioned and the procedure is concluded simply by placing a Surgicel on the incision site.

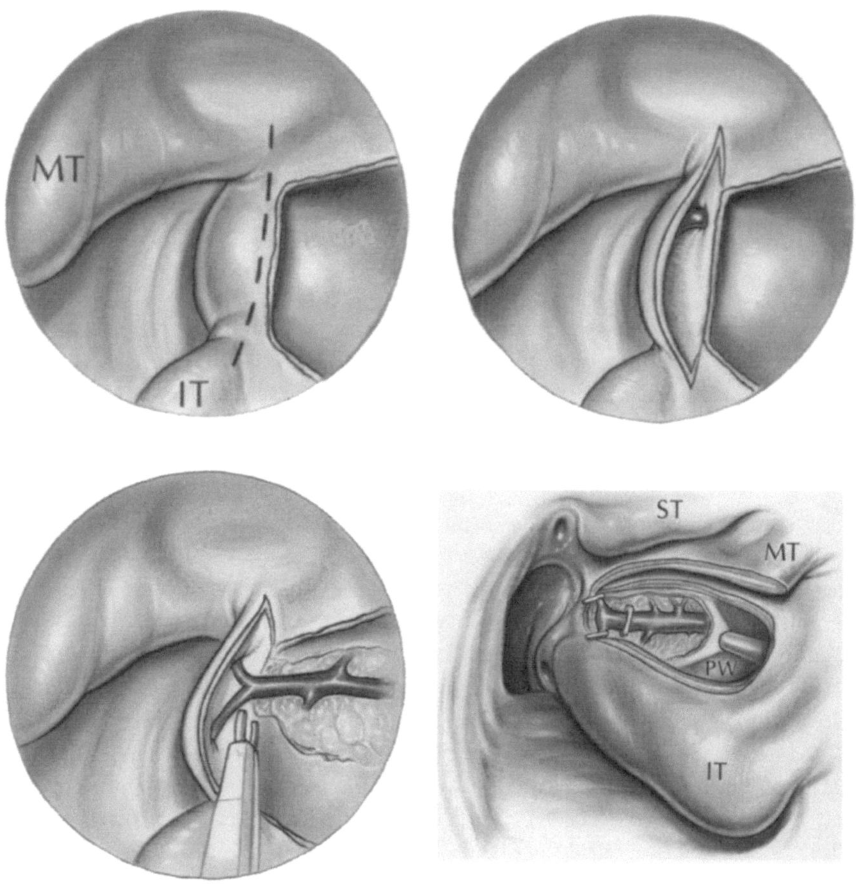

Fig. 5. Endoscopic ligation of sphenopalatine artery. Left side. A.The mucosa immediately posterior to the attachment of the middle turbinate is elevated to expose the branches of the sphenopalatine artery. B. The bone of the sphenopalatine foramen is removed to expose the main artery. C. The artery and its main branches are ligated with microclips. D. The mucosal flap is covered for the last step of the surgery. (Snyderman & Carau, 1997) MT; middle turbinate, IT; inferior turbinate, ST; superior turbinate.

After the operation, the patient's activity should be restricted for several days. After discharge from the hospital, activity and diet are gradually returned to normal. Full activity, including exercise, should be avoided for 2 weeks after the procedure. Extreme care must be exercised when suctioning over the area of the ligation during dressing, to avoid accidentally suctioning off one of the clips. All of the complications associated with endoscopic sinus surgery are possible with this endoscopic ligation procedure, though the risks of those are lower in this setting than for routine endoscopic sinus surgery.

5.4.4 External carotid artery ligation

External carotid artery ligation is performed at site afar from nasal cavity, so rebleeding from collateral vessels from internal carotid artery or contralateral carotid artery is reported upto 45% of patients. Therefore, limited cases of epistaxis from peripheral collateral vessels from external carotid artery are indicated for external carotid artery ligation.

Horizontal incision between hyoid and superior border of thyroid cartilage is made, subplatysmal flap elevation is performed and sternocleidomastoid muscle is retracted posteriorly to visualize internal jugular vein, which is retracted to identify external carotid artery. More than two branches should be identified to confirm external carotid artery from internal carotid artery, and then external carotid artery is ligated.

5.5 Arterial embolization

One of the options for severe posterior epistaxis is intraarterial embolization. Selective arterial embolization has advantages that duration of in-hospital stay is short, procedure can be performed under local anesthesia, vessels that are laborious for surgical approach can be treated, and success rate is high in surgical failure cases of arteriovenous communication. This procedure is usually performed under local anesthesia in the arteriography suite of the hospital, a catheter is placed into the groin and threaded through the femoral artery, into the aorta, into the carotid artery and finally into the internal maxillary artery. A test injection is performed to identify the bleeding site. If there is no communication between internal maxillary artery and internal carotid artery or vertebral artery, various materials are used for embolization, including gelfoam, coils, balloons, and polyvinyl alcohol particles. Injection of the materials is repeated until blood flow at the bleeding sites decreases or stops. If bleeding have recurred short after the embolization, the source of the bleeding is anterior or posterior ethmoid artery, which are branches of internal carotid artery, so surgical approach to these vessels might be needed, and collateral vessel bleeding from facial artery is occurred, reembolization should be performed. More than half of cases of rebleeding long after the treatment are reported to be hereditary hemorrhagic telangiectasia.

Embolization is a useful and highly successful technique for controlling posterior epistaxis. However, in all large series of carotid artery catherization, there is an incidence of serious cerebrovascular accident (CVA) resulting in permanent neurologic deficit. The incidence of this varies with the skill of the radiologist in performing the procedure, with an overall average of about 4%. As it is a relatively high rate for such a major complication, the use of embolization for control of epistaxis is still controversial.

5.6 Septoplasty

Septoplasty is helpful to manage epistaxis in selected cases with severe septal deviation or septal mass. This procedure is needed in cases that bleeding focus is behind the septal spur or management approach is hindered by septal deviation. As most haemorrhages occur from the septum, raising a mucoperichondral flap during septal surgery can be beneficial as this will decrease blood flow to the mucosa, which often in itself stems bleeding. It is also performed to block the blood supply in Kiesselbach plexus, or to remove hemorrhagic nodule or septal turbinate. Surgery is also used to correct a deviated septum or remove a septal spur, which may be the cause of epistaxis. This occurs either by altering air flow through the nose or in severe cartilage deformities, by persistent mucosal irritation. As it is one of the most common procedures that are performed by rhinologists, detailed operation skills are not described in this chapter. (Pope & Hobbs, 2005)

5.7 Anonymous

5.7.1 Fibrin glue

Fibrin glue is developed from human plasma cryoprecipitate and binds itself to damaged vessels. The technique entails spraying a thin layer of glue over the bleeding site and can be repeated as needed. On one randomized trial has reported that complications of local swelling, nasal mucosa atrophy, and excessive nasal discharge were lower than the electrocautery, silver nitrate, and nasal packing group. The rebleed rate was 15%, which is comparable to electrocautery. (Pope & Hobbs, 2005)

5.7.2 Hot water irrigation

Hot water irrigation was first described by Guice in 1878 as an effective method of treating severe, life-threatening epistaxis. Hot water irrigation is performed in continuous posterior epistaxis cases. The affected nasal cavity is continuously irrigated during 3 minutes with 500 ml water heated to 50°C after packing the posterior choanae with balloon catheter. Tap water is administered via a water irrigator. The patient is then seated upright with their face pointed downward over a basin, to allow outflow of water from the affected nasal cavity into the basin. This method produces vasodilation and edema of the nasal mucosa without the risk of necrosis. This mucosal edema leads to local compression of the bleeding vessels, while at the same time triggering and probably accelerating the clotting cascade. (Novoa & Schlegel-Wagner, 2011)

5.8 Management of Hereditary Hemorrhagic Telangiectasia

The management of HHT depends on several independent factors. These include the number and location of the intranasal lesions, the severity and frequency of epistaxis, the number and location of gastrointestinal, brain and pulmonary lesions, the number of blood transfusions attributable to the epistaxis, the effect of the epistaxis on the patient's quality of life and the previous treatments attempted.

Medical therapy for HHT, in addition to that outlined earlier for epistaxis in general, has focused on the use of estrogen and progesterone. This treatment was based on the observation that epistaxis tended to decrease during pregnancy among affected individuals. Antifibrinolytic therapy using aminocaproic acid has also been discussed. None of these medical treatments has proven effective in completely relieving epistaxis in the long term, but some benefits have been claimed.

Because of the failure of these methods, numerous other modalities have been attempted, including sclerotherapy, brachytherapy, electrocautery, arterial ligation, embolization, septodermoplasty, closure of the nasal cavities, and laser coagulation. The clear implication of all of these reports is that there remains no cure for HHT and, despite all treatment attempts, recurrent epistaxis is possible. In light of these facts, the author suggests that treatment should be designed to minimize the bleeding while avoiding complications. For this reason, extreme measures, such as brachytherapy, embolization, and invasive surgery, should be avoided.

As regards laser treatment of HHT, there is controversy over which type of laser is best. Carbon dioxide, ND:YAG, pulsed dye laser, diode and KTP lasers have all been used for this purpose, with the KTP laser now gaining consensus as the most popular device. It has been suggested that laser can easily ablate the periphery of larger lesions to reduce central blood flow, but that direct laser focused on the center of a lesion causes extensive bleeding and makes further treatment difficult. (Joshi et al., 2011)

Septodermoplasty involves removal of nasal mucosa from the anterior part of the nasal cavity and replacement by a split skin graft. This technique has been found to have good initial outcomes in patients with HHT patients, which unfortunately decline over time due to contraction and revascularization of the graft. The technique has also been found to be associated with nasal crusting and halitosis.

Closure of the nasal cavity, the so called Young's procedure is a radical technique involving closure of the nasal vestibule. Although it provides long term relief in patients with moderate to severe epistaxis secondary to HHT, the disadvantages (dry mouth, loss of smell and complete nasal obstruction) are often not tolerated by patients. Upon reviewing the procedure, Young himself found that many patients had to have the procedure reversed because of these problems. Young's procedure is best reserved for cases of HHT unresponsive to other treatment modalities.

Radiofrequency coblation is a relatively new technique which is being increasingly used in ENT surgery. Coblation has been demonstrated to promote good healing and to preserve surrounding normal tissue. Despite low temperatures, small blood vessels are sealed by this process. Radiofrequency coblation can therefore theoretically achieve both ablation and hemostasis of telangiectatic and arteriovenous malformations, using the same instrument. The use of coblation for hereditary haemorrhagic telangiectasia epistaxis is a much more conservative procedure, which can be safely repeated without significant complications. (Joshi et al., 2011)

Elevated plasma levels of vascular endothelial growth factor (VEGF) play a key pathogenic role in HHT. Bevacizumab, an anti-VEGF monoclonal antibody, prevents the binding of VEGF to VEGF receptor on endothelial cells, thus blocking cellular proliferation and angiogenesis. As a result, bevacizumab has been used as a potential treatment of recurrent epistaxis. Previous studies have demonstrated marked improvement of epistaxis with intravenous administration of bevacizumab. Intranasal treatment with bevacizumab, by either submucosal injection or topical nasal spray, has recently been reported to be a safe alternative to intravenous treatment. (Brinkerhoff et al., 2011)

6. Conclusion

Over the past decade, there has been a significant development in the options available for the management of epistaxis. Traditional strategies like nasal packing have been supplemented by modern technology using the latest optic and electrical devices. Treatment should ideally use a systematic protocol; starting with simple procedures that can be undertaken in the clinic environment and proceeding to endoscopic techniques for more difficult cases.

7. References

Brinkerhoff, BT, Choong, NW, Treisman, JS & Poetker, DM (2011). Intravenous and topical intranasal bevacizumab (Avastin) in hereditary hemorrhagic telangiectasia. *American Journal of Otolaryngology* Vol. No., (Sep 12), pp., ISSN 0196-0709

Cho, JS (2009).Epistaxis. In: *Otorhinolarngology head and neck surgery*, surgery, KsoO-Han, pp. 1048-1057, Ilchokak, ISBN 978-89-337-0559-9, Seoul

Fuchizaki, U, Miyamori, H, Kitagawa, S, Kaneko, S & Kobayashi, K (2003). Hereditary haemorrhagic telangiectasia (Rendu-Osler-Weber disease). *The Lancet* Vol. 362, No. 9394, (Nov 1), pp. 1490-1494, ISSN 0140-6736

Guttmacher, AE, Marchuk, DA & White, RI, Jr. (1995). Hereditary hemorrhagic telangiectasia. *The New England Journal of Medicine* Vol. 333, No. 14, (Oct 5), pp. 918-924, ISSN 0028-4793

Herkner, H, Laggner, AN, Mullner, M, Formanek, M, Bur, A, Gamper, G, Woisetschlager, C & Hirschl, MM (2000). Hypertension in patients presenting with epistaxis. *Annals of Emergency Medicine* Vol. 35, No. 2, (Feb), pp. 126-130, ISSN 0196-0644

Joshi, H, Woodworth, BA & Carney, AS (2011). Coblation for epistaxis management in patients with hereditary haemorrhagic telangiectasia: a multicentre case series. *The Journal of Laryngology & Otology* Vol. No., (Aug 16), pp. 1-5, ISSN 1748-5460

Novoa, E & Schlegel-Wagner, C (2011). Hot water irrigation as treatment for intractable posterior epistaxis in an out-patient setting. *The Journal of Laryngology & Otology* Vol. No., (Sep 5), pp. 1-3, ISSN 1748-5460

Pope, LE & Hobbs, CG (2005). Epistaxis: an update on current management. *Postgraduate Medical Journal* Vol. 81, No. 955, (May), pp. 309-314, ISSN 0032-5473

Snyderman, CH & Carau, RL (1997). Endoscopic Ligation of the Sphenopalatine Artery For Epistaxis. *Operative Techniques in Otolaryngology Head and Neck Surgery* Vol. 8, No. 2, (Jun 1997), pp. 85-89, ISSN 1043-1810

Viducich, RA, Blanda, MP & Gerson, LW (1995). Posterior epistaxis: clinical features and acute complications. *Annals of Emergency Medicine* Vol. 25, No. 5, (May), pp. 592-596, ISSN 0196-0644

3

Endoscopic Dacryocystorhinostomy

Chris de Souza[1], Rosemarie de Souza[2*] and Jayesh Nisar[3]
[1]*Lilavati Hospital, Holy Family Hospital and Tata Memorial Hospital*
[2]*TNMC Medical College and the BYL Nair Hospital*
[3]*Gala Eye Hospital and Jain Health Center*
Mumbai
India

1. Introduction

Early cases of dacryocystitis occur because of inflammation of the mucous membrane with resulting malfunction in the subepithelial cavernous body with occlusion of the lacrimal passage. Repeated attacks of dacryocystitis leads to structural epithelial changes, with loss of mucin, loss of TFF peptide producing goblet cells and columnar epithelial cells. Remodeling of the helical arrangement of the subepithelial connective tissue fibers leads to total fibrous closure. This then leads to epiphora.Primary acquired nasolacrimal duct obstruction (PANDO) is a syndrome of unknown origin.

2. Diagnostics

Two basic causes of tearing exist. Epiphora that is associated with blockage of the lacrimal system and excessive lacrimation (hyperlacrimation) which is a less common cause. Hyperlacrimation is caused by corneal irritation. Unilateral hyper lacrimation is caused by trigeminal sensory nerve stimulation.

Epiphora is tearing caused by a reduced tear transport mechanism or a defective tear drainage outflow. Epiphora can on occasion be caused by a combination of both.

2.1 Goals of diagnostics are the following

1. To distinguish epiphora from hyperlacrimation.
2. Determine pathological process that is the cause.
3. To distinguish anatomical and functional disorders.
4. To evaluate the location of the block, its extent and to decide on the appropriate approach which is usually surgical.

2.2 The diagnostic tests are divided into the following

a. Anatomical tests for investigation of morphological disorders and location of the site of obstruction as in punctal and canalicular pathologies, nasolacrimal duct obstruction (PANDO) and nasal pathologies.

* Corresponding Author

b. Functional (physiological) tests for drainage of tears under normal conditions as in lacrimal pump insufficiency due to incorrect eyelid closure,, ectropion , enteropion etc.
c. Secretion: tests for assessment of secretion.

2.3 The clinical tests are the following

Anatomical tests include palpation of the lacrimal sac, examination of the eyelids and condition of the puncta, syringing (irrigation), diagnostic probing, dacrycystography, nasal examination, and CT scanning and MRI.

Physiological tests are:- Fluorescein dye disappearance, scintigraphy Jones dye I, saccharin test.

Tests of secretion include:- Schirmirs tests, Bengal rose test, tear film break up and tear lysozyme test.

3. Surgery

3.1 Endoscopic DCR surgery versus external DCR?

Endoscopic DCR has gained wide spread acceptance and is now considered the surgical approach of choice **(1)**, **(2)**.

The reasons why the external approach has declined is because (a) There is a facial scar following External DCR and (b) It is difficult to revise.

Endoscopic DCR is attractive because

1. The results are equal to if not better than External DCR.
2. There is no facial scar.
3. It can be revised easily.
4. It can be performed on patients of all ages.
5. It can easily be learnt and can be done safely and reliably.
6. Small fibrotic lacrimal sacs which cannot be operated upon by the external approach can be operated upon using the endoscopic approach.
7. Complications like bleeding are much less.
8. Endoscopic DCRs take much less operating time.

3.2 The role of stents

Stents can be used for small fibrotic lacrimal sacs to make sure that the neo-ostium remains patent **(3)**. The authors prefer to reserve stents for this situation only because (1) Removal causes the opening to close, (2) The possibility of corneal opacity should the stent move its position. Surgery was successful as long as the stent was in situ. When stents were removed the sac obstructed again. Therefore the authors decided to leave the stents in situ indefinitely as long as there were no problems caused by the stent. An exact time frame for removal of the stents could not be given to patients.

4. The use of 5 fluorouracil and mitomicin

The authors have found that these substances do not add to the success of patency in their series.

The authors in their series of over one thousand consecutive endoscopic DCRs found that the best technique for achieving consistently good reliable results was the removal of the medial wall of the lacrimal sac allowing it to heal in close conjunction with the mucosa of the nasal cavity. This was possible in a majority of cases as the lacrimal sac was large. When the lacrimal sac was small fibrosed and cicatrized stents were needed to maintain patency.

4.1 Surgical technique

The surgeons preferred to operate under local anesthesia. An external block was given with .5% bupivacaine. The nasal cavity was anesthetized and decongested with 4% xylocaine cotton patties.

The area of the Agger Nasi air cells was infiltrated with 2% xylocaine with 1 in 200,000 adrenaline solution.

The flap anterior to the Middle turbinate was elevated. The periosteum was also elevated.

The lacrimal bone was drilled out with a large diamond polishing burr. A large osteotomy was performed until the entire limits of the lacrimal sac was seen and clearly identified. Once the lacrimal sac was clearly identified its medial wall was excised. Methyline blue was carefully and gently flushed from both puncta to ascertain clear passage through both puncta.

Once this was achieved then the medial wall of the lacrimal sac was removed. The medial wall was removed in such a way that it lies flush with the osteotomy. The nasal mucosa was then trimmed so that no bone was left bare. This step in particular is important because it has reduced the formation of granulomas. Care was taken such that the nasal flap did not cover the opening created in the lacrimal sac.

A pack was placed which can be removed 12 hours later.

The patient is instructed not to blow his nose. Careful nasal toilette ensures removal of crusts/ debris. This nasal toilette also prevents the occurrence of synechiae. The puncta are not flushed as the authors believe that this could result in trauma to the puncta which in turn could result in stenosis of the puncta.

4.2 Goals of surgery

1. Cessation of Epiphora
2. Patency of the neo-ostium
3. There should be no further attacks of dacryocystitis.

4.3 Results

The authors reported their results in a series of 1450 consecutive endoscopic DCRs using 4 different techniques from January 1994 to December 2007 **(4)**.

In one set of patients they merely incised and drained the lacrimal sacs, in another they inserted grommets. In a third set they removed the medial wall of the LS and in a fourth set they inserted stents. All the data was then analyzed statistically.

It was found that the best results were achieved with removal of the medial wall allowing the LS to get marsupialized. Stenting the LS also provided good results but had the disadvantage of causing corneal opacities especially if the stent moved from its position**(5)**.

Inserting grommets or incising and draining the LS gave poor results. Removal of the medial wall of the LS allowing it to fistulize into the nasal cavity was statistically more successful and was found to be statistically significant.

5. Conclusions and summary

1. Endoscpic DCR is a safe and valid procedure
2. Results with endoscopic DCRs are excellent.
3. It can be revised easily.
4. It is cost effective
5. It is not associated with major complications.
6. Removal of the medial wall allowing the lacrimal sac to marsupialize into the nasal cavity is the best way to ensure long term patency.
7. Stenting is also effective but on occasion can cause corneal opacities especially when it is loosened.

6. References

Feretis M, Newton JR, Ram B et al: Comparison of external and endonasal dacryocystorhinostomy. *Journal of Laryngology and Otology* 2008:20:1-5.

Yigit O, Samancioglu M, Taskin U et al: External and endoscopic dacryocystorhinostomy in chronic dacryocystitis; comparison of results. *European Archives of Otorhinolaryngology* 2007: 264:879-885.

Welsh MG, Katowitz JA: Timing of silastic tubing removal after intubation for congenital nasolacrimal duct obstruction. *Opthal Plastic Reconstr Surger.* 1989:5:43-48.

De Souza CE, Nissar J: Experience with endoscopic dacryocystorhinostomy using four methods. *Otolaryngology- Head and Neck Surgery*2010:142:389-393.

Smirnov G, Tuomilehto H, TerasvirtaM et al; Silicone tubing is not necessary after primary endoscopic dacryocystorhinostomy: a prospective randomized study.*American Journal of Rhinology* 2008: 22: 214-217.

4

Endoscopic Dacryocystorhinostomy

Farhad Farahani
Hamedan university of Medical Sciences
Iran

1. Introduction

Endoscopic DCR has gained a lot of attention among otolaryngologists since the outcomes are comparable to the external approach. Advances in surgical technique and a better understanding of the anatomy have resulted in improvement of outcomes.

The main goal of this chapter is to acquaint readers with the anatomy and function of lacrimal system, the newly emerged technique of endoscopic DCR and its related topics.

In this chapter, the anatomy of the lacrimal system will be discussed in detail. Then, the conditions needing surgical manipulation will be noted in addition to assessing the patients with such problems. Surgical indications and techniques of DCR will be explained. Some topics such as the advantages, results and complications of the surgery and the role of Mytomycin C are included, too.

2. Anatomy

2.1 Lacrimal gland and excretory system

2.1.1 Lacrimal gland

The main lacrimal gland is located in a shallow depression along the superior lateral orbit. There is fibroadipose tissue between the gland and the orbit. The gland is divided into 2 parts by a lateral expansion of the levator apeunorosis. An isthmus of glandular tissue occasionally exists between the palpebral lobe and the main orbital gland[1].

Many accessory lacrimal glands can be found along the inner surface of the eyelids. A variable number of thin-walled excretory ducts, blood vessels, lymphatics, and nerves pass from the main orbital gland into these accessory lacrimal glands. The ducts continue downward, and about 12 of them empty into the conjunctival fornix approximately 5 mm above the superior margin of the upper tarsus. Because the lacrimal excretory ducts pass through the palpebral portion of the gland, biopsy of the lacrimal gland is usually performed on the main part to avoid sacrificing the ducts[1].

The lacrimal glands are exocrine glands, and they produce a serous secretion. The body of each gland contains 2 cell types:

- acinar cells, which line the lumen of the gland

- myoepithelial cells, which surround the parenchyma and are covered by a basement membrane

The lacrimal artery, a branch of the ophthalmic artery, supplies the gland. The lacrimal gland receives secretomotor cholinergic, vasoactive intestinal polypeptide (VIP)-ergic,and sympathetic nerve fibers in addition to a sensory innervation via the lacrimal nerve (CN V1). Cyclic adenosine monophosphate is the second messenger for VIP and β-adrenergic stimulation of the gland; cholinergic stimulation acts through an inositol 1,4,5-triphosphate-activated protein kinase C. The gland also contains α_1-adrenergic receptors. Extremely complex, the gland's neuroanatomy governs both reflex and psychogenic stimulation[1].

2.1.2 Accessory glands

The accessory lacrimal glands of Krause and Wolfring are located at the proximal lid borders or in the fornices and are cytologically identical to the main lacrimal gland, receiving a similar innervation. They account for about 10% of the total lacrimal secretory mass[1].

2.1.3 Lacrimal excretory system

The lacrimal excretory (drainage) system includes the upper and lower puncta, the lacrimal canaliculi, the lacrimal sac, and the nasolacrimal duct. It is important to note that the first 2 mm of canaliculi are perpendicular to the lid margin but the distal 8 mm are parallel to the

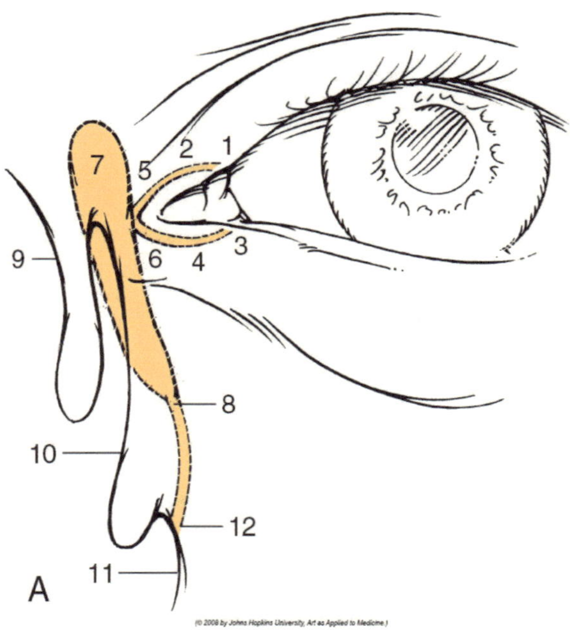

Fig. 1. Anatomy of the left lacrimal apparatus
1.superior punctum 2.superior canaliculus 3.inferior punctum 4.inferior canaliculus 5.medial canthal ligament 6.common canaliculus 7.lacrimal sac 8. Lacrimal duct 9.middle turbinate 10.lacrimal bone 11.inferior turbinate 12.Hasner's valve

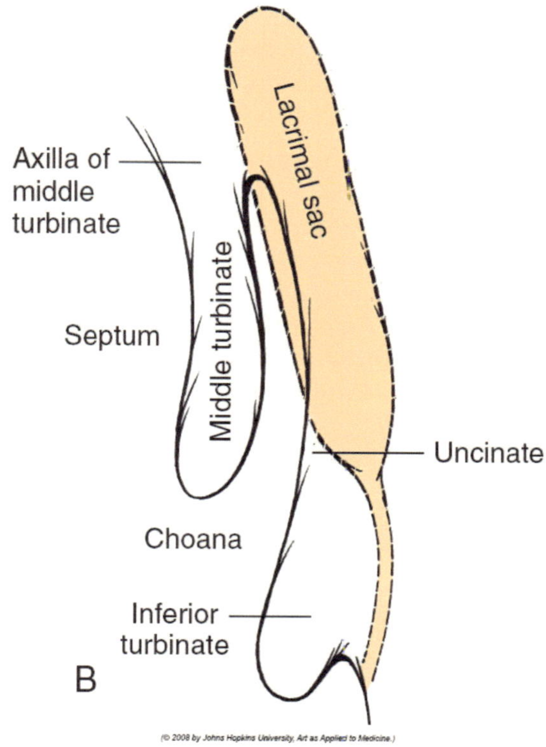

Fig. 2. Position of lacrimal sac as seen during endonasal visualization

lid. In 90% of people, the two canaliculi join to make a common canaliculus before entering the lacrimal sac. The lacrimal sac is placed in an oval-shaped fossa measuring 15 mm in height and 10 mm in width. This fossa is bounded by anterior and posterior lacrimal crests which fuse at a suture line that crosses the lacrimal fossa in a vertical manner. The lacrimal sac opens into nasolacrimal canal which is formed by the maxillary, lacrimal, and inferior turbinate bones. The nasolacrimal duct passes through this osseous canal for approximately 12 mm. Then it turns into a membranous duct for 5 mm before entering the inferior meatus[2]. The duct orifice is often covered by Hasner's valve to prevent reflux of secretions. In about 30% of full-term neonates, the outlet of the nasolacrimal duct is closed for up to 6 months. Occasionally, probing may be necessary to achieve patency.

The lacrimal puncta and the canaliculi are lined with stratified squamous nonkeratinized epithelium that merges with the epithelium of the eyelid margins. Near the lacrimal sac, the epithelium changes into 2 layers: a superficial columnar layer and a deep, flattened cell layer. Goblet cells and occasional cilia are present. In the canaliculi, the substantia propria consists of collagenous connective tissue and elastic fibers. The wall of the lacrimal sac resembles adenoid tissue and has a rich venous plexus and elastic fibers.

3. Etiologies and predisposing factors of lacrimal obstruction

Patients with obstruction of lacrimal system usually complain of excessive tearing or epiphora. When dacryocystitis occurs, purulent drainage or inflammation can be noticed in the medial canthal region. It is important to ask patients about any nasal airway obstruction, drainage or epistaxis, which may suggest intranasal causes of lacrimal obstruction, such as polyps or neoplasms. Sometimes, the nasolacrimal duct is injured secondary to prior sinus surgery, particularly a large maxillary antrostomy.

Lacrimal excretory system foreign bodies are rare but they can impair draining function and might be presented as epiphora, recurrent attacks of acute dacryocystitis and in some patients, chronic dacryocystitis[3]. Exogenous foreign bodies in most patients lodge in lacrimal sac or nasolacrimal duct after external manipulation[3]. Foreign bodies in some patients have endogenous origin and in the form of dacryoliths may lead to lacrimal flow obstruction[3]. In both forms, surgical removal of foreign bodies is necessary[3]. Classic surgical approach is external dacryocystorhinostomy (DCR) but in recent years with rapid improvement of endoscopic techniques intranasal approaches introduce themselves as an effective substitute for external DCR[3]. These approaches are helpful for preoperative diagnosis and effective for surgical removal of lacrimal foreign bodies.

We had an experience with foreign bodies which was published in Iranian journal of ophthalmology. In our case, the lacrimal sac foreign body was a piece of silicon tube that was used as a stent in previous external DCR. On retrospective enquiry we found that at the time of silicon tube removal, it was pulled forcefully out through the lacrimal canaliculi and when it was impacted at the given site it was cut and the remaining part could not be found through the nose. The presenting signs and symptoms of this case were completely similar to the failed DCR procedure, so she was referred to our department for more evaluation. Anterior rhinoscopy is normal in many of such cases, so we should emphasize on the role of the nasal endoscopy as a safe and rapid diagnostic method. In the nasal endoscopy, the condition of rhinostomy site can be evaluated and any foreign body, granulation tissue, scar formation or synechia between middle turbinate and lateral nasal wall can be found and appropriate treatment plan can be established[3].

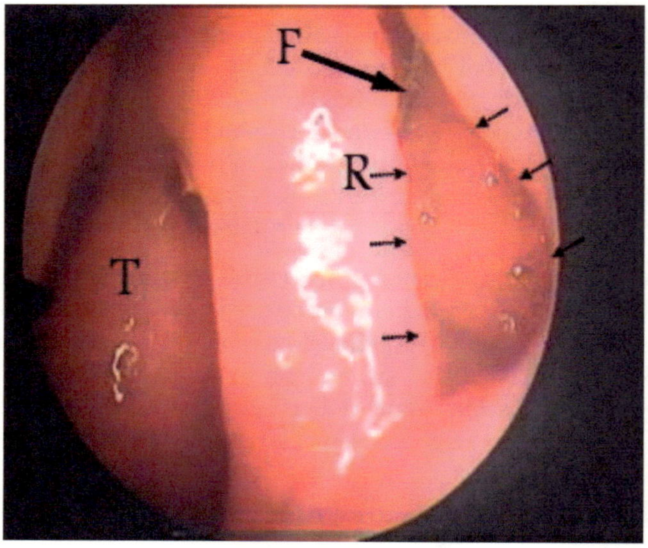

Fig. 3. Rhinostomy site with foreign body T: Middle turbinate, R: Previous rhinostomy site, F: Foreign body

Dacryoliths (lacrimal stones) or "calculi" of the nasolacrimal ducts were described by Cesoni in as early as 1670[4], and have been reported to occur in between 6 and 18% of patients with nasolacrimal duct obstruction who undergo dacryocystorhinostomy (DCR). Dacryoliths may occur in any part of the nasolacrimal system, albeit most commonly in the lacrimal sac. Several predisposing factors have been suggested, such as increased occurrence in females, patient age below 50 years, association with cigarette smoking and facial-sinonasal trauma, and increased frequency subsequent to previous occurrence of dacryocystitis. However, other studies have indicated increased frequency in males and patients aged above 50 years. Therefore, it seems that both genders are involved to nearly the same extent. Dacryoliths usually become symptomatic when they obstruct the nasolacrimal system. This can result in epiphora, acute dacryocystitis, protrusion of the lacrimal canthal region, and partial closure of the lacrimal passage (recognized during syringing by the ophthalmologist). Interestingly, dacryoliths occur more often in patients with partial and incomplete closure of the lacrimal passage (i.e., patients with epiphora despite patent lacrimal passages on syringing). Scanning electron microscopy has shown that dacryoliths are composed of lobes and lobules built on an amorphous core material[5]. Atomic absorption spectrophotometric investigations demonstrate that dacryoliths consist almost entirely of organic proteins and, to a much lesser extent, of inorganic material[5]. According to Lew et al., lacrimal fluid from patients with dacryoliths contains a reduced amount of lysozyme and a lower calcium concentration than normal lacrimal fluid. It is important to recognize that daryoliths are not calcified or composed of any other "hard" substances. Some stones reveal hyphae-like structures, although no fungi were recovered by culturing[5].

4. Assessment of the patient

4.1 Physical examination

A comprehensive ophthalmologic examination is mandatory in the primary evaluation of every patient with lacrimal system obstruction. An examination with the slit lamp can reveal the normal or abnormal tear film over the conjunctiva and if the thickness of the tearfilm is more than usual, it can be a sign of lacrimal drainage system obstruction. In addition, the ocular surface, eyelid structures, visual acuity, extraocular motility, and visual field should be tested and documented before surgery.

Gentle pressure over the sac produces reflux of mucopurulent material suggestive of lower sac obstruction (regurgitation test).

Irrigation test is another useful test in assessing patients. In this test, an appropriate lacrimal syringe is passed through the inferior lacrimal punctum and 2-5 ml of sterile distilled water is injected and pushed though the inferior canaliculus. If the water passes easily into the nose and the patient senses that, the patency of the system is confirmed. Otherwise, it is one of the most reliable signs of lacrimal system obstruction. Some authors recommend that after either external or endoscopic DCR, this test can be performed indicating the patency of the system.

Nasal examination, especially nasal endoscopy, should be obligatory for every lacrimal obstruction patient. The examination of the lacrimal area with the nasal speculum and headlight provides only a poor view of this region and is not sufficient; Endoscopy provides a clear diagnostic look for nasal polyps, imporant anatomic variations, tumors, and other pathological endonasal conditions such as septal deviation.

Diagnostic nasal endoscopy is performed with a rigid endoscope or flexible endoscope which can be used without any difficulties in small children, too.

The rigid endoscopes are 4-mm in diameter, with 0 or 30° viewing angle. The 2.7-mm diameter endoscope can be advantageous, especially in children and some adults with narrow nasal cavities. The inferior and the middle meatus are better viewed if some decongestants are introduced into the nose.

4.2 Radiologic evaluation

Radiological tests should be done before DCR which include dacryocystography (DCG), nuclear lacrimal scintigraphy (dacryo scintillography), computed tomography (CT), and magnetic resonance imaging (MRI).

Dacryocystography is an anatomical investigation and is indicated if there is a block on syringing in the lacrimal system, and thus it can help in creating an image of how the internal anatomy of the lacrimal system looks.

Scintigraphy is a functional test and is useful in assessing the site of a delayed tear transit, i.e., it is useful only if the lacrimal system is patent on syringing.

Both CT and MRI are used very seldom and are reserved only for some patients with preceded trauma, facial surgery, tumor, or in whom sinus diseases are suspected.

4.3 Dacryocystography

Dacryocystography is a method in which injection of the radio-opaque water-soluble fluid is instilled into either lower or upper canaliculus taking magnified images. The digital subtraction technique is preferred because it gives an image of better quality. A DCG better evaluates the lacrimal sac and duct anatomy, but it evaluates worse canalicular anatomy. It outlines diverticulae and fistulae, and shows intrasac pathology (dacryoliths or tumor) and the sac size. A DCG is not routinely performed. It is seldom necessary with a complete obstruction in the non-traumatic situation. It can be especially useful in patients with previous trauma to localize the position of bone fragments or, after previously unsuccessful lacrimal surgery, to determine the size of the sac. With patency to syringing, the DCG helps to determine whether the stenosis is in the common canaliculus or sac, and it can rule out the presence of a lacrimal sac diverticulum[6]. A DCG can often find drainage abnormalities present in patients with "functional obstruction"[6].

4.4 Nuclear lacrimal scintigraphy

Nuclear lacrimal scintigraphy is a simple, non-invasive physiological test that evaluates patency of the lacrimal system. Scintigraphy uses a radiotracer (technetium-99m pertechnetate), which is very easily detectable with a gamma camera. While a DCG is usually preferred especially in a complete obstruction, scintigraphy is useful only in those patients whose lacrimal system is patent to syringing in the presence of constant epiphora. The test is more physiological than DCG, anatomical information is lacking, and fine anatomical details are not available in comparison with DCG[7]. Correlation of the anatomical study (DCG) and functional study (scintigraphy) may be necessary in planning surgery[8]; However, it is important to bear in mind that a normal result is considered to be a contraindication to any surgical intervention[7]. Nuclear lacrimal scan has been found to be helpful especially in difficult cases with incompletely obstructed pathways in which DCG could not be interpreted in a satisfactory manner to determine whether surgery should be undertaken or not[9].

4.5 Computed tomography and MRI

Computed tomography (CT) can be helpful in assessing the structures intimately associated with the nasolacrimal drainage system. The CT scanning is used mainly when an extrinsic disease is suspected and is of great help to the patients with paranasal sinus or facial pathology associated with the lacrimal system (tumor, rhinosinusitis, facial trauma, following facial surgery, etc.)[10].

Magnetic resonance is not used in practice in lacrimal diagnostics and is reserved only for the special cases, e.g., for differentiation of masses of the lacrimal sac[8].

5. Surgical indications

DCR is the treatment of choice for those patients who present with persistent epiphora or chronic dacryocystitis from nasolacrimal duct obstruction. The obstruction is usually due to a primary acquired condition of unknown etiology. The other causes are trauma, infection, neoplasm, and lacrimal stones.

6. Surgical technique

Dacryocystorhinostomy can be performed both externally and as an endoscopic approach. The external approach is commonly done by ophthalmologists. In external approach, an incision is made between the medial canthus and the nasal dorsum. Then the lacrimal sac is exposed and elevated from the lacrimal fossa. The lacrimal bone with an almost diameter of 1 cm is drilled. Hence, two anterior and posterior lacrimal flaps are created which are sutured to the flaps made from nasal mucosa. Finally, two silicone tubes (Budkin's tubes) are passed through the superior and inferior canaliculi and fixed in the nose.

The endoscopic approach, however, has gained much attention among ENT surgeons. Endoscopic DCR can be performed under either local or general anesthesia. It is recommended to have a video camera attached to the endoscope so that the assistant surgeon can observe the maneuvers on a video monitor.

The patient is placed in a supine position with the head slightly elevated to decrease the venous pressure at the operation site. To decongest the mucosa, vasoconstrictors are applied through pledgets in the nose. Then, injections composing of 1% lidocaine and 1:100000 epinephrine must be performed. Usually, superior to the axilla and anterior to the uncinate process are injected.

Sometimes, an endoscopic septoplasty is needed to reduce the complexity of the procedure[11, 12]. If required, appropriate injections in the septum must be done, too. The septoplasty is usually limited and just the superior and anterior portions of the bony septum are corrected.

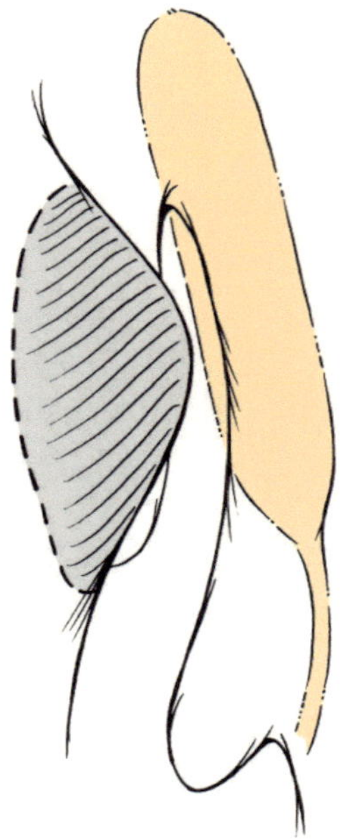

Fig. 4. High endoscopic septoplasty. Ideal area of removal is indicated by a dashed line.

A 30-degree scope is used through the procedure to have adequate visualization around the frontal process of the maxilla. A DCR flap must be created considering the lacrimal sac in mind. The superior incision must be 5mm posterior and 10mm superior to the axilla. It is brought 10mm anterior to the middle turbinate to be able to marsupialize the lacrimal sac fully. The inferior incision would be at the insertion of the inferior turbinate.

An elevator is used to make a subperiosteal plane along the incisions towards the frontal process of the maxilla. The flap must be mobilized over the frontal process of the maxilla until the lacrimal bone is identified. The best place to identify the lacrimal bone is the region adjacent to the inferior horizontal incision just above the inferior turbinate. Superiorly, the flap is elevated on to the insertion of the middle turbinate and posteriorly, it is elevated past the lacrimal bone onto the uncinate process. When the flap is completely elevated, its inferior pedicle is cut off the superior aspect of the inferior turbinate and its insertion to the uncinate.

A round knife is used then to identify the junction of frontal process and lacrimal bone and to flake off the lacrimal bone. The posterioinferior aspect of the lacrimal sac and adjacent nasolacrimal duct would be exposed this way. Then, a punch is used to remove the frontal process of maxilla. Superiorly, the bone thickens and it would be difficult for the punch to grip the bone. Therefore, drilling with a DCR diamond bur may be required. Care must be taken to ensure that excessive pressure is not placed on the sac wall. When the lacrimal sac is opened, it will lie flat on the lateral nasal wall. It would be marsupialized. By removing the bone from the posterolateral region of the lacrimal sac, the mucosa of the agger nasi cell will be exposed. There is a pyramid-shaped bone between the anterior aspect of the agger nasi cell and the lacrimal sac which must be completely removed. The agger nasi mucosa is opened by a sickle knife.

The next step would be checking the lacrimal puncta and dilating them by a probe if required. A sinus endoscope would be helpful for lighting the region. By passing the lacrimal probe, its metallic part can be seen within the translucent sac wall.

Then the mucosal flap is positioned to approximate nasal mucosa to the lacrimal mucosa. The common canaliculus should be visible in the lateral sac wall. Then, stenting of the system would be done. If the lacrimal probes pass easily without any resistance in the canaliculus and the common canaliculus valve of Rosenmuller, lacrimal probes need not be placed. However, if there is tightness of common canaliculus, stents should be placed through the superior and inferior canaliculi and brought out of the common canaliculus. It must be considered that the sac should stay open without the stenting action of the tubes.

Finally, the end of the tubes can be knotted and cut. The nose can be packed lightly. If there is minimal risk of epistaxis, no packing is needed.

7. Revision endoscopic dacryocystorhinostomy

The principles are similar to those of primary DCR. As far as the bone along the lateral nasal wall has already been removed, endoscopic revision DCR is much easier than the primary procedure. The important point in revision DCR is the size of the lacrimal sac.

If the sac is normal in size, the rate of success is high (89%)[11, 12]. If there is scarring and cicatrizaion of the sac, the success rate is lower because only a small amount of lacrimal mucosa can be marsupialized.

In severe stenosis and scarring of the lacrimal sac, the agger nasi mucosa can be used as a free graft to create functional mucosa surrounding the common canaliculus-sac junction.

8. Postoperative care

If nasal packing is placed at the end of surgery, it is removed the following morning. Patients must irrigate their nose with saline at least twice a day. The patient must be visited one week later and intranasal debris must be removed then.

The silastic tubing is removed 1-12 months after surgery. According to our experience, we recommend removing the tube in about 4 weeks after surgery. Exposed tubing at the medial canthus is cut with scissors and the stent is withdrawn through the nose. In revision cases with scarring the stent can be left in the place for 6 months or even longer.

During surgery sufficient opening from the lacrimal sac into the nose is made, but the final size of the healed surgical ostium is 1 to 2 mm in diameter on average.

9. Complications

Complications of endonasal DCR surgery can be divided into intraoperative and early or late postoperative. Early postoperative (up to one month) complications include hemorrhage, crusting, perirhinostomy granuloma, and transnasal synechiae; 1 - 6 months side effects of surgery include surgical failure from impacted tubes, rhinostomy scarring, granuloma, and synechiae. Most of these later complications occur between one and three months after surgery[13].

In endonasal surgery, complications are greater with inexperienced surgeons. The complications of endoscopic DCR are similar to those for endoscopic sinus surgery. Excessive bleeding during surgery precludes visualization and accounts for major intraoperative complications such as blindness and cerebrospinal fluid leakage. If excessive bleeding is encountered in endoscopic surgery, the procedure must either be terminated or converted to an open DCR. Severe postoperative epistaxis occurs in less than 5% of cases. Bleeding usually occurs within one week of surgery and is caused by a branch of the sphenopalatine artery supplying the remnant of a partially resected middle turbinate.

Sometimes, during bone removal to uncover the lacrimal sac, orbital fat is exposed. This fat should not be disturbed, otherwise orbital contents such as blood vessels, nerves, and the medial rectus muscle would be injured.

Nasal or orbital infection following DCR is rare. Nevertheless, perioperative antibiotics are administered to avoid this complication.

One of the most common causes of surgical failure for both endoscopic and external DCR is postoperative adhesions. These adhesions usually cause obstruction of the surgically created ostium. In order to decrease this complication, surgical trauma to the turbinate mucosa should be avoided and the anterior end of the turbinate should be resected so that it is not near the ostium. Correction of the deviated septum also reduces the likelihood of postoperative adhesion formation.

10. Advantages of endoscopic DCR

The advantages of intranasal endoscopic DCR in comparison to classic external DCR are as follows[13]:

1. Providing better visualization.
2. Avoiding the external scar and damage to the angular vein.
3. Preserving the normal function of lacrimal pump.
4. Identification of the sac and correct placement of the opening between the sac and the nasal cavity
5. Immediate correction of surgical mistakes such as immediate control of brisk epistaxis after anterior ethmoidal artery trauma by its direct cauterization
6. Reduction of surgery time
7. Diagnosis and treatment of coexistent intranasal disturbances.

11. Outcomes of surgery

The result of surgery, no matter the technique, depends on the type of obstruction. In a study by Tsirbas and Wormald, 95% of anatomic obstructions and 81% of fuctional obstructions became asymptomatic. Although the rate of getting asymptomatic in functional obstructions is lower, still most of them state that their situation is improved.

In one of our studies, the success rate of endoscopic DCR with mechanical devices was 91.4% in 6 months followup and 88.5% in a year followup. Intraoperaive bleeding in 88.6% of patients was mild to moderate and epistaxis during the first three days after surgery was noted in 21% of patients which was mild. In 3% of patients, the intranasal bleeding was moderate. 18% of patients had moderate pain in the first three days and 6%of them had that much pain in days 4 to 7 [13].

12. Mytomycin C and DCR

Mitomycin C is a chemotherapeutic antibiotic isolated from the broth of *streptomyces caespitosus*. Mitomycin C is an alkylating agent that is widely used systemically for the treatment of malignancies, and has also gained popularity as a topical adjunctive in the treatment of ocular surface neoplasia. The ability of this drug to modify the normal wound healing pathway by inhibiting fibroblast and endothelial cell growth and replication has made it an attractive adjunct in glaucoma and pterygium surgery, as well as in DCR surgery[14].

The primary cause of failure in DCR surgery is closure of the surgical osteotomy due to fibrosis, scarring, and granulation tissue. The intraoperative application of the anti-metabolite mitomycin C to the surgical anastamosis can theoretically inhibit such closure, and has been previously shown to increase the ostium size. Mitomycin C application varies in different published articles according to duration, manner and procedures[14].

Liao et al. by a randomized trial of 88 eyes undergoing external DCR, showed a significant increase in the number of symptom-free cases from 70.5% to 95.5% with the use of mitomycin C at 10-months follow-up and You and Fang showed increases in both ostium patency and size with the use of mitomycin C during external DCR at a mean follow-up of 3 years. Based on our study, it appeared that patients with nasolacrimal obstruction who underwent endoscopic DCR did not benefit from adjunctive topical application of mitomycin C. However, we suggest further multi-central trials for comparing results in different hospital settings[14].

13. Setup of endoscopic DCR

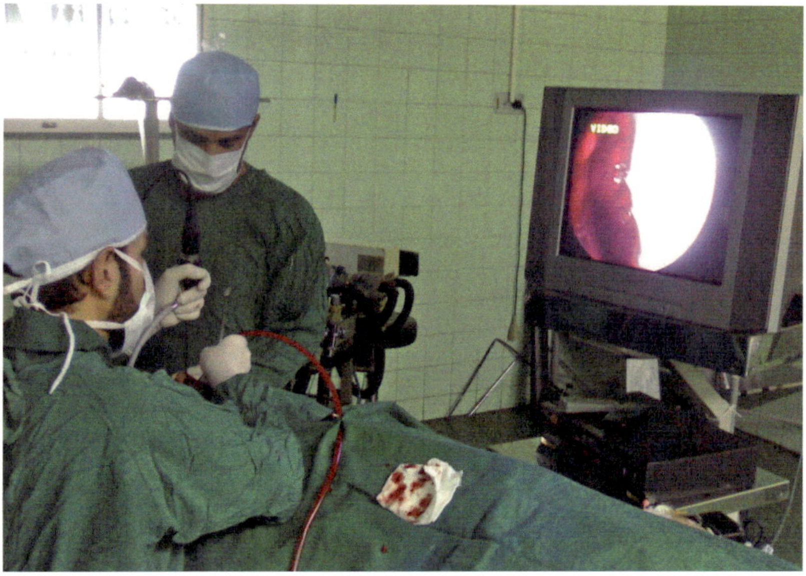

Fig. 5.

14. Acknowledgement

I would like to thank Dr. Neda Baghbanian, resident of otolaryngology- head and neck surgery, for her kind cooperation in writing this chapter.

15. References

[1] Eye MD association,American academy of ophthalmology, 2007-2008,31-34.
[2] Lang J. Clinical anatomy of the nose, nasal cavity and paranasal sinuses, New York: Thieme Medical; 1989; 99-102.
[3] Farahani F, Bazzazi N., Hashemian F. 2010, Failed Dacryocystorhinostomy due to retained silicone tube : a case report, Iranian Journal of ophthalmology;22(4).
[4] Linberg JV (2001) Discussion of lacrimal sac dacryoliths. Ophthalmology 108:1312-1313.
[5] Orhan M, Onerci M, Dayanir V, Orhan D, Irkec T, Irkec M (1996) Lacrimal sac dacryolith: a study with atomic bsorption spectrophotometry and scanning electron microscopy. Eur J Ophthalmol 6:478–480.
[6] Hurwitz JJ, Molgat Y (1994) Nasolacrimal drainage system evaluation. Ophthalmol Clin N Am 7:393–406.
[7] Hurwitz JJ (1996) The lacrimal system. Lippincott-Raven Publishers, Philadelphia.
[8] Olver J (2002) Colour atlas of lacrimal surgery. Butterworth-Heinemann, Oxford.
[9] Hurwitz JJ, Molgat Y., 1992, May23–24, Radiological test of lacrimal drainage. Diagnostic value versus cost-effectiveness. Lacrimal system. Symposium on the Lacrimal System, Brussels, 15–26.
[10] Komínek P, Červenka S, Müllner K (2003) The lacrimal diseases. Diagnosis and treatment. Maxdorf, Prague.
[11] Tsirbas A, Wormald PJ:, 2006, Mechanical endonasal dacryocystorhinostomy with mucosal flaps Otolaryngol Clin North Am; 39:1019-1036.
[12] Wormald PJ., 2006, Powered endoscopic dacryocystorhinostomy Otolaryngol Clin North Am; 39:539-549.
[13] Farahani F, Hashemian F, Fazlian MM., 2007, Endoscopic dacryocystorhinostomy for primary nasolacrimal duct obstruction. Saudi Med J;28(10):1611-3.
[14] Farahani F, Ramezani A., 2008, Effect of intraoperative mitomycin C application on recurrence of endoscopic dacryocystorhinostomy. Saudi Med J;29(9):1354-6.

5

Treatment of Allergic Rhinitis: ARIA Document, Nasal Lavage, Antihistamines, Cromones and Vasoconstrictors

Jesús Jurado-Palomo[1], Irina Diana Bobolea[2],
María Teresa Belver González[2], Álvaro Moreno-Ancillo[1],
Ana Carmen Gil Adrados[3] and José Manuel Morales Puebla[4]
[1]*Department of Allergology, Nuestra Señora del Prado General Hospital, Talavera de la Reina*
[2]*Department of Allergology, Hospital La Paz Health Research Institute (IdiPAZ), Madrid*
[3]*Centro de Salud La Solana, Talavera de la Reina*
[4]*Department of Otorhinolaryngology, University General Hospital, Ciudad Real*
Spain

1. Introduction

Throughout history, various classifications of rhinitis have emerged, many of which originated from expert groups. We would have to go back to 1994 to find the "*International Consensus Report on Diagnosis and Management of Rhinitis*" (International Rhinitis Management Working Group, 1994), which was subsequently modified in the 2000 "*Consensus statement on the treatment of allergic rhinitis. EAACI Position paper*" (Van Cauwenberge et al, 2000). Of particular interest is the "*Executive Summary of Joint Task Force Practice Parameters on Diagnosis and Management of Rhinitis*" of 1998 (Dykewicz & Fineman, 1998). In 2001, a group of experts, the "*Allergic Rhinitis and its Impact on Asthma (ARIA) Workshop Expert Panel*", met to develop guidelines on the diagnosis and treatment of rhinitis, which also dealt with other inflammatory processes interrelated/associated with asthma. The acronym "ARIA" comes from "Allergic Rhinitis and its Impact on Asthma". ARIA is a document from a non-governmental organisation of the World Health Organization (WHO), endorsed by numerous scientific societies, such as the International Association of Allergology and Clinical Immunology (IAACI) and the World Allergy Organization (WAO) (Bousquet et al, 2001).

It was established as an educational program as the "Guidelines for recommendations for the diagnosis and comprehensive handling of patients with rhinitis", associated with asthma and other interrelated processes (sinusitis, conjunctivitis and otitis).

2. The "United airway" concept

Asthma is a chronic inflammatory disorder of the airways in which many cells and cellular elements play a role. The chronic inflammation is associated with airway hyperresponsiveness that leads to recurrent episodes of wheezing, shortness of breath, chest tightness, and coughing. These episodes are associated with widespread and variable airflow obstruction within the lung, which is often reversible either spontaneously or with treatment (Global Initiative for Asthma, Update 2010).

There is increasing evidence that asthma is a complex syndrome made up of a number of disease variants, so-called asthma phenotypes, with different underlying pathophysiologies. Limited knowledge of the mechanisms of these disease subgroups is possibly the greatest obstacle in understanding the causes of asthma and improving treatment, and can explain the failure to identify consistent genetic and environmental correlations to asthma (Lötvall et al, 2011). It has been proposed that the asthma syndrome should be divided into distinct disease entities with specific mechanisms, which have been called "asthma endotypes." An "endotype" is considered to be a subtype of a condition defined by a distinct pathophysiological mechanism (Lötvall et al, 2011).

The ARIA document acknowledged the concept of a "single airway" or "one airway, one disease", in recognition of the indisputable epidemiological and etiopathogenic relationship that exists between asthma and allergic rhinitis (AR). Both are "a single disease whose basis is the chronic inflammatory process of the airway, a premise that must determine the diagnostic and treatment strategy (Bousquet et al, 2008).

The prevalence of allergic rhinitis in developed countries is between 10%-20%, almost three times the prevalence of asthma (Gergen & Turkettaub, 1991; Lester et al, 2001; Mannino et al, 2002). The concept "allergy; systemic disease" with clinical manifestations in various organs makes "one single airway" more accessible. This way, allergic rhinitis, rhinosinusitis, rhinitis with bronchial hyperresponsiveness, asthma, etc., may be reflections of different stages of the same chronic inflammatory disease of the airway.

In our settings, it is important to note that 20.4% of patients visit an allergist for the first time for rhinitis and asthma symptoms, as highlighted by the "2005 Allergological Study" (Spanish Society of Allergology and Clinical Immunology, 2006). Rhinoconjunctivitis (in allergy clinic settings), which was the main reason for visits in the 1992 Allergological Study (2,279 patients who represented the 57.4% of the sample) (Spanish Society of Allergology and Clinical Immunology, 1995), remains so in the 2005 Allergological Study (2,771 patients who represented the 55.5% of the sample) (Spanish Society of Allergology and Clinical Immunology, 2006). These absolute rates and figures reflect the importance of this disorder. In a study of 650 asthmatics from a health area of the Community of Madrid, 50% had an association with allergic rhinitis (Espinosa de los Monteros et al, 1999).

2.1 Why a new "ARIA document Update 2008" (Bousquet et al, 2008) and "Update 2010" (Brozek JL et al, 2010)?

However, during the period between the first edition in 2001 (Bousquet et al, 2001) and the present (2012), the appearance of numerous studies have caused it to be revised, giving a dynamic and current outlook on the problem both from epidemiologic and therapeutic viewpoints. Thus, the most notable aspect is the inclusion of anti-leukotrienes (Philip G et al, 2004) and the first mention of Omalizumab (Anti-IgE). Successive meetings of experts, along with numerous studies of controlled clinical trials and evidence-based medicine, will produce new up-to-date revisions of this document (Bousquet et al, 2008) (Figure 1).

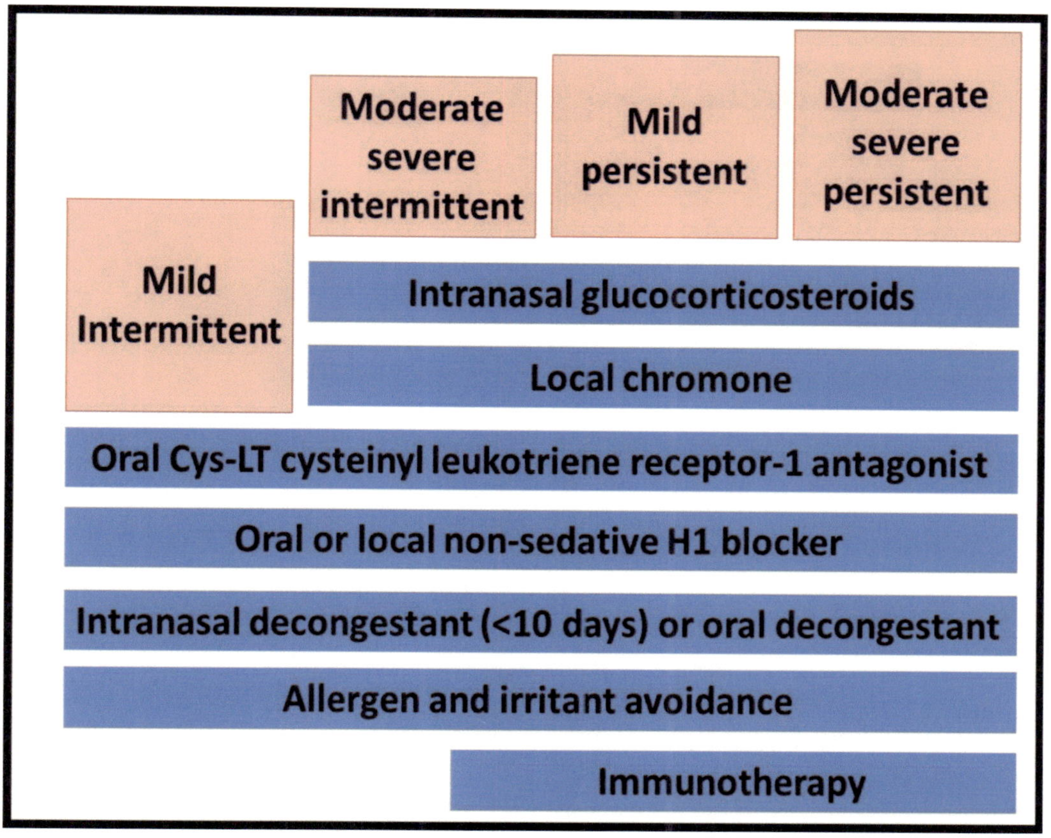

Fig. 1. Classification steps for the severity / persistence of allergic rhinitis symptoms with various therapy steps.

The update to the ARIA document is necessary because:

a. During the period 2001-2012, knowledge of epidemiology, diagnosis, management and comorbidity of patients with allergic rhinitis broadened due to the considerable number of publications.
b. The ARIA Recommendations that were proposed by an expert group must be validated in terms of classification and management.
c. New evidence-based medicine systems will guide and include recommendations for safety, expenditure and efficacy of various treatments.
d. Gaps in the understanding of the first ARIA document:
   - Certain aspects of treatment, such as complementary and alternative medicine.
   - Description of the relationship between upper and lower airways in developing countries.
   - The role of rhinitis in athletes.
   - The link between rhinitis and asthma in preschool aged children.

The rhinitis management (algorithm of the ARIA-Update recommendations 2008 and 2010) are shown in Figure 2.

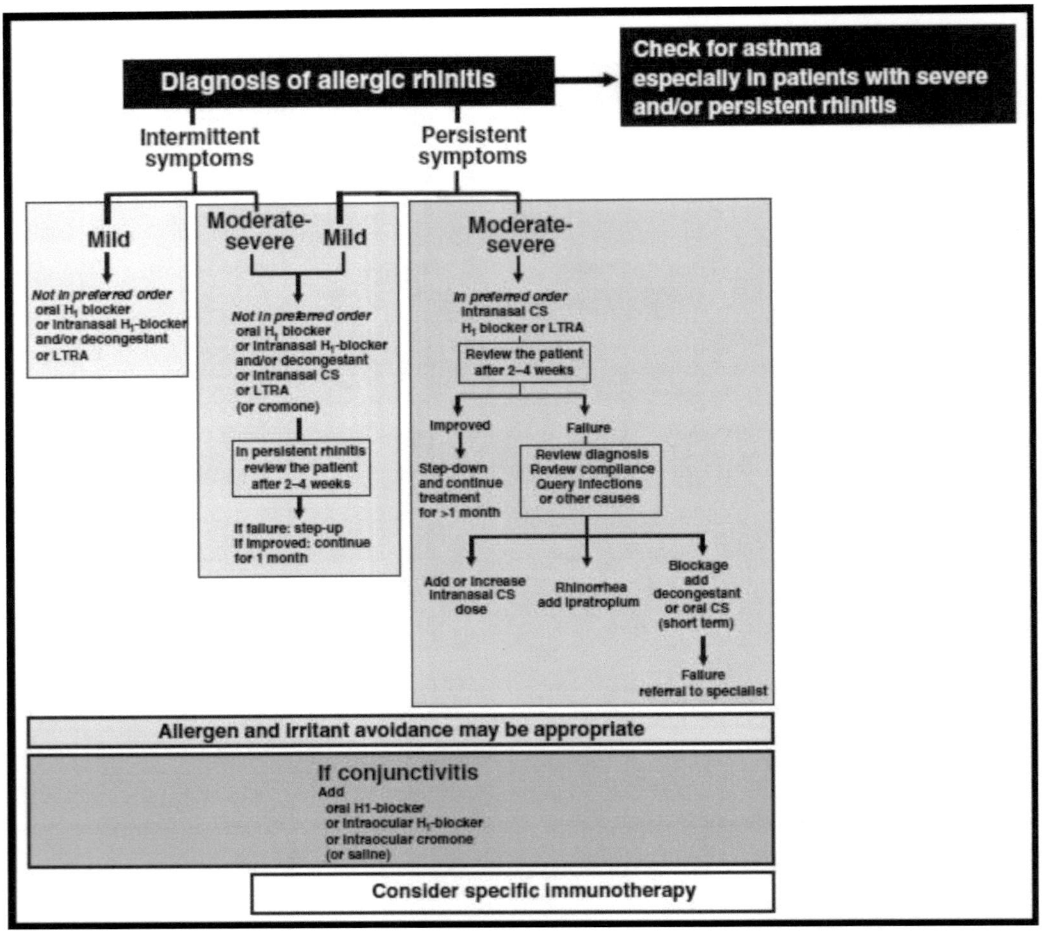

Fig. 2. Rhinitis management (algorithm of the ARIA-Update recommendations 2008 and 2010) (Bousquet et al, 2008; Brozek et al, 2010).

The **initial primary goal** of "education and implementation of the handling of allergic rhinitis based on the dissemination of information that exists about it, its relationship with asthma, as well as allowing scientific evidence (increasingly up-to-date) to be used for control, which results in the benefiting of more than 600 million patients who suffer from this pathology" has been supplemented by the following news:

Developments of the 2008- and 2010-ARIA document (Brozek et al, 2010):

- Confirm the clinical validity of the new allergic rhinitis classification.
- Better understand the impact of allergic rhinitis on patient quality of life starting with the management of rhinitis.
- Perform a review based on the scientific evidence of all available treatments (published trials), including anti-leukotrienes and omalizumab.
- Emphasize studies that highlight the relationship between rhinitis and asthma.
- Suggest a plan for implementing the recommendations in Europe (in collaboration with the EAACI).

- Provide an initial view of the magnitude of the problem with the first strategies in developing countries.

The following Figure 3 presents the degrees of evidence of the various studies in terms of each type of treatment (Shekelle et al, 1999; Custovic & Wijk, 2005; Bousquet et al, 2006; Passalacqua et al, 2006; Passalacqua & Durham, 2007).

Intervention	SEASONAL RHINITIS		PERENNIAL RHINITIS (mostly applies for studies ≤ 4 weeks)		PERSISTENT RHINITIS
	Adults	Children	Adults	Children	
H1-Antihistamines					
- oral	A	A	A	A	A
- intranasal	A	A	A	A	No data
- intraocular	A	A	B	B	No data
Glucocorticosteroids:					
- intranasal	A	A	A	A	No data
- oral	A	B	B	B	No data
- intramuscular	A	B	B	B	No data
Cromones:					
- intranasal	A	A	A	B	No data
- intraocular	A	A	B	B	No data
NAAGA topical	B	C	C	C	No data
Antileukotriene	A	A over 6 years			No data
Decongestants					
- intranasal	C	C	C	C	No data
- oral	A				No data
- oral + H1-antihistamine	A	B	B	B	No data
Anticholinergic			A	A	No data
Homeopathy	D	D	D	D	No data
Acupuncture	D	D	D	D	No data
Phytotherapy	B	D	D	D	No data
Other CAM	D	D	D	D	No data
Specific immunotherapy: rhinoconjunctivitis					
- subcutaneous	A	A	A	A	No data
- sublingual	A	A	A	A	No data
- intranasal	A				No data
Specific immunotherapy: asthma					
- subcutaneous	A	A	A	A	
- sublingual	A	A	A	A	
Anti-IgE	A	A over 12 years	A	A over 12 years	No data
Allergen avoidance:					
- house dust mites	D	D	D	D	No data
- other indoor allergens	D	D	D	D	No data
- total avoidance of occupational agent			A (for asthma)		No data
- partial avoidance of latex			B		No data

Fig. 3. Level of evidence of different interventions in allergic rhinitis (AR) (Bousquet et al, 2008).

The recommendations follow criteria which may differ from country to country, and in Europe and at WHO another Shekelle method was commonly used (Shekelle et al, 1999) (Figure 3).

Strength of recommendation:

A: Category I evidence (meta-analysis of randomized-controlled trials (RCT); or at least one RCT).
B: Category II evidence (at least one controlled study without randomization; or at least one other type of study) or extrapolated recommendation from category I evidence
C: Category III evidence (nonexperimental descriptive studies) or extrapolated recommendation from category I or II evidence.
D: Category IV evidence (expert committee reports or opinions or clinical experience of respected authorities) or extrapolated recommendation from category I, II or III evidence.

2.3 Controversy in the treatment of allergic rhinitis

Rhinitis, or inflammation of the nasal mucosa, is currently recognised as a major cause of morbidity, which significantly deteriorates quality of life (ISAAC Steering Committee, 1998). Although the prevalence of rhinitis is highly variable, we can conclude that between 15% and 20% of the population suffers from rhinitis, based on various studies that are influenced by the questionnaires used and the geographical area in which they are carried out (Broder et al, 1974a; Broder et al, 1974b; Sibbald & Rink, 1991; Spanish Society of Allergology and Clinical Immunology, 1995; Spanish Society of Allergology and Clinical Immunology, 2006). Early intervention with appropriate treatment may improve patient quality of life and productivity, as well as prevent its evolution to asthma (European Academy of Allergology and Clinical Immunology, 1998). A few years ago, the goal of rhinitis treatment was to improve symptoms. Currently, the goal is to block pathophysiological mechanisms that cause chronic inflammation and that leave patients vulnerable to respiratory airway infections.

The therapeutic approach to allergic rhinitis (AR) entails comprehensive treatment of the allergic inflammation of the airways (ARIA). The selection and combination of the therapeutic arsenal is achieved by taking into account current clinical practice guidelines, and by individualising the treatment for each patient, depending on the frequency of discomfort (intermittent or persistent AR) and its repercussion on the quality of life (mild or moderate/severe AR) (Bousquet et al, 2001). Treatment cost-effectiveness must also be assessed, as well as safety and the fact that we are dealing with a chronic disease.

The protocol for managing rhinitis, according to the 1994 Consensus (International Rhinitis Management Working Group, 1994), proposes a phased approach for the treatment of both allergic and non-allergic rhinitis. The above protocol is not very clear about the indications for immunotherapy, which in the final summary is indicated exclusively for seasonal AR. The European Academy of Allergy and Clinical Immunology (EAACI) Position Paper for treatment of AR published in 2000 and created from consensus between experts of the Academy (van Cauwenberge et al, 2000), reviewed 185 articles on rhinitis, focusing exclusively on therapeutic issues. The proposed treatment guidelines in this review, differentiated for seasonal and perennial AR in children and adults, are too rigid. The indication for immunotherapy is envisioned in very advanced phases of the therapeutic range, and also in an undefined manner. The therapeutic approach in ARIA (Bousquet et al, 2001) is phased and not as rigid as in other consensus. Treatment guidelines are open and do not list directives, and quality of life is assessed through the use of questionnaires. The recommendations for treatment depend on symptom severity along with repercussions on patient quality of life.

For the first time, therapy is approached using evidence-based medical criteria, reviewing controlled randomised studies, and performed according to the prior classification of seasonal and perennial rhinitis. These recommendations are based on meta-analysis studies regarding drug treatment and immunotherapy, and on a clinical practice guideline drawn up after an analysis of evidence available to date, based on the opinion of experts regarding the elimination of the antigen.

Of note are considerations regarding drug administration routes, and their advantages/disadvantages and indications/contraindications. There is special attention given to the intranasal route.

In 1995, the first manual portable controlled-dose inhaler, called the "Medihaler", was introduced, which was the result of studies carried out in the Richer Co. laboratories (British Society for Allergy and Clinical Immunology, 2000). In the USA, a smaller inhaler was developed that was easier to handle than nebulizers and avoided the use of sedative antihistamines, which alter cognitive and motor functions. The inhaler was developed for the asthmatic daughter of Dr. G. Maison, chairman of the laboratories. The inhaler had a pressurized canister and metering valve. The use of topical medication in rhinitis has been developed to reduce systemic side effects as much as possible.

2.3 Allergen avoidance

Although there is disagreement as to the efficacy of eliminating the antigen, it must always be carried out using environmental control measures.

2.4 Therapeutics groups in the "ARIA-pharmaceutical"

Although there is disagreement as to the efficacy of eliminating the antigen, it must always be carried. In recent years, the pharmaceutical industry has researched new administration routes. It appears that the nose is a magnificent channel for drugs that until recently could only be administered systemically.

There are eight major therapeutic groups in the "ARIA-pharmaceutical market" available use (Table 1).

Drugs	Generic names	Mechanism of action	Side effects	Comments
Local H1-antihistamines (intranasal, intraocular)	Azelastine Levocabastine Olopatadine	Blockage of H1 receptor. Some antiallergic activity for azelastine.	Minor local side effects. Azelastine: bitter taste.	Rapidly effective (minor than 30 minutes) on nasal or ocular symptoms.
Intranasal glucocorticosteroids	Beclomethasone dipropionate Budesonide Ciclesonide Flunisolide Fluticasone	Potently reduce nasal inflammation. Reduce nasal hyperactivity.	Minor local side effects. Wide margin for systemic side effects. Growth concerns with BDP only. In young children	The most effective pharmacologic treatment of allergic rhinitis. Effective on nasal congestion.

Drugs	Generic names	Mechanism of action	Side effects	Comments
	propionate Fluticasone furoate Metasone furoate Triamcinolone acetonide		consider the combination of intranasal and inhaled drugs.	Effective on smell. Effect observed after 12 hours but maximal effect after a few days
Leukotriene antagonists	Montelukast Pranlukast Zafirlukast	Blockage of CystLT receptor.	Excellent tolerance.	Effective on rhinitis and asthma. Effective on all symptoms of rhinitis and on ocular symptoms.
Local cromones (intranasal, intraocular)	Cromoglycate Nedocromil NAAGA	Mechanism of action poorly known.	Minor local side effects.	Intraocular cromones are very effective. Intranasal cromones are less effective and their effect is short lasting.
Intranasal anticholinergics	Ipratropium	Anticholinergic block almost exclusively rhinorrhea	Minor local side effects. Almost no systemic anticholinergic activity.	Effective on allergic and non-allergic patients with rhinorrhea.
Oral decongestants	Ephedrine Phenylephrine Phenylpropanolamine Pseudoephedrine Oral H1-antihistamine decongestants combinations	Sympathomimetic drugs. Relieve symptoms of nasal congestion.	Hypertension. Palpitations. Restlessness. Agitation. Tremor. Insomnia. Headache. Dry mucous membranes. Urinary retention. Exacerbation of glaucoma or thyrotoxicosis.	Use oral decongestants with caution in patient with heart disease. Oral H1-antihistamine-decongestant combination products may be more effective than either product alone but side effects are combined.
Intranasal decongestants	Oxymethazoline Xylomethazoline Others	Sympathomimetic drugs. Relieve symptoms of nasal congestion	Same side affects as oral decongestants but less intense. Rhinitis medicamentosa is a rebound phenomenon occurring with prolonged use (over 10 days)	Act more rapidly and more effectively than oral decongestants. Limit duration of treatment to minor 10 days to avoid rhinitis medicamentosa.
Oral/intramuscular glucocorticosteroids	Dexamethasone Hydrocortisone Methylprednisolone Prednisolone Prednisone Triamcinolone	Potently reduce nasal inflammation. Reduce nasal hyperreactivity.	Systemic side effects common in particular for intramuscular drugs. Depot injections may cause local tissue atrophy.	When possible, intranasal glucocorticosteroids should replace oral or intramuscular drugs. However a short course of oral glucocorticosteroids may be needed of moderate /severe symptoms.

Table 1. Therapeutic groups in the "ARIA-pharmaceutical market" (Bousquet et al, 2008).

Topical nasal drugs acts as both a preventive and a curative medication for rhinitis. It is very important that the application be performed appropriately, with the goal of achieving uniform distribution of the drug throughout the nasal mucosa, especially if rhinorrhoea is abundant.

3. Nasal lavage

Nasal lavage is a non-pharmacological treatment of rhinitis. Most authors agree that this is a well-tolerated, effective and inexpensive treatment.

3.1 Efficacy in AR

Georgitis showed that the use of saline solution in nasal irrigation reduces inflammatory mediators (nasal histamine, prostaglandin D2 and leukotriene C4), while at the same time decreasing nasal symptoms (Georgitis, 1994). It observed that performing nasal lavage is important in the treatment of allergic rhinosinusitis.

Subiza et al, published one of the best and most complete articles in the JACI, which indicated that the action of nasal lavages is simple and known: cleaning of nasal secretions, with anti-inflammatory effect and reduction in basophils and other anti-inflammatory cells. It is a complementary technique for intranasal corticosteroids, but is effective and convenient. Saline irrigation of the nose and sinuses during the pollen season inhibits the IgE response to grass pollen (Subiza et al, 1999).

According to Tomooka et al, patients who use nasal lavage twice a day for 3-6 week periods have statistically significant improvement (23 of the 30 symptoms on The Quality of Well Being scale questionnaires improve or disappear) (Tomooka et al, 2000).

Garavello et al state that the use of nasal irrigation with hypertonic saline serum (3 times a day) decreases the consumption of antihistamines and significantly improves rhinitis, starting from the third week of treatment, and clearly in the fourth and fifth, with a significant reduction in the use of oral antihistamines (Garavello et al, 2003). The study was performed on 20 children, whose ages were not reported, with seasonal AR and sensitisation to *Parietaria judaica*. Irrigation with hypertonic serum was performed on 10 of the children 3 times at day during the entire pollen season (6 weeks). The other 10 were not administered lavages and were used as controls.

Degirmencioglu et al showed that saline irrigation with isotonic or hypertonic solutions improve symptoms during the pollen season (Degirmencioglu et al, 2004).

3.2 Usefulness in sinusitis and chronic rhinitis

Lavages with isotonic and hypertonic saline serum are one of the mainstays of treatment of rhinosinusal disease, as they are safe, inexpensive and effective. The weight of evidence is such that the Allergy Foundation published an International Consensus article in *Allergy* (International Rhinitis Management Working Group, 1994) recommending the routine performance of these lavages for rhinitis.

Different clinicians confirmed that nasal irrigations with a saline solution along with nasal steroids are the basis of treatment for chronic sinusitis (Aukema & Fokkens, 2004).

Nevertheless, is cautioned that nasal irrigation with saline solutions could no longer be considered a mere adjunct treatment of rhinosinusitis (Brown & Graham, 2004). Despite being effective and safe, it is underused.

Metson lends support to the conviction that saline irrigation improves breathing and adds, more importantly, that it lengthens the time between relapses (Metson, 2004). Daily saline irrigation improves the quality of life of patients with sinusitis, decreasing symptoms and the use of medication (Rabago et al, 2002).

Nasal irrigation is a simple and inexpensive treatment that improves symptoms of a variety of sinonasal diseases, reduces the use of resources and helps minimise resistance to antibiotics (Papsin & McTavish, 2003). Also, nasal lavage improves endoscopic imaging of nasal mucosa and the quality of life of patients with chronic rhinosinusitis (Taccariello et al, 1999). The nasal lavage increases mucociliary flow, dilutes thick secretions, relieves irritated mucous membranes, eliminates crusts and foreign bodies, facilitates the healing of mucous membranes, reducing the need for blowing and improving the sense of smell. The sinus irrigation by itself prevented the need for surgery in 58% of patients with chronic sinusitis over a year (Hartog et al, 1997)

4. Antihistamines

Histamine is one of the main mediators of allergic reactions occurring as a result of contact between the allergen and the nasal mucosa. Its actions are not limited to triggering of the signs and symptoms of the early phase of the allergic reaction but are also implicated in the release of multiple proinflammatory cytokines, with a vasoactive effect that favors arrival in the nasal zone of a range of cellular elements that characterize allergic inflammation.

Antihistamines inhibit the effects of histamine at H1 receptors. Histamine is a physiologically active, endogenous substance that binds to and activates histamine H1 and H2 receptors in the respiratory tract (including the nose), the gastrointestinal tract, brain, adrenal medulla, skin vasculature, and the heart (Golightly & Greos, 2005).

4.1 Oral antihistamines

The antihistamines exert a number of effects upon the histamine receptor. On one hand, it is now clear that all known antihistamines act as reverse agonists, inactivating the intracellular actions of the receptor. On the other hand, antiinflammatory effects have been demonstrated for these drugs, explained by modulation of nuclear factor NF-κB, such as the inhibition of ICAM-1 expression or action upon the bradykinins (Leurs et al, 2002).

Antihistamines are classified (Handley et al, 1998) as first generation (sedating, including chlorpheniramine, diphenhydramine, promethazine, and hydroxyzine) and newer. The newer antihistamines are sometimes referred to as second generation (relatively nonsedating, including terfenadine, astemizole, loratadine, cetirizine, and levocetirizine) and third generation (including fexofenadine, norastemizole, and descarboethoxyloratadine) (Table 2).

Antihistamine drugs are the most commonly used pharmaceutical group. The effective use of anti-H1 (in its oral, intranasal and ophthalmic presentations) for the treatment of AR

Chemical class	Functional class	
	First (old) generation	Second (new) generation
Alkylamines	Brompheniramine, chlorpheniramine, dexchlorpheniramine, dimenthindene, pheniramine, triprolidine	Acrivastine
Piperazines	Buclizine, cyclizine, hydroxyzine, meclizine, oxatomide	Cetirizine, levocetirizine
Piperidines	Azatadine, cyproheptadine, diphenylpyraline, ketotifen	Astemizol, bepotastine, bilastine, desloratadine, ebastine, fexofenadine, levocabastine, loratadine, mizolastine, rupatadine, terfenadine, alcaftadine
Ethanolamines	Carbinoxamine, clemastine, dimenhydrinate, diphenhydramine, doxylamine, phenyltoloxamine	
Ethylenediamines	Antazoline, pyrilamine, tripelennamine	
Phenothiazines	Methdilazine, promethazine	
Others	Doxepin*	Azelastine, emedastine, epinastine, olopatadine

* Doxepin has dual H_1- and H_2- antihistamine activities and is classified as a tricyclic antidepressant.

Table 2. H1-antihistamines: chemical and functional classification (modified: Simons, 2004; Simons & Akdis, 2009; Simons & Simons, 2011).

(seasonal or perennial) in children or adults is backed by significant evidence from published clinical trials (ARIA).

In the new classification of rhinitis and in the clinical practice guidelines promoted in the ARIA document, oral anti-H1 is recommended for use in intermittent and persistent mild AR, and combined with topical corticosteroids in persistent moderate/severe AR. It shows good response in seasonal AR, where symptoms mediated by histamines predominate and ocular symptoms are common. In persistent AR, in which congestion is significant, anti-H1 has a moderate effect.

Oral antihistamines may cause subclinical side effects not noticed by the patient (somnolence, decreased coordination, etc.). This does not happen with the new non-sedating antihistamines, but generally up to 50% of patients self-medicate (Storms, 1997).

Treatment with antihistamines in AR is almost universally accepted. In fact, the treatment of seasonal AR in children: The results of placebo-controlled trials of cetirizine (Allegra et al, 1993; Masi et al, 1993; Ciprandi et al, 1997a; Ciprandi et al, 1997b; Pearlman et al, 1997) and fexofenadine (Wahn et al, 2003) demonstrated significant improvements in symptoms with the study drug compared with placebo. Active-control studies compared cetirizine (Charpin et al, 1995) and loratadine (Boner et al, 1989) to first-generation antihistamines, with no significant differences between groups.

Various studies were identified which examined the efficacy of newer antihistamines among children with perennial AR (Baelde & Dupont, 1992; Jobst et al, 1994; Charpin et al, 1995; Pearlman et al, 1997; Sienra-Monge et al, 1999; Ciprandi et al, 2001; Yang et al, 2001; Lai et al, 2002; Wahn et al, 2003; Ciprandi et al, 2004; Hsieh et al, 2004). In three studies with active controls, cetirizine improved symptoms compared with placebo arms and compared with ketotifen and oxatomide (Lai et al, 2002). Cetirizine was comparable to montelukast in one study (Hsieh et al, 2004), but similar in efficacy in another (Chen et al, 2006). Three fair-quality, placebo-controlled studies (Baelde & Dupont, 1992; Jobst et al, 1994; Ciprandi et al, 2001) found cetirizine efficacious for nasal symptoms, particularly at a dosage of 10 mg daily (either at bed time or divided doses twice daily) for children 6 to 12 years.

4.2 Topical (intranasal) antihistamines

Up until the late 80s, antihistamines had not yet been developed for local application. In the last 20 years, several clinical trials have been carried out on local application of various new generation antihistamines. Their marketing and use started almost 15 years ago.

4.2.1 Azelastine

Azelastine hydrochloride was initially researched for use in bronchial asthma, and is currently used in the symptomatic treatment of seasonal AR and for acute exacerbations of perennial AR. It is administered in an aqueous solution as a nasal spray, and was initially administered orally.

Clinical evaluation of its efficacy and side effects were carried out in several multicentre studies (Weiler & Meltzer, 1997). It does not affect driving ability or handling of machinery, but may occasionally irritate the mucous membrane and cause epistaxis.

One of the first studies with azelastine was published by Dorow, who performed two studies with pollen-allergic patients. The first study compared azelastine with a double-blind placebo in 16 patients over one week. Significant improvement was noted in the group using the drug, with a decrease in sneezing ($P<.01$) and nasal pruritus ($P<.01$). There were no significant improvements in nasal congestion and hydrorrhoea (Dorow et al, 1993).

The second study was a double-blind comparison of 36 patients treated with either azelastine or budesonide for 15 days. There were no significant differences between the groups.

Weiler studied the effects of pre-treatment with azelastine in nasal provocation with grass pollens. Mean percent improvements in the total symptom complex severity scores for azelastine were statistically significant ($P\leq.05$) or showed a trend toward statistical significance ($P<.05$ or $P\leq.10$) versus placebo from the second through the first ten hours after the initial dose and for each of the last five hours of the second day, demonstrating a rapid onset of action and sustained efficacy over the 2-day study period (Weiler & Meltzer, 1997).

Grossman performed a double-blind study of 199 patients with perennial AR for 8 weeks, obtaining significant improvement when compared to placebo (Grossman et al, 1994). Other studies have compared azelastine nasal spray with other oral antihistamines, finding that its efficacy is similar and that it has fewer side effects.

Conde Hernandez et al compared the safety and efficacy of two antihistamines, azelastine in nasal spray and oral ebastine, for 14 days. Authors found no significant differences between the two treatments, considering both to be effective in the treatment of seasonal AR (Conde Hernández et al, 1995a; Conde Hernández et al, 1995b).

Berlin et al compared the efficacy of topical nasal corticosteroids with antihistamines in nasal spray (azelastine), and found that the results with topical nasal corticosteroids were clearly superior for managing nasal symptoms of rhinitis. The authors recommended topical nasal corticosteroids as a first-line treatment of perennial AR (Berlin et al 2000).

4.2.1 Levocabastine

The first antihistamine developed for nasal application, levocabastine is a highly selective histamine antagonist of the H1 receptor, and acts immediately (Janssens et al, 1991). Since it is eliminated through the kidneys, it should be used with caution in renal patients. It does not sedate or boost the effects of alcohol. The dose is 2 applications of 0.5 mg each every 12 hours in each nostril. It is more powerful than chlorpheniramine (Dechant & Goa, 1991) and similar to other oral antihistamines [loratadine (Swedish GP Allergy Team, 1994) and terfenadine (The Livostin Study Group, 1993)] and disodium cromoglycate (Fisher, 1994).

In 1995, a study was published on 21 patients with AR sensitised to mites. The patients were treated with topical levocabastine, and a reduction of inflammatory mediators and nasal hyperreactivity was observed. The authors concluded that it was an effective antagonistic of H1 receptors, with immediate clinical response and few anti-inflammatory properties (de Graaf-in´t Veld et al, 1995). Previously in 1991, other spanish authors showed the efficacy of levocabastine in seasonal AR using a double-blind study (Palma-Carlos et al, 1991).

5. Mast cell membrane stabilising drugs

Applied topically, these drugs are very useful in mild and moderate AR, as they lack systemic effects and are very well tolerated. To achieve effectiveness, appropriate application methods must be used so that an even distribution of the medication is achieved, especially if there is abundant rhinorrhoea (Okuda et al, 1985). The main drugs being used are:

5.1 Disodium cromoglycate

Derived from the natural chromone Khellin, disodium cromoglycate (DSCG) is extracted from the *Ammi visnaga* plant, and was synthesised by Fisons (Cox, 1967).

It is a dual chromone joined by a flexible chain. The chromone chain has a hydrogen atom substituted by a sodium atom. It is a white powder that is barely water-soluble.

It is administered by inhalation because it is absorbed poorly orally. It has a plasma half-life of 80 minutes, and it reaches maximum levels in 20 minutes.

- *Mechanism of action:* DSCG has a stabilising effect on the mast cell membrane, preventing the release of the chemical mediators responsible for allergic reactions:

histamines and eosinophil/neutrophil chemotactic factors. It has no effect on basophils (Okuda et al, 1985). It increases the intracellular level of cyclic AMP, inhibiting phosphodiesterase and regulating the calcium retention mechanism.

- *Side effects:* Side effects are very infrequent. Symptoms may include epistaxis and dryness of nasal mucous, sometimes accompanied by sneezing. It is a safe drug, since no significant side effects have been reported in long-term treatments.

The dose is 20-40 mg every 6 hours in each nostril. Therapeutic non-compliance with the dosage is the main cause for the lack of spectacular results.

It is effective in the treatment of AR, especially in patients with high IgE (Okuda et al, 1985). It works to prevent sneezing and rhinorrhoea, but not obstruction.

DSCG performs better than placebo in studies on pollen-sensitized patients. In a double-blind study that included 104 patients and took place over 6 weeks, authors found significant improvement with minimal side effects (Handelman et al, 1977).

It is important to note that during administration:

- The container should be protected from light.
- The aqueous solution should not remain open for more than 30 days.
- Patient collaboration and discipline is necessary, since application every 6 hours is essential.
- The treatment must not be abandoned due to sneezing during administration, since it is usually temporary and lasts only a short time.
- The drug is mainly preventive and does not, therefore, provide control for patients with severe symptoms.

5.2 Nedocromil sodium

A pyrano quinoline dicarboxylic acid, nedocromil sodium has a half-life of 90 minutes, and is eliminated by the liver and kidneys. It acts extracellularly because it does not pass through the lipid membranes due to its physicochemical properties. It acts by blocking the chloride channels that are responsible for cellular activity. It inhibits the release of histamine, leukotriene C4, prostaglandin D2 and chemotactic factors.

Although its mechanism of action is similar to DSCG, nedocromil sodium acts on other types of cells: eosinophils, neutrophil, macrophages, platelets and monocytes (Kaulbach et al, 1992).

Side effects are rare, similar to those of DSCG, although nausea, vomiting, dizziness and headaches have been reported. It is administered by inhalation in doses of 4 mg twice a day. This lower frequency of administration is an advantage over DSCG. Studies demonstrated its clinical efficacy in allergic rhinitis.

5.3 N-acetylaspartylglutamate acid

The magnesium salts of N-acetylaspartylglutamate (NAAGA) acid are effective in the treatment of seasonal allergic rhinitis.

Althaus performed a multicentre double-blind study for 4 weeks in pollen-allergic patients. Sixty-three patients were treated with NAAGA, 63 others with cromolyn sodium and 64 with placebo. The efficacy of NAAGA compared to placebo (P<.001) and to cromolyn sodium (P<.03) was demonstrated. Terfenadine was used as a rescue medication, requiring greater use for placebo than for NAAGA (P<.0001) (Althaus & Pichler, 1994).

6. Vasoconstrictors (α-adrenergics)

Vasoconstrictors are sympathomimetic drugs may act on α-receptors, causing vasoconstriction, or on β-receptors (vasodilation). The use of α-adrenergics in rhinitis is based on its ability to cause vasoconstriction, reducing blood flow in vessels and reducing secretions.

They are widespread in Spain, and should not be administered without medical supervision.

Those that are used topically are imidazole derivatives: oxymetazoline, naphazoline and xylometazoline. They should not be administered for more than 7 days as their prolonged use causes the onset of a rebound effect by secondary hyperaemia. This effect occurs a few hours after administration and may be interpreted by the patient as a sign of illness, which may make them increase the dose.

Vasoconstrictors have a significant effect on nasal obstruction, but continued use may cause drug-induced rhinitis, creating a dependence on nasal drops. Administration to children less than 1 year of age is dangerous.

Based on their study, Graf and Juto recommended avoiding the use of oxymetazoline in nasal spray for more than 10 days due to it causing hyperreactivity in the nasal mucosa, thus increasing susceptibility to histamines (Graf & Juto, 1994). These authors showed the lack of rebound with xylometazoline in nasal spray, when used at the recommended dosage, even over twice the recommended time period (Graf & Juto, 1995).

In the same time, other authors demonstrated the benefit of oxymetazoline above all, and xylometazoline somewhat less, in the topical treatment of nasal inflammation of rhinitis, due to its antioxidant properties (Westerveld et al, 1995).

Graf et al, in a study of oxymetazoline, benzalkonium chloride and placebo in nasal spray, found that prolonged use (more than recommended) induced an increase in nasal hyperreactivity and the feeling of nasal obstruction, developing into secondary drug-induced rhinitis. This may be related to the presence of benzalkonium in decongestant nasal sprays, which can produce or exacerbate drug-induced rhinitis (Graf & Hallen, 1996). Other authors performed a 4 to 8-week study with oxymetazoline and showed that it was safe, if used once a day, preferably at night (Yoo et al, 1997).

Moreover, it was confirmed that oxymetazoline and xylometazoline were beneficial in the treatment of upper respiratory tract inflammation, due to their dose-dependent inhibitory effects on nitric oxide synthase activity (Westerveld et al, 2000)

Stubner studied the efficacy of cetirizine associated with pseudoephedrine, comparing it to xylometazoline at 0.1% in nasal spray. With the exception of nasal obstruction, which improved quickly with xylometazoline nasal spray, the rest of the rhinitis symptoms (mainly the reduction of nasal secretions) clearly improved with the combination of anti-Hl and pseudoephedrine (Stubner et al, 2001).

Wellington compared the efficacy of the cetirizine-pseudoephedrine combination (5/120), administered twice a day with 100 micrograms of intranasal budesonide for 23 weeks. The study found that the cetirizine-pseudoephedrine combination was clearly more effective than monotherapy, significantly reducing the score symptoms for both allergic and perennial rhinitis, and was also well tolerated (Wellington & Jarvis, 2001).

7. Conclusions

Considering the reviewed data, and unifying the above-mentioned opinions on the treatment of AR, we provide the following guidelines:

- Aetiological treatment based on a correct aetiological diagnosis should always be achieved.
- Nasal lavage is a concomitant, non-pharmacological and economical treatment, useful in the treatment of AR and especially indicated in chronic rhinosinusitis.
- New generation antihistamines are the treatment of choice in AR and perhaps the only choice for intermittent mild rhinitis.
- Vasoconstrictors should only be used for a short time when combined with antihistamines and/or intranasal corticosteroids when nasal obstruction is not controlled.

8. References

Allegra L, Paupe J, Wieseman HG, Baelde Y. Cetirizine for seasonal allergic rhinitis in children aged 2-6 years. (1993) *Pediatr Allergy Immunol*, Vol.4, No.3 (August 1993), pp. 157-161, Print ISSN 0905-6157, Electronic ISSN 1399-3038.

Althaus MA, Pichler WJ. Nasal application of a gel formulation of N-acetyl-aspartyl glutamic acid (NAAGA) compared with placebo and disodium cromoglycate in the symptomatic treatment of pollinosis. (1994) *Allergy*, Vol.49, No.3 (March 1994), pp. 184-188, Print ISSN 0105-4538, Electronic ISSN: 1398-9995.

Aukema AA, Fokkens WJ. Chronic rhinosinusitis: management for optimal outcomes. (2004) *Treat Respir Med*, Vol.3, No.2 (March-April 2004), pp. 97-105, Print ISSN 1176-3450.

Baelde Y, Dupont P. Cetirizine in children with chronic allergic rhinitis. *Drug Investigation.* 1992;4(6):466-472.

Berlin JM, Golden SJ, Teets S, Lehman EB, Lucas T, Craig TJ. Efficacy of a steroid nasal spray compared with an antihistamine nasal spray in the treatment of perennial allergic rhinitis. (2000) *J Am Osteopath Assoc*, Vol.100, No.7 Suppl (July 2000), pp. S8-S13, Print ISSN 0098-6151.

Boner AL, Miglioranzi P, Richelli C, Marchesi E, Andreoli A. Efficacy and safety of loratadine suspension in the treatment of children with allergic rhinitis. (1989) *Allergy*, Vol.44, No.6 (August 1989), pp. 437-441, Print ISSN 0105-4538, Electronic ISSN 1398-9995.

Bousquet J, Khaltaev N, Cruz AA, Denburg J, Fokkens WJ, Togias A, Zuberbier T et al. Allergic Rhinitis and its Impact on Asthma (ARIA) 2008 update (in collaboration with the World Heatlth Organization, GA(2)LEN and AllergGen). (2008) *Allergy*, Vol.63, No.86 Suppl (April 2008), pp. 8-160, Print ISSN 0105-4538, Electronic ISSN 1398-9995.

Bousquet J, Van Cauwenberge P, Aït Khaled N, Bachert C, Baena-Cagnani CE, Bouchard J, et al. Pharmacologic and anti-IgE treatment of allergic rhinitis ARIA update (in collaboration with GA2LEN). (2006) *Allergy*, Vol.61, No.9 (September 2006), pp. 1086-1096, Print ISSN 0105-4538, Electronic ISSN 1398-9995.

Bousquet J, Van Cauwenberge P, Khaltaev N; ARIA Workshop Group; World Health Organization. ARIA workshop group. World Health Organization. Allergic Rhinitis and its impact on asthma Workshop Report. (2001) *J Allergy Clin Immunol*, Vol.108, No.5 Suppl (November 2001), pp. S147-S334, Print ISSN 0091-6749, Electronic ISSN 1097-6825.

British Society for Allergy and Clinical Immunology. Rhinitis Management Guidelines: British Society for Allergy and Clinical Immunology ENT Sub-Committee. 2000. CRC Press, ISBN: 1853179698.

Broder I, Higgins MW, Mathews KP, Keller JB. Epidemiology of asthma and allergic rhinitis in a total community, Tecumseh, Michigan. 3. Second survey of the community. (1974) *J Allergy Clin Immunol*, Vol.53, No.3 (March 1974), pp. 127-138, Print ISSN 0091-6749, Electronic ISSN 1097-6825.

Broder I, Higgins MW, Mathews KP, Keller JB. Epidemiology of asthma and allergic rhinitis in a total community, Tecumseh, Michigan. IV. Natural history. (1974) *J Allergy Clin Immunol*, Vol.54, No.2 (August 1974), pp. 100-110, Print ISSN 0091-6749, Electronic ISSN 1097-6825.

Brown CL, Graham SM. Nasal irrigations: good or bad? (2004) *Curr Opin Otolaryngol Head Neck Surg*, Vol.12, No.1 (February 2004), pp. 9-13, Print ISSN 1068-9508, Electronic 1531-6998.

Brozek JL, Bousquet J, Baena-Cagnani CE, Bonini S, Canonica GW, Casale TB, et al. Global Allergy and Asthma European Network; Grading of Recommendations Assessment, Development and Evaluation Working Group. Allergic Rhinitis and its Impact on Asthma (ARIA) guidelines: 2010 revision. (2010) *J Allergy Clin Immunol*, Vol.126 ,No.3 (September 2010), pp. 466-476, Print ISSN 0091-6749, Electronic ISSN 1097-6825.

Charpin D, Godard P, Garay RP, Baehre M, Herman D, Michel FB. A multicenter clinical study of the efficacy and tolerability of azelastine nasal spray in the treatment of seasonal allergic rhinitis: a comparison with oral cetirizine. (1995) *Eur Arch Otorhinolaryngol*, Vol.252, No.8 (August 1995), pp. 455-458, Print ISSN 0937-4477, Electronic ISSN 1434-4726.

Chen ST, Lu KH, Sun HL, Chang WT, Lue KH, Chou MC. Randomized placebo controlled trial comparing montelukast and cetirizine for treating perennial allergic rhinitis in children aged 2-6 yr. (2006) *Pediatr Allergy Immunol*, Vol.17, No.1 (February 2006), pp. 49-54, Print ISSN 0905-6157, Electronic ISSN 1399-3038.

Ciprandi G, Tosca MA, Milanese M, Ricca V. Cetirizine reduces cytokines and inflammatory cells in children with perennial allergic rhinitis. (2004) *Eur Ann Allergy Clin Immunol*, Vol.36, No.6 (June 2004), pp. 237-240, Print ISSN 1764-1489.

Ciprandi G, Tosca M, Passalacqua G, Canonica GW. Long-term cetirizine treatment reduces allergic symptoms and drug prescriptions in children with mite allergy. (2001) *Ann Allergy Asthma Immunol*, Vol.87, No.3 (September 2001), pp. 222-226, Print ISSN 1081-1206, Electronic ISSN 1534-4436.

Ciprandi G, Tosca M, Ricca V, Passalacqua G, Fregonese L, Fasce L et al. Cetirizine treatment of allergic cough in children with pollen allergy. (1997) *Allergy*, Vol.52, No.7 (July 1997), pp. 752-754, Print ISSN 0105-4538, Electronic ISSN 1398-9995.

Ciprandi G, Tosca M, Ricca V, Passalacqua G, Riccio AM, Bagnasco M, et al. Cetirizine treatment of rhinitis in children with pollen allergy: evidence of its antiallergic activity. (1997) *Clin Exp Allergy*, Vol.27, No.10 (October 1997), pp. 1160-1166, Print ISSN 0954-7894, Electronic ISSN 1365-2222..

Conde Hernández DJ, Palma Aguilar JL, Delgado Romero J. Comparison of azelastine rinitis. (1995) *Curr Med Resp Opin*, Vol.13, No.3 (March 1995), pp. 299-304, Print ISSN 0300-7995, Electronic ISSN 1473-4877.

Conde Hernández J, Palma Aguilar JL, Delgado Romero J. Investigation on the efficacy and tolerance of azelastine (HCL) nasal spray versus ebastine tablets in patients with seasonal allergic rhinitis. (1995) *Allergol Immunopathol (Madr)*, Vol.23, No.2 (March-April 1995), pp. 51-57, Print ISSN 0301-0546, Electronic ISSN: 1578-1267.

Cox JS. Disodium cromoglycate (FPL 670) ('Intal'): a specific inhibitor of reaginic antibody-antigen mechanisms. (1967) *Nature*, Vol.216, No.5122 (December 1967), pp. 1328-1329, Print ISSN 0028-0836.

Custovic A, Wijk RG. The efectiveness of measures to change the indoor enviroment in the treatment of allergic rhinitis and asthma: ARIA update (in collaboration with GA(2)LEN. (2005) *Allergy*, Vol.60, No.9 (September 2005), pp. 1112-1115, Print ISSN 0105-4538, Electronic ISSN 1398-9995.

de Graaf-in 't Veld T, Garrelds IM, van Toorenenbergen AW, Mulder PG, Gerth van Wijk R, Boegheim JP. Effect of topical levocabastine on nasal response to allergen challenge and nasal hyperreactivity in perennial rhinitis. (1995) *Ann Allergy Asthma Immunol*, Vol.75, No.3 (September 1995), pp. 261-266, Print ISSN 1081-1206.

Dechant KL, Goa KL. Levocabastine. A review of its pharmacological properties and therapeutic potential as a topical antihistamine in allergic rhinitis and conjunctivitis. (1991) *Drugs*, Vol.41, No.2 (February 1991), pp. 202-224, Print ISSN 0012-6667.

Degirmencioglu H, Karadag A, Acvi Z, Kurtaran H, Catal F. Is hypertonic saline better than normal saline for allergic rhinitis in children? (2004) *Pediatr Allergy Immunol*, Vol.15, No.2 (April 2004), pp. 190, Print ISSN: 0905-6157. Electronic ISSN: 1399-3038.

Dorow P, Aurich R, Petzold U. Efficacy and tolerability of azelastine nasal spray in patients with allergic rhinitis compared to placebo and budesonide. (1993) *Arzneimittelforschung*, Vol.43, No.8 (August 1993), pp. 909-912, Print ISSN 0004-4172, Electronic ISSN 1616-7066.

Dykewicz MS, Fineman S. Executive Summary of Joint Task Force Practice Parameters on Diagnosis and Management of Rhinitis. (1998) *Ann Allergy Asthma Immunol*, Vol.81, No.5 Pt 2 (November 1998), pp. 463-468, Print ISSN 1081-1206, Electronic ISSN 1534-4436.

Espinosa de los Monteros MJ, González A, Rodríguez F, Gabriel R, Ancochea J. Análisis descriptivo (características clínicas y funcionales) de la población asmática de un área sanitaria. (1999) *Arch Bronconeumol*, Vol.35, No.11 (December 1999), pp. 518-524, Print ISSN 0300-2896, Electronic ISSN 1579-2129.

European Academy of Allergology and Clinical Immunology. The impact of allergic rhinitis on quality of life and other airway diseases. Summary of a European conference. (1998) *Allergy*, Vol.53, No.41 Suppl (January 1998), pp. 1-31, Print ISSN 0105-4538, Electronic ISSN: 1398-9995.

Fisher WG. Comparison of budesonide and disodium cromoglycate for the treatment of seasonal allergic rhinitis in children. (1994) *Ann Allergy*, Vol.73, No.6 (December 1994), pp. 515-520, Print ISSN 0003-4738.

Garavello W, Romagnoli M, Sordo L, Gaini RM, Di Berardino C, Angrisano A. Hypersaline nasal irrigation in children with symptomatic seasonal allergic rhinitis: a randomized study. (2003) *Pediatr Allergy Immunol*, Vol.14, No.2 (April 2003), pp. 140-143, Print ISSN: 0905-6157. Electronic ISSN: 1399-3038.

Georgitis JW. Nasal hyperthermia and simple irrigation for perennial rhinitis. Changes in inflammatory mediators. (1994) *Chest*, Vol.106, No.5 (November 1994), pp. 1478-1492, Print ISSN 0012-3692, Electronic ISSN 1931-3543.

Gergen P, Turkettaub P. The association of allergen skin test reactivity and respiratory disease among whites in the US population Data from the Second National Health & Nutrition Examination Survey, 1976-1980. (1991) *Arch Intern Med*, Vol.151, No.3 (March 1991), pp. 487-492, Print ISSN 0003-9926, Electronic ISSN 1538-3679.

Global Initiative for Asthma (GINA). Global strategy for asthma management and prevention: NHLBI/WHO workshop report. Bethesda: National Institutes of Health, National Heart, Lung and Blood Institute. Updated 2010. Available at http://www.ginasthma.com

Golightly LK, Greos LS. Second-generation antihistamines: actions and efficacy in the management of allergic disorders. (2005) *Drugs, Vol.65, No.3 (March* 2005), pp. 341-384, Print ISSN 0012-6667.

Graf P, Hallén H. Effect on the nasal mucosa of long-term treatment with oxymetazoline, benzalkonium chloride, and placebo nasal sprays. (1996) *Laryngoscope*, Vol.106, No.5 Pt 1 (May 1996), pp. 605-609, Print ISSN: 0023-852X, Electronic ISSN: 1531-4995.

Graf P, Juto JE. Histamine sensitivity in the nasal mucosa during four-week use of oxymetazoline. (1994) *Rhinology*, Vol.32, No.3 (September 1994), pp. 123-126, Print ISSN 03000-0729.

Graf P, Juto JE. Sustained use of xylometazoline nasal spray shortens the decongestive response and induces rebound swelling. (1995) *Rhinology*, Vol.33, No.1 (March 1995), pp. 14-17, Print ISSN 03000-0729.

Grossman J, Halverson PC, Meltzer EO, Shoenwetter WF, van Bavel JH, Woehler TR, et al. Double-blind assessment of azelastine in the treatment of perennial allergic rhinitis. (1994) *Ann Allergy*, Vol.73, No.2 (August 1994), pp. 141-146, Print ISSN 0003-4738.

Handelman NI, Friday GA, Schwartz HJ, Kuhn FS, Lindsay DE, Koors PG et al. Cromolyn sodium nasal solution in the prophylactic treatment of pollen-induced seasonal allergic rhinitis. (1977) *J Allergy Clin Immunol*, Vol.59, No.3 (March 1977), pp. 237-242, Print ISSN 0091-6749, Electronic ISSN 1097-6825.

Handley DA, Magnetti A, Higgins AJ (1998). Therapeutic advantages of third generation antihistamines. (1998) *Expert Opin Investig Drugs*, Vol.7, No.7 (August 1998), pp. 1045-1054, Print ISSN 1354-3784, Electronic ISSN 1744-7658.

Hartog B, van Benthem PP, Prins LC, Hordijk GJ. Efficacy of sinus irrigation versus sinus irrigation followed by functional endoscopic sinus surgery. (1997) *Ann Otol Rhinol Laryngol*, Vol.106, No.9 (September 1997), pp. 759-766, Print ISSN 0003-4894.

Hsieh JC, Lue KH, Lai DS, Sun HL, Lin YH. A comparison of cetirizine and montelukast for treating childhood perennial allergic rhinitis. (2004) *Pediatr Allergy and Immunol*, Vol.17, No.1 (January 2004), pp. 59-69 , Print ISSN 0905-6157, Electronic ISSN 1399-3038.

International Rhinitis Management Working Group. International Consensus Report on the diagnosis and management of rhinitis. (1994) *Allergy*, Vol.49, No.19 Suppl (June 1994), pp.1-34, Print ISSN 0105-4538, Electronic ISSN: 1398-9995.

ISAAC Steering Committee. Worldwide variation in prevalence of symptoms of asthma, allergic rhinoconjunctivitis, and atopic eczema: ISAAC. The International Study of

Asthma and Allergies in Childhood (ISAAC) Steering Committee. (1998) *Lancet*, Vol.351, No.9111 (April 1998), pp. 1225-1232, Print ISSN 0140-6736, Electronic ISSN 1474-547X.

Janssens MM, Vanden Bussche G. Levocabastine: an effective topical treatment of allergic rhinoconjunctivitis. (1991) *Clin Exp Allergy*, Vol.21, No.2 Suppl (May 1991), pp. 29-36, Print ISSN 0954-7894, Electronic ISSN: 1365-2222.

Jobst S, van den Wijngaart W, Schubert A, van de Venne H. Assessment of the efficacy and safety of three dose levels of cetirizine given once daily in children with perennial allergic rhinitis. (1994) *Allergy*, Vol.49, No.8 (September 1994), pp. 598-604, Print ISSN 0105-4538, Electronic ISSN 1398-9995.

Kaulbach HC, Igarashi Y, Mullol J, White MV, Kaliner MA. Effects of nedocromil sodium on allergen-induced rhinitis in humans. (1992) *J Allergy Clin Immunol.* Vol.89, No.2 (February 1992), pp. 599-619, Print ISSN 0091-6749, Electronic ISSN 1097-6825.

Lai DS, Lue KH, Hsieh JC, Lin KL, Lee HS. The comparison of the efficacy and safety of cetirizine, oxatomide, ketotifen, and a placebo for the treatment of childhood perennial allergic rhinitis. (2002) *Ann Allerg Asthma Immunol*, Vol.89, No.6 (December 2002), pp. 589-598, Print ISSN 1081-1206, Electronic ISSN 1534-4436.

Lester LA, Rich SS, Blumenthal MN, Togias A, Murphy S, Malveaux F, et al. Ethnic differences in asthma and associated phenotypes: collaborative study on the genetics of asthma. (2001) *J Allergy Clin Immunol*, Vol.108, No.3 (September 2001), pp. 357-362, Print ISSN 0091-6749, Electronic ISSN 1097-6825.

Leurs R, Church MK, Taglialatela M. H1-antihistamines: inverse agonism, anti-inflammatory actions and cardiac effects. (2002) *Clin Exp Allergy*, Vol.32, No.4 (April 2002), pp. 489-498, Print ISSN 0954-7894, Electronic ISSN 1365-2222.

Lötvall J, Akdis CA, Bacharier LB, Bjermer L, Casale TB, Custovic A, et al. Asthma endotypes: a new approach to classification of disease entities within the asthma syndrome. (2011) *J Allergy Clin Immunol*, Vol.127, No.2 (February 2011), pp. 355-360, Print ISSN 0091-6749, Electronic ISSN 1097-6825.

Mannino D, Homa D, Akinbami L, Moorman J, Gwynn C, Redd S. Surveillance of asthma – United States, 1980-1999. *MMWR Surveill Summ*, Vol.51, No.1 (March 2002), pp. 1-13, Print ISSN 1546-0738, Electronic ISSN 1545-8636.

Masi M, Candiani R, van de Venne H. A placebo-controlled trial of cetirizine in seasonal allergic rhino-conjunctivitis in children aged 6 to 12 years. (1993) *Pediatr Allergy Immunol*, Vol.4, No.4 Suppl (April 1993), pp. 47-52, Print ISSN 0905-6157, Electronic ISSN 1399-3038.

Metson R. When sinus trouble won't stay away. For people with chronic sinusitis, nasal irrigation and surgery offer avenues for fewer relapses and better breathing. (2004) *Health News*, Vol.10, No.5 (May 2004), pp. 12-13, Print ISSN 1081-5880.

Okuda M, Ohmishi M, Ohisuka H. The effects of cromolyn sodium on the nasal mast cell. (1985) *Ann Allergy*, Vol.55, No.5 (November 1985), pp. 721-723, Print ISSN 0003-4738.

Palma-Carlos AG, Chieira C, Conde TA, Cordeiro JA. Double-blind comparison of levocabastine nasal spray with sodium cromoglycate nasal spray in the treatment of seasonal allergic rhinitis. (1991) *Ann Allergy*, Vol.67, No.4 (October 1991), pp. 394-398, Print ISSN 0003-4738.

Papsin B, McTavish A. Saline nasal irrigation: Its role as an adjunct treatment. (2003) *Can Fam Physician*, Vol.49, No.1 (February 2003), pp. 168-173, Print ISSN 0008-350X, Electronic ISSN 1715-5258.

Passalacqua G, Bousquet PJ, Carlsen KH, Kemp J, Lockey RF, Niggeman B, et al. ARIA update: I. Systematic review of complementary and alternative medicine for rhinitis and asthma. (2006) *J Allergy Clin Immunol*, Vol.117, No.5 (May 2006), pp. 1054-1062, Print ISSN 0091-6749, Electronic ISSN 1097-6825.

Passalacqua G, Durham SR; Global Allergy and Asthma European Network. Allergic rhinitis and its impact on asthma update: allergen immunotherapy. (2007) *J Allergy Clin Immunol*, Vol.119, No.4 (April 2007), pp. 881-891, Print ISSN 0091-6749, Electronic ISSN 1097-6825.

Pearlman DS, Lumry WR, Winder JA, Noonan MJ. Once-daily cetirizine effective in the treatment of seasonal allergic rhinitis in children aged 6 to 11 years: a randomized, double-blind, placebo-controlled study. (1997) *Clin Pediatr (Phila)*, Vol.36, No.4 (April 1997), pp. 209-215, Print ISSN 0009-9228, Electronic ISSN 1938-2707.

Philip G, Nayak AS, Berger WE, Leynadier F, Vrijens F, Dass SB, Reiss TF. The effect of montelukast on rhinitis symptoms in patients with asthma and seasonal allergic rhinitis. (2004) *Curr Med Res Opin*, Vol.20, No.10 (October 2004), pp. 1549-1558, Print ISSN 0300-7995, Electronic ISSN 1473-4877.

Rabago D, Zgierska A, Mundt M, Barrett B, Bobula J, Maberry R. Efficacy of daily hypertonic saline nasal irrigation among patients with sinusitis: a randomized controlled trial. (2002) *J Fam Pract*, Vol.51, No.12 (December 2002), pp. 1049-1055, Print ISSN 0094-3509, Electronic ISSN 1533-7294.

Shekelle PG, Woolf SH, Eccles M, Grimshaw J. Clinical guidelines: developing guidelines. (1999) *BMJ*, Vol.318, No.7183 (February 1999), pp. 593-596, Print ISSN 0959-8138, Electronic ISSN 1468-5833.

Sibbald B, Rink E. Epidemiology of seasonal and perennial rhinitis: clinical presentation and medical history. (1991) *Thorax*, Vol.46, No.12 (December 1991), pp. 895-901, Print ISSN 0040-6376, Electronic ISSN 1468-3296.

Sienra-Monge JJ, Gazca-Aguilar A, Del Rio-Navarro B. Double-blind comparison of cetirizine and loratadine in children ages 2 to 6 years with perennial allergic rhinitis. (1999) *Am J Ther*, Vol.6, No-3 (May 1999), pp. 149-155, Print ISSN 1075-2765, Electronic ISSN 1536-3686.

Simons FER. Advances in H1-antihistamines. (2004) *N Engl J Med*, Vol.351, No.21 (November 2004), pp. 2203-2217, Print ISSN 0028-4793, Electronic ISSN 1533-4406.

Simons FER, Akdis CA. Histamine and H1-antihistamines. In: Adkinson NF Jr, Bochner BS, Busse WW, Holgate ST, Lemanske RF Jr, Simons FER, editors. Middleton's allergy: principles and practice. 7th ed. St Louis: Mosby (an affiliate of Elsevier Science); 2009. p. 1517-48. ISBN: 978-0-323-05659-5.

Simons FE, Simons KJ. Histamine and H1-antihistamines: celebrating a century of progress. (2011) *J Allergy Clin Immunol*, Vol.128, No.6 (December 2011), pp. 1139-1150, Print ISSN 0091-6749, Electronic ISSN 1097-6825.

Spanish Society of Allergology and Clinical Immunology. Estudio Alergológica 92. Factores Epidemiológicos, Clínicos y Socioeconómicos de las enfermedades alérgicas en España. Sociedad Española de Alergología e Inmunología Clínica y Alergia e Inmunología Abello SA, editores. Madrid: NILO Industria Gráfica. 1995. ISBN 10 : 84-605-2749-2 / ISBN 13 : 978-84-605-2749-7.

Spanish Society of Allergology and Clinical Immunology. Estudio Alergológica 2005. Factores Epidemiológicos, Clínicos y Socioeconómicos de las enfermedades alérgicas en España en 2005. Sociedad Española de Alergología e Inmunología Clínica y Alergia-Schering Plough. editores. Madrid: Egraf, S.A. 2006. ISBN: 84-7989-428-8.

Storms W. Tratamiento de la rinitis alérgica: efectos de la rinitis alérgica y de los antihistamínicos sobre el funcionamiento. *Allergy and Asthma Proc.* 1997;XI,5:1-3. ISSN 1088-5412, Electronic ISSN: 1539-6304.

Stübner UP, Toth J, Marks B, Berger UE, Burtin B, Horak F. Efficacy and safety of an oral formulation of cetirizine and prolonged-release pseudoephedrine versus xylometazoline nasal spray in nasal congestion. (2001) *Arzneimittelforschung*, Vol.51, No.11 (November 2001), pp. 904-010, Print ISSN 0004-4172.

Subiza J, Barjau MC, Rodríguez R, Gavilán MJ. Inhibition of the seasonal IgE increase to *Dactylis glomerata* by daily sodium chloride nasal-sinus irrigation during the grass pollen season. (1999) *J Allergy Clin Immunol*, Vol.104, No.3 Pt 1 (September 1999), pp.711-712, Print ISSN 0091-6749, Electronic ISSN 1097-6825.

Swedish GP Allergy Team. Topical levocabastine compared with oral loratadine for the treatment of seasonal allergic rhinoconjunctivitis. (1994) *Allergy*, Vol.49, No.8 (September 1994), pp. 611-615, Print ISSN 0105-4538, Electronic ISSN: 1398-9995.

Taccariello M, Parikh A, Darby Y, Scadding G. Nasal douching as a valuable adjunct in the management of chronic rhinosinusitis. (1999) *Rhinology*, Vol.37, No.1 (March 1999), pp. 29-32, Print ISSN 03000-0729.

The Livostin Study Group. A comparison of topical levocabastine and oral terfenadine in the treatment of allergic rhinoconjunctivitis. (1993) *Allergy*, Vol.48, No.7 (October 1993), pp. 530-534, Print ISSN 0105-4538, Electronic ISSN: 1398-9995.

Tinkelman DG, Kemp J, Mitchell DQ, Galant SP. Treatment of seasonal allergic rhinitis in children with cetirizine or chlorpheniramine: A multicenter study. (1996) *Pediatric Asthma, Allergy and Immunology* , Vol.10, No. (January 1996), pp. 9-17.

Tomooka LT, Murphy C, Davidson TM. Clinical study and literature review of nasal irrigations. (2000) *Laringoscope*, Vol.110, No.7 (July 2000), pp. 1189-119, Print ISSN 0023-852X, Electronic ISSN 1531-4995.

Van Cauwenberge P, Bachert C, Passalacqua G, Bousquet J, Canonica G, Durham S et al. Consensus statement on the treatment of allergic rhinitis. EAACI Position paper. (2000) *Allergy*, Vol.55, No.2 (February 2000), pp. 116-134, Print ISSN 0105-4538, Electronic ISSN 1398-9995.

Wahn U, Meltzer EO, Finn AF Jr, Kowalski ML, Decosta P, Hedlin G, et al. Fexofenadine is efficacious and safe in children (aged 6-11 years) with seasonal allergic rhinitis. (2003) *J Allergy Clin Immunol*, Vol.111, No.4 (April 2003), pp. 763-769, Print ISSN 0091-6749, Electronic ISSN 1097-6825.

Weiler JM, Meltzer EO. Azelastine nasal spray as adjunctive therapy to azelastine tablets in the management of seasonal allergic rhinitis. (1997) *Ann Allergy Asthma Immunol*, Vol.79, No.4 (October 1997), pp. 327-332, Print ISSN 1081-1206, Electronic ISSN 1534-4436.

Wellington K, Jarvis B. Cetirizine/pseudoephedrine. (2001) *Drugs*, Vol.61, No.15 (April 2001), pp. 2231-2240; Discussion 2241-2242, Print ISSN 0012-6667.

Westerveld GJ, Scheeren RA, Dekker I, Griffioen DH, Voss HP, Bast A. Anti-oxidant actions of oxymethazoline and xylomethazoline. (1995) *Eur J Pharmacol*, Vol.291, No.1 (September 1995), pp. 27-31, Print ISSN 0014-2999.

Yang YH, Lin YT, Lu MY, Tsai MJ, Chiang BL. A double-blind, placebo-controlled, and randomized study of loratadine (Clarityne) syrup for the treatment of allergic rhinitis in children aged 3 to 12 years. (2001) *Asian Pac J Allergy Immunol*, Vol.19, No.3 (September 2001), pp. 171-175, Print ISSN 0125-877X.

Yoo JK, Seikaly H, Calhoun KH. Extended use of topical nasal decongestants. (1997) *Laryngoscope*, Vol.107, No.1 (January 1997), pp. 40-43, Print ISSN: 0023-852X, Electronic ISSN: 1531-4995.

6

Treatment of Allergic Rhinitis: Anticholinergics, Glucocorticotherapy, Leukotriene Antagonists, Omalizumab and Specific-Allergen Immunotherapy

Jesús Jurado-Palomo[1], Irina Diana Bobolea[2], María Teresa Belver González[2], Álvaro Moreno-Ancillo[1], Ana Carmen Gil Adrados[3] and José Manuel Morales Puebla[4]

[1]*Department of Allergology, Nuestra Señora del Prado General Hospital, Talavera de la Reina*

[2]*Department of Allergology, Hospital La Paz Health Research Institute (IdiPAZ), Madrid*

[3]*Centro de Salud La Solana, Talavera de la Reina*

[4]*Department of Otorhinolaryngology, University General Hospital, Ciudad Real*

Spain

1. Introduction

Throughout history, various classifications of rhinitis have emerged, many of which originated from expert groups. We would have to go back to 1994 to find the "*International Consensus Report on Diagnosis and Management of Rhinitis*" (International Rhinitis Management Working Group, 1994), which was subsequently modified in the 2000 "*Consensus statement on the treatment of allergic rhinitis. EAACI Position paper*" (Van Cauwenberge et al, 2000). Of particular interest is the "*Executive Summary of Joint Task Force Practice Parameters on Diagnosis and Management of Rhinitis*" of 1998 (Dykewicz & Fineman, 1998). In 2001, a group of experts, the "*Allergic Rhinitis and its Impact on Asthma (ARIA) Workshop Expert Panel*", met to develop guidelines on the diagnosis and treatment of rhinitis, which also dealt with other inflammatory processes interrelated/associated with asthma. The acronym "ARIA" comes from "Allergic Rhinitis and its Impact on Asthma". ARIA is a document from a non-governmental organisation of the World Health Organization (WHO), endorsed by numerous scientific societies, such as the International Association of Allergology and Clinical Immunology (IAACI) and the World Allergy Organization (WAO) (Bousquet et al, 2001).

It was established as an educational program as the "Guidelines for recommendations for the diagnosis and comprehensive handling of patients with rhinitis", associated with asthma and other interrelated processes (sinusitis, conjunctivitis and otitis).

In this chapter, we revised others modalities of treatment for AR; anticholinergics, glucocorticotherapy, leukotriene antagonists, omalizumab and specific-allergen immunotherapy.

2. Anticholinergics

Ipratropium bromide is an anticholinergic compound related to atropine. It is poorly absorbed, but has high topical activity. It inhibits secretion for at least 4 hours, without the appearance of systemic symptoms.

Mechanism of action: It is capable of significantly reducing rhinorrhoea by acting selectively on the muscarinic receptors, which, when activated by acetylcholine released by the parasympathetic nervous system, induce the secretion of mucus by the nasal seromucous glands.

Systemic cholinergic collateral effects rarely appear, but include changes in vision, tachycardia, urinary retention and dry mouth. However, it should be administered with caution to patients with glaucoma or prostatic hypertrophy.

Ipratropium bromide is used in aqueous solution for topical nasal use in doses of two inhalations of 0.02 mg each three times a day in each nostril. The recommended dose should not be increased if there is no improvement.

It has been used for allergic (Kaiser et al, 1995) and non-allergic (Bronsky et al, 1995) perennial rhinitis, and acts by improving hydrorrhoea, with a maximum peak 1-4 hours after administration. It has barely any effect on nasal obstruction and sneezing, and its most frequent side effects are epistaxis, nasal dryness and headache (Kaiser et al, 1995; Bronsky et al, 1995).

3. Glucocorticotherapy

In the literature review we performed, we found only one published article that covers the treatment of seasonal AR with systemic corticosteroids (Myging et al, 2000). They report that they could find only 5 studies published between 1960 and 1993 on systemic corticosteroids and AR, compared to more than 100 published studies on topical corticosteroids. There are several publications that compare topical corticosteroids with each other and with other drugs.

According to the 1994 Consensus (International Rhinitis Management Working Group, 1994), first-line therapy for the handling of seasonal AR in moderate cases with intermittent symptoms are antihistamines, and intranasal corticosteroids in severe cases with daily symptoms. In case of exacerbations during the pollen season, it is currently common practice to administer a short cycle of oral or intramuscular corticosteroids. It seems that systemic corticosteroids are highly effective for nasal blockage, but not so much for rhinorrhoea and sneezing. One high oral dose of 30 mg daily seems effective in controlling all nasal symptoms. Subcutaneous atrophy has been reported at the injection site, as well as local reactions, changes of pigmentation, etc.

The lack of reliable comparative studies and the fear of severe side effects have pushed studies and treatment towards therapy with inhaled corticosteroids.

3.1 Systemic glucocorticosteroids

Brown et al published the first placebo-controlled study of the use of systemic corticosteroids for the treatment of AR. They report that the use of 3 injections of 240 mg of methylprednisolone in one-week intervals, achieved significant improvement of symptoms (Brown et al, 1960).

In the decade of the 70´s, other authors prescribed 2 injections of 80 mg of methylprednisolone with 14-day intervals to 8 patients with seasonal AR. Cortisol levels decreased after the injection, and patients began to recover and return to normal after 3 weeks (Ganderton & James, 1970).

McMillin scheduled an 80 mg injection of triamcinolone acetonide to 18 patients with severe AR, and measured morning plasmatic cortisol levels for 21 days. Although the levels descended on several occasions, the initial values were recovered after 3 weeks (Mc Millim, 1971).

In the decade of the 80´s, various clinicians studied the results of administering an injection of 5 mg of betamethasone dipropionate, another of 3 mg of betamethasone phosphate, with 3 mg of betamethasone acetate, and a third of 40 mg of methylprednisolone. These injections were administered to 60 patients with significant AR, who were divided into 3 groups depending on the type of injection (Ohlander et al, 1980)

Methylprednisolone and beclomethasone dipropionate (BDP) reduced the production of endogenous cortisol for at least 14 days, while the combination of phosphate and betamethasone acetate did not suppress plasma cortisol in 12 days. Glycaemia increased in the 3 groups in the first two days following the injection.

Hedner et al, prescribed an injection of 80 mg of methylprednisolone to 14 patients with AR. Baseline cortisol and plasma cortisol response to hypoglycaemia had moderate but significant reductions at 2 weeks, although they returned to normal in 4 weeks (Hedner & Persson, 1981).

Almost in parallel, Borum et al performed two trials in 24 patients with AR. In the first, they gave an injection of 80 mg of methylprednisolone at the start of the pollen season, and in the second, they gave it at the peak of the pollen season (Borum et al, 1987). In the first group, the effect lasted the entire season (at least 5 weeks), with all symptoms disappearing. In the second group, the injection had a rapid effect on nasal obstruction, which disappeared and did not return in the remaining 5 weeks of pollen season. Rhinorrhoea and sneezing did not disappear as noticeably as in the first group and reappeared in a few weeks. The use of rescue anti-Hl, however, was clearly inferior in both groups, compared to placebo.

Laursen et al studied the effect of a 5 g injection of betamethasone dipropionate and 2 mg of betamethasone, immediately before the start of the birch pollen season (study was performed in Denmark). They found that these patients had fewer symptoms, especially nasal obstruction, than patients treated with placebo, with the effect lasting 4 weeks (Laursen et al, 1987).

In 1988, the following year, these same authors performed a double-blind placebo-controlled trial with 30 adults with rhinoconjunctivitis (RC) who were allergic to seasonal birch pollen (Laursen et al, 1988). The patients were treated with 100 micrograms of BDP in each nostril twice a day for 4 weeks. Patients received either a placebo or an injection of 5 mg of BDP and 2 mg of betamethasone phosphate, immediately before the start of the birch pollen season. The authors concluded that an injection of BDP and betamethasone phosphate immediately before the birch pollen season produced a significant reduction in rhinoconjunctivitis symptoms, compared to placebo and topical steroid treatment.

That same year, other authors found a significant reduction in plasma cortisol 3 weeks after an injection of 80 mg of methylprednisolone, but not during treatment with 200 micrograms of intranasal budesonide. They found no differences between the two therapies in terms of nasal obstruction, but there was a tendency to favour topical treatment with budesonide in terms of sneezing and rhinorrhoea (Pichler et al, 1988).

Brooks et al, treated 31 patients with rhinitis for 5 days with placebo or methylprednisolone in daily doses of 6, 12 or 24 mg, divided into 3 daily doses. They achieved significant improvement in nasal obstruction with 6 mg, and with all symptoms except for sneezing with 24 mg (Brooks et al, 1993)

Based on the literature, systemic corticosteroids seem to have a significant effect on nasal obstruction, but less so on sneezing and rhinorrhoea. These studies demonstrated a reduction in cortisol plasma levels after an IM injection of corticosteroids. The effect is greatest at 3 days and disappears after 3 weeks.

We have not found any published study on whether systemic corticosteroids should be added due to a lack of improvement with topical corticosteroids or other drugs.

3.2 Topical (intranasal) glucocorticosteroids

Several studies have shown the inhibitory efficacy of topical corticosteroids in the delayed response of allergic reactions. Symptoms that occur 2-11 hours after nasal provocation by an allergen are completely eliminated with their administration. Initially, it was thought that topical corticosteroids did not inhibit the early response; however, there is clear evidence that they also act on symptoms immediately. Studies have shown their efficacy in reducing both specific and non-specific nasal hyperreactivity.

It has been shown that the effective dose of antihistamines (loratadine oral) can be reduced with the use of fluticasone in nasal spray, in the treatment of seasonal AR. The conclusion is that the efficacy and decreased inflammation is greater with fluticasone (decreases eosinophilic cationic proteins and the number of eosinophils, and improves scores on quality-of-life questionnaires).

A reduction has been shown in the number of subepithelial cells (CD3+, CD4+, CD8+) in patients treated with topical corticosteroids. Recent studies have demonstrated a reduction in the expression of adhesion molecules (ICAM-l) in patients treated over long periods of time. Their anti-inflammatory effects are increased by the decrease in chemotaxis and the activation of eosinophils. In terms of symptoms, this translates into decreased obstruction, pruritus, sneezing and rhinorrhoea. Currently, various compounds are used.

3.2.1 Beclometasone dipropionate

Introduced in 1973 for topical nasal treatment, beclometasone dipropionate (BDP) is a potent local steroid, with absorption at therapeutic doses. It was the first steroid that proved effective in the topical treatment of hay fever.

BDP acts by penetrating the cell membrane and binding with cytoplasmic receptors. The compound formed is transferred to the nucleus, where it binds to the DNA molecule. It seems to act by emptying histamine deposits, reducing the number of mast cells and inhibiting their synthesis of histamines. It lowers the number of eosinophils, lessening the release of cytotoxic proteins, and reduces mucosal oedema by decreasing vascular permeability.

BDP may cause non-serious local side effects, such as epistaxis, nasal pruritus and, rarely, mycotic infection, but it is doubtful that it causes mucosal atrophy in long-term treatments.

It is used in nasal spray, with a standard dose of 100 micrograms every 6 hours. It has an anti-inflammatory effect 5000 times more powerful than hydrocortisone.

Cockcroftf performed a study for 42 days on patients with AR. At 35 days, there was a decrease in clinical symptoms in 86% (*P*<.05) of patients who had been treated with BDP, compared to 13% who had received placebos (Cockcroft et al, 1976)

In a 4-week study, Peluchi compared azelastine at doses of 0.56 mg/day with BDP at doses of 200 micrograms/day and placebo. Both drugs were effective, reducing eosinophilia more in patients who had received the corticosteroid (Peluchi et al, 1995).

3.2.2 Budesonide

A non-halogenated corticosteroid, budesonide is an anti-inflammatory drug 2-3 times more powerful than BDP (Bryson & Faulds, 1992). It has a half-life of 2 hours, and is inactivated in the liver by oxidative metabolism after systemic absorption. It has the same mechanism of action as BDP, and may cause temporary epistaxis, nasal pruritus and sneezing as collateral effects.

The average recommended dose is 100 micrograms every 12 hours in each nostril. Prophylactic administration protects against immediate allergic reactions. Therefore, treatment of seasonal rhinitis should be started before exposure to the allergen.

Cimetidine influences the pharmacokinetics and pharmacodynamics of budesonide after concomitant oral and intravenous administration, although it is of little clinical significance.

3.2.3 Fluticasone propionate

A fluorinated glucocorticoid with significant topical activity, fluticasone propionate (FP) (Flixonase; GlaxoSmithKline, London, UK) is structurally similar to cortisol, with certain variations that increase its lipophilic properties and its potency of action. It has high selectivity and affinity for glucocorticoid receptors.

FP possesses an anti-inflammatory potency twice than that of BDP which is linked to its effect on various cellular elements and the mediators of the inflammation (Barnes, 1992). It reduces the number of activated eosinophils in the nose during antigenic stimulation in allergic individuals.

FP significantly reduces the number of T lymphocytes, and reduces the number of non-activated basophils, neutrophils and eosinophils. Meltzer studied nasal eosinophilia in 497 patients treated with fluticasone or placebo, and found a decrease (*P*<.01) in patients treated with fluticasone (Melzer et al, 1990).

The lipolytic character of topical corticosteroids is significant, since it leads to increased drug retention in the tissues. The recommended dose is 200 mg/day (two applications of 50 µg per nostril, once a day). For children between the ages of 4-11 years, half the dose is recommended. Side effects are similar to those of the other inhaled corticosteroids described above (LaForce et al, 1994).

FP is eliminated from systemic circulation at a rate approximately equal to hepatic blood flow. It is metabolised through hydrolysis with the formation of 17-ß-carboxylic metabolic acid, which has insignificant anti-inflammatory and systemic activity due to incomplete absorption in the gastrointestinal tract and to extensive metabolism during the first hepatic step.

Comparative studies of BDP at similar doses have shown that both steroids have a similar efficacy for controlling nasal symptoms, in all cases superior to that of placebo. The speed of action is greater in fluticasone, as evidenced by the fact that significant improvement in symptoms is seen by the second day of treatment, while the delay in the onset of improvement for those treated with BDP was three days (Scadding et al, 1994).

Same authors found that after nasal provocation with an allergen, treatment with FP decreased obstruction in 45%, sneezing in 73%, pruritus in 78% and hydrorrhoea in 80% (Scadding et al, 1994).

Kaszuba demonstrated the efficacy of antihistamines (loratadine oral) with the use of fluticasone in nasal spray, in the treatment of seasonal AR. The conclusion was that the efficacy and decreased inflammation was greater with FP (decreased ECP, the number of eosinophils and improved scores on quality-of-life questionnaires) (Kaszuba et al, 2001).

3.2.4 Fluticasone furoate

Fluticasone furoate (FF) (Avamys; GlaxoSmithKline, London, UK) is the most recent intranasal glucocorticosteroid available for the treatment of AR (allergic rhinitis). It possesses a distinctive combination of pharmacodynamic and physico-chemical properties, which confers a high affinity for the glucocorticosteroid receptor and a potent anti-inflammatory activity. This allows its effectiveness in treating both nasal and ocular symptoms to be complemented by a favorable safety and tolerance profile. In addition, the new nasal delivery device was designed according to the needs experienced and expressed by patients, which assures an optimal dispensation that promotes its extensive use. (Allen et al, 2007; Rosenblut et al, 2007; Baumann et al, 2009).

The compliance of the patients in treatment with intranasal corticosteroids may be influenced by both the sensorial properties of the drug and the delivery device. FF has been formulated to release a low volume (50 µl) in the form of a fine mist, with a favorable profile of sensory characteristics in terms of reduction in odor, in the posterior aftertaste, and in the retro-nasal dripping down the throat (Mahadevia et al, 2004; Meltzer et al, 2008).

In addition to the greater affinity for the glucocorticosteroid receptor, FF shows a high selectivity for the same as compared to other intranasal glucocorticosteroids; for each FF molecule which binds to the mineralocorticoid receptor, other 800 will bind to the glucocorticosteroid receptor, which considerably limits the potential undesirable side effects.

FF has demonstrated superior efficacy when compared to placebo in the treatment of nasal symptoms of seasonal allergic rhinitis in adults and children, and demonstrated a significant improvement in overall relief of associated eye symptoms. Symptomatic relief of allergic rhinitis begins 8 hours after administration and lasts for 24 hours (Máspero et al, 2008; Nathan RA et al, 2008; Vasar et al, 2008; Baroody et al, 2009; Meltzer et al, 2009).

The efficacy of FF administered for 4 weeks versus placebo has also been assessed in adolescents and adults with perennial allergic rhinitis, with significant improvement in nasal symptoms and extraocular manifestations (such as pharyngeal or palatal itching) and in the RQLQ scores (Keith & Scadding, 2009; Keith & Scadding, 2010).

The recommended dose of FF in Spain for patients older than 12 years is 110 µg, which equals two sprays in each nostril once a day. It may be reduced to one spray in each nostril once symptoms are controlled. For children between 6 and 12 years of age, the recommended dose is one spray in each nostril once daily (55 µg), but can be increased to two sprays if it fails to control the symptoms. In Europe FF is not approved in children less than 6 years of age (GlaxoSmithKline, 2011).

FF (like the rest of intranasal corticosteroids) has proven effective for controlling nasal symptoms in allergic rhinitis. But unlike other intranasal corticosteroids, which show contradictory effects on ocular symptoms, FF is the only intranasal corticosteroid that demonstrates a consistent positive effect on ocular symptoms in seasonal allergic rhinitis in a large number of patients from different studies, across different pollen seasons and geographical locations (Keith & Scadding, 2009; Keith & Scadding, 2010).

3.2.5 Flunisolide

Introduced in 1978, flunisolide is a poorly water-soluble drug, which is therefore dissolved in propylene glycol and water (Horan & Johnson, 1978; Schulz et al, 1978). Rhinoscopy is recommended once a year for prolonged treatment.

3.2.6 Mometasone furoate

A corticosteroid available worldwide in dermatological preparations, mometasone furoate (MF) has been classified as a powerful corticosteroid according to European Union directives. It has few systemic side effects when applied topically to the skin. Solutions of MF in aqueous suspension are prepared for subsequent administration with a nasal nebulizer, and have been marketed for several years now. The absorption rate for MF is 8%, and absolute bioavailability has been estimated at less than 1% of the adjusted dose, due to hepatic metabolism.

MF, a potent, topically active, synthetic, 17-heterocyclic corticosteroid was originally introduced for the treatment of dermatological conditions (Lundbland et al, 2001). MF aqueous nasal spray (Nasonex; Schering-Plough, Inc., Kenilworth, NJ, USA) was shown to be effective in several inflammatory conditions of the upper respiratory tract, including AR (van Drunen et al, 2005) and non-AR (Lundbland et al, 2001), nasal polyps (Small et al, 2005; Stjarne et al, 2006), adenoidal hypertrophy (Berlucchi et al, 2007) and uncomplicated rhinosinusitis (Meltzer et al, 2005). Safety and pharmacokinetic evaluations of MF have shown a lack of systemic activity when applied to the nasal mucosa, even in pediatric patients (Zitt et al, 2007). There is no clinical evidence that MF nasal spray suppresses the function of the hypothalamic-pituitary-adrenal axis when the drug is administered at clinically relevant doses (100-400 μg/day) (Small et al, 2005), and there are no reports of any influence on children´s growth (Schenkel et al, 2000; Meltzer et al, 2005). Histological studies after long-term use of MF nasal spray have shown no signs of atrophy of the nasal mucosa (Minshall et al, 1998).

3.3 Side effects, safety and tolerance of glucocorticosteroids

We performed a literature review of articles published between 1994 and 2012, and found numerous articles that studied the effectiveness, side effects, safety and tolerance of inhaled corticosteroids, and then compared them with each other and with other drugs. We have summarised these articles below.

Edwards compared BDP with hydrocortisone, prednisolone, dexamethasone and betamethasone, which cause suppression of the hypothalamic-pituitary-adrenal cortex axis and adverse systemic reactions. The undesirable action of the topical corticosteroid is reduced at the application site (Edwards, 1995)

It is metabolised quickly and has longer duration of action. The study concluded by declaring the safety and efficacy of intranasal treatment with BDP as an indicated treatment for patients with AR.

Other authors tested the usefulness and efficacy of topical corticosteroids, with a reduction in the number of Langerhans cells in nasal mucosa, as well as the number of eosinophils. Moreover, they demonstrated the corticosteroids' efficacy, since these reduced three of the major symptoms of AR: sneezing, rhinorrhoea and nasal blockage (Mygind & Dahl, 1996).

Howland tested the advantages of FP in nasal spray over oral antihistamines in the treatment of seasonal AR, in doses of 200 micrograms once a day. After a follow-up of one year, the study found no side effects on bone mineralisation, subcapsular cataracts, glaucoma or the pituitary axis (Howland, 1996).

The same year they published a similar study in another journal: Efficacy of 200 micrograms of FP in aqueous nasal spray once a day. The study observed mild local topical effects and no indirect effects after systemic absorption (Howland et al, 1996).

Other clinicians observed that intranasal FP is an effective treatment for AR, is well tolerated and is indicated over other treatments using intranasal corticosteroids, antihistamines or intranasal cromolyn sodium, when administered once a day. It has better cost-effectiveness than the antihistamines loratadine and terfenadine (Wiseman & Benfield, 1997).

Finally, it confirmed that topical nasal corticosteroids decrease nasal blockage more effectively than antihistamines (Mygind et al, 1977).

The topical corticosteroids, such as triamcinolone, are the most powerful and effective agents in the treatment of AR, and have little systemic absorption (Naclerio, 1998). Oral antihistamines do not always control nasal congestion. Vasoconstrictors can cause drug-induced rhinitis, if used for a prolonged period of time, which is typical. Anti-leukotrienes need more studies; cromolyn sodium is effective in AR, but less so than topical corticosteroids.

Storms concluded that the benefits of FP exceed the risk in studies on the treatment of asthma and AR, using intranasal doses of 200 micrograms once a day. There were no cases of adrenal suppression or osteoporosis due to its use (Storms, 1998).

Corren stated that the use of intranasal corticosteroids has been shown to be an effective and safe form of therapy for AR. In terms of side effects, MF and FP seem to be safer and have less potential for systemic effects, even in cases of prolonged use and use in children, making them the ideal drugs for allergic rhinitis (Corren, 1999)

Lumry considered MF and FP as the best drugs for the treatment of AR, although there is lesser systemic involvement with mometasone. A case has been reported of suppression of nocturnal cortisol levels with FP, indicating suppression of the hypothalamic-pituitary-adrenal axis (Lumry, 1999).

Other authors tested the superiority of treatment with intranasal FP (200 micrograms once a day) over levocabastine in nasal spray and placebo nasal spray. The antihistamine improved symptoms of nasal blockage and rhinorrhoea. The placebo improved symptoms of sneezing, nasal blockage, rhinorrhoea and pruritus (Di Lorenzo et al, 1999). Furthermore, it is recommended the use of triamcinolone as the intranasal corticosteroid of choice in AR at a recommended dose of 220 micrograms once a day (Gawchik & Saccar, 2000).

Allen, from his perspective as an endocrinologist, observed that intranasal corticosteroids have been established as the first-line treatment of AR. They are safe and have few reported side effects due to excessive and prolonged doses, or to several concomitant inhaled corticosteroids (Allen, 2000).

However, Szefler warned that topical administration of corticosteroids may reduce the total required dose of corticosteroid for treating patients with minimal side effects (Szefler, 2001). This has prompted the development of intranasal corticosteroids as treatment for allergic and perennial rhinitis.

It has been shown that intranasal MF does not cause adverse side effects, and can even be used in children, as it does not affect bone growth. Therefore, we can say that the side effects of intranasal corticosteroids are minimal at the recommended doses.

Transrud stated that intranasal corticosteroids accepted as first-line treatment of AR are safe and effective. They reduce nasal congestion, pruritus, rhinorrhoea and sneezing that occur in the early and late phases of the allergic response. They join other studies that demonstrated an almost complete prevention of late phase symptoms. Adverse reactions are usually limited to nasal mucosa, along with headache and epistaxis in 5%-10% of patients (Trangsrud et al, 2002).

Wang reported that there was no difference between the efficacy of anti-Hl and topical corticosteroids in the treatment of AR, with both drugs recommended despite their different pharmacological characteristics. The greater benefit of topical corticosteroids is in its longer lasting anti-inflammatory action, compared with the speed of action of anti-Hl (Wang, 2002).

Finally, it is confirmed the greater efficacy of an intranasal treatment with FP over oral loratadine and a leukotriene inhibitor (montelukast) in seasonal AR. The results were significantly better in the fluticasone group in the reduction of nasal symptoms (Saengpanich et al, 2003).

Other authors showed that both intranasal corticosteroids and intranasal antihistamines were effective topical therapies in the treatment of AR (Salib & Howarth, 2003). Intranasal therapy represents a better form of treatment in AR, with a highly favourable risk/benefit ratio. It is the preferred route of administration of corticosteroids in the treatment of the disease, as well as an important option compared to therapy with antihistamines, especially when quick symptom relief is needed.

Using meta-analysis, Waddell compared the efficacy of intranasal corticosteroids and oral antihistamines in the treatment of AR, and found a clear benefit in favour of intranasal corticosteroids. However, there is no clear evidence that one corticosteroid spray is more effective and safer than another in the treatment of rhinitis. It has not been demonstrated that either FP, MF or triamcinolone are more effective, or they are more expensive than BDP, budesonide and dexamethasone (Waddell et al, 2003).

Conversely, it was demonstrated that intranasal FP, in doses of 200 micrograms once a day, improves ocular symptoms in patients with AR, without the need for adding oral antihistamines or topical eye drops (De Wester, 2003).

Towards the end of 2003, Borish stated that an effective therapy in the treatment of rhinitis is that which is direct and decreases inflammation and its systemic manifestations. Antihistamines quickly resolve nasal symptoms, but not inflammation, at least not significantly. Oral corticosteroids are highly effective, but have significant systemic side effects. Local intranasal corticosteroids act on the level of local inflammatory processes of rhinitis, reducing local inflammatory cells, but without direct involvement of other tissues (Borish, 2003). Anti-leukotrienes have systemic anti-inflammatory effects and an acceptable safety profile.

They compared the efficacy of antihistamines versus intranasal corticosteroids in AR, with the studies favouring corticosteroids. Antihistamines also do not seem to be superior in the treatment of conjunctivitis associated with AR (Nielsen & Dahl, 2003).

Other author warned that it would be best to avoid allergens during pregnancy (Keleç, 2004). If cromolyn is not tolerated or is ineffective, first- or second-generation anti-H1 (cetirizine and loratadine) may be used. Intranasal corticosteroids may be added for treatment of significant nasal obstruction. There are no studies on the use of new intranasal corticosteroids (FP, FF, flunisolide, triamcinolone, MF) during the first trimester of pregnancy. Kim confirmed that intranasal corticosteroids are safe and effective for treating AR in adults (Kim et al, 2004). The administration of budesonide aqueous nasal spray for 6 weeks is well tolerated and safe, with no suppression of the pituitary-adrenal axis, even in children aged 2 to 5 years with AR.

Patel et al stated that the use of betamethasone suppresses the adrenal axis, which does not happen with MF nasal spray. The concentration of cortisol in morning saliva is a tool for monitoring adrenal function (Patel et al, 2004).

Gradually, it has been established that AR and asthma often coexist and represent 2 manifestations of the same disease, which has recently been called CARAS (combined allergic rhinitis and asthma syndrome) (Taramarcaz & Gibson, 2004). The benefit of using intranasal corticosteroids in CARAS has been shown, although there is still a lack of studies. Currently, the best practice is to treat conventional asthma with bronchial corticosteroids (inhaled) with or without ß-agonists and adding intranasal corticosteroids to avoid symptoms specific to rhinitis.

4. Oral Cys-LT cysteinyl leukotriene receptor-1 antagonist

Allergic rhinitis is a common airways hypersensitivity disease. Histamine and leukotrienes are involved in the pathogenesis of allergic rhinitis. Conventional treatments include topical steroids and antihistamines. Due to the adverse effects of these treatments, new drugs like leukotriene receptor antagonists are being investigated for the treatment of allergic rhinitis (Modgill et al, 2010).

The cysteinyl leukotrienes (LTC4, LTD4, LTE4) are products of arachidonic acid metabolism and are released from various cells, including mast cells and eosinophils. These eicosanoids bind to cysteinyl leukotriene (CysLT) receptors. The CysLT type-1 (CysLT1) receptor is found in the human airway (including airway smooth muscle cells and airway macrophages) and on other pro-inflammatory cells (including eosinophils and certain myeloid stem cells). CysLTs have been correlated with the pathophysiology of asthma and AR. In asthma, leukotriene-mediated effects include airway edema, smooth muscle contraction, and altered cellular activity associated with the inflammatory process. In allergic rhinitis, CysLTs are released from the nasal mucosa after allergen exposure during both early- and late-phase reactions and are associated with symptoms of allergic rhinitis (Lipworth, 1999).

There are two different LT inhibitors/modifiers:

- LT receptor antagonists [LTRAs; montelukast (Singulair®, Merck Sharp & Dohme Inc, NJ, USA), zafirlukast (Accolate®,AstraZeneca farmacéutica, Madrid, Spain), and pranlukast (Azlaire®, Schering Plough Inc, NJ, USA).
- 5-Lypoxigenase inhibitor of LT synthesis [zileuton® (Zyflo®)].

Montelukast and zafirlukast block binding of cysteinil LTs to the cysLT1 receptor in the extracellular space. Zileuton inhibits 5-lipoxygenase and therefore all LT synthesis within inflammatory cells. By blocking the actions of LTs, it promotes bronchodilation and decreases the inflammatory response. Anti-LTs also have been used successfully by some authors to control allergic diseases such as AR, atopic dermatitis, chronic urticaria and allergic conjunctivitis. The FDA has approved montelukast for the treatment of AR (Scow et al, 2007).

4.1 Montelukast

Montelukast is indicated for the prophylaxis and chronic treatment of asthma in adults and pediatric patients 12 months of age and older; for prevention of exercise-induced bronchoconstriction in patients 15 years of age and older; and for the relief of symptoms of seasonal allergic rhinitis in patients 2 years of age and older and perennial allergic rhinitis in patients 6 months of age and older (this last indication is available in the USA but not in Spain) (Merch, Sharp & Dohme, 2011).

For AR, montelukast should be taken once daily. Efficacy was demonstrated for seasonal AR when montelukast was administered in the morning or the evening without regard to time of food ingestion. The time of administration may be individualized to suit patient needs. The following doses for the treatment of symptoms of seasonal AR are recommended: 10 mg for adults and adolescents 15 years of age and older; 5 mg for pediatric patients 6 to 14 years of age; and one 4 mg for pediatric patients 2 to 5 years of age (Merch, Sharp & Dohme, 2011).

Safety and effectiveness in pediatric patients younger than 2 years of age with seasonal AR have not been established. The following doses for the treatment of symptoms of perennial allergic rhinitis are recommended: 10 mg for adults and adolescents 15 years of age and older; 5 mg for pediatric patients 6 to 14 years of age; 5 mg for pediatric patients 2 to 5 years of age; 4 mg for pediatric patients 6 to 23 months of age. Safety and effectiveness in pediatric patients younger than 6 months of age with perennial AR have not been established.

Montelukast is an orally active compound that binds with high affinity and selectivity to the CysLT1 receptor (in preference to other pharmacologically important airway receptors, such as the prostanoid, cholinergic, or β-adrenergic receptor). Montelukast inhibits physiologic actions of LTD4 at the CysLT1 receptor without any agonist activity.

The efficacy of montelukast for the treatment of persistent and seasonal AR was investigated in different studies and clinical trials.

Evidence in persistent AR:

- Montelukast alone or in combination with antihistamines (desloratadine or levocetirizine) gave a gradual increase in nasal symptom improvement within 6 weeks of treatment in patients with persistent AR (Ciebiada et al, 2011).
- A multicenter, randomized, double-blind, placebo-controlled study was conducted in the US among 1992 patients to evaluate montelukast for treatment of perennial AR. The study was conducted during the winter, and all patients had positive skin tests for at least 2 perennial allergens. The investigators conclude that montelukast provides statistically significant symptomatic relief of persistent AR over 6 weeks of treatment (Patel et al, 2005).
- A randomized, double-blind, placebo-controlled, parallel-group study was performed to compare the effects of oral montelukast 4 mg once daily at bedtime with those of oral cetirizine 5 mg once daily at bedtime for 12 weeks in 60 children with perennial AR. The results revealed that both montelukast and cetirizine were significantly efficacious compared with placebo in nasal airway resistance, eosinophil percentage in nasal smears, Pediatric Rhinoconjunctivitis Quality of Life Questionnaire (PRQLQ), Total Symptom Score (TSS) and all symptom items except nasal itching, throat itching and tearing. For nasal itching, only cetirizine was significantly efficacious (Chen et al, 2006).

Evidence in persistent AR:

- Weinstein et al analyzed data from 4 phase III clinical trials to determine the onset of action of montelukast in seasonal allergic rhinitis. The 4 trials were double-blind, parallel-group, multicenter studies conducted in Fall 1999 (Study 1), Spring 2000 (Study 2), Fall 2000 (Study 3), and Spring 2001 (Study 4). Over the entire 2 weeks treatment period, pooled data indicated that montelukast was significantly better than placebo in decreasing symptom scores. The authors conclude that in patients with seasonal allergic rhinitis, montelukast reduces daytime and nighttime symptoms by the 2nd day of once-daily therapy (Weinstein et al, 2005).
- A multicenter, randomized, double-blind, placebo-controlled, parallel-group study was performed to compare the effects of montelukast 10 mg once daily at bedtime with those of loratadine 10 mg once daily at bedtime for 2 weeks during the allergy season in 1302 patients with seasonal AR. Quality of life scores (including measures of activity, sleep, nasal symptoms, eye symptoms, other symptoms, practical problems, and

emotions) also improved significantly in the montelukast and loratadine groups (P=0.003 and P≤0.001, respectively, versus placebo) (Philip et al, 2002).

- A multicenter, randomized, double-blind, double-dummy, placebo- and active-controlled study was performed in the US and Canada to evaluate the effects of montelukast 10 mg once daily in 1214 patients with spring seasonal AR. Therapy with montelukast significantly improves assessments of symptom severity as well as quality-of-life parameters for patients with seasonal AR (van Adelsberg et al, 2003).

4.2 Zafirlukast

Donnelly et al performed a study with 164 patients who were administered increasing doses of oral Zafirlukast (10, 20, 40, 100 mg and placebo). They found a significant decrease in nasal obstruction, sneezing and rhinorrhoea in patients who received doses starting from 20 mg (Donnelly et al, 1995)

5. Omalizumab (anti-IgE monoclonal antibody)

Several therapeutic anti-IgE antibodies, able to reduce free IgE levels and to block the binding of IgE to FcεRI without cross-linking IgE and triggering degranulation of IgE-sensitized cells have been developed. At present omalizumab is the only monoclonal antibody (mAb) - based drug approved for the treatment of asthma. A new mAb specific for human IgE has been shown to possess a unique set of binding specificities. This mAb, 8D6, binds to a conformational epitope on the CH3 domain of human IgE and can compete with omalizumab for binding to IgE. Like omalizumab, it does not bind to IgE already bound to the high-affinity IgE Fc receptor (FcεRI) on basophils and mast cells. It also does not cause activation and degranulation of IgE-pulsed, human FcεRI-expressing rat basophilic leukemic cells (RBL SX-38). This mAb can inhibit IgE binding to recombinant α chain of human FcεRI in ELISA and to human FcεRI-expressing RBL SX38 cells in fluorescence flow cytometric analysis. However, unlike omalizumab, 8D6 can bind to IgE already bound by the low-affinity IgE Fc receptors (FcεRII, or CD23). Since earlier investigators have shown that anti-CD23 mAbs can inhibit the synthesis of IgE in lymphocyte culture in vitro and can down-regulate IgE production in treated patients, 8D6 may offer pharmacological mechanisms in addition to those mediated by omalizumab, for controlling IgE in patients with allergic diseases. (Shiung et al, 2001).

Chu et al, have explored the effects of IgE sequestration versus IgE suppression by comparing omalizumab to FcγRIIb-optimized anti-IgE antibodies in humanized mouse models of immunoglobulin production. By using a murine anti-IgE antibody as a template, the authors humanized, increased IgE binding, and modified its Fc domain to increase affinity for FcγRIIb. Relative to omalizumab, this new mab, XmAb7195, has a 5-fold higher affinity for human IgE and more than 400-fold higher affinity for FcγRIIb. In addition to sequestering soluble IgE, XmAb7195 inhibited plasma cell differentiation and consequent human IgE production through coengagement of IgE B-cell receptor with FcγRIIb. In peripheral blood mononuclear cells-engrafted mice, XmAb7195 reduced total human IgE (but not IgG or IgM) levels by up to 40-fold relative to omalizumab (Chu et al, 2012).

Omalizumab represents an important clinical advance in the management of allergic diseases and can be considered to be safe in children with seasonal allergic rhinitis undergoing specific immunotherapy simultaneously (Kamin et al, 2010). Rush IT (RIT) carries a greater risk of acute allergic reactions (including anaphylaxis) than standard subcutaneous IT. In RIT, the accelerated dosing schedule can cause early increases in total and specific IgE concentrations that could predispose individuals to allergic reactions. The effect of omalizumab on the safety and efficacy of RIT was studied in adult patients with ragweed-AR. (Table 1).

Study	Patients and type of AR	Type of study	Comments
Casale et al, 1997	240 patients with ragweed AR	comparison omalizumab-placebo	Decrease dose-dependent in serum free IgE correlation between symptoms and IgE levels
Ädelroth et al, 2000	251 patients with birch pollen AR	comparison omalizumab-placebo	Decrease serum free IgE levels with omalizumab association between free IgE levels and clinical outcome mean daily NSSS, concomitant medication use, RRQoL was significantly better with omalizumab
Casale et al, 2001	536 patients with ragweed AR	comparison omalizumab-placebo	Significant association between IgE reduction, nasal symptoms and rescue medication use; significantly lower NSSS, lower need for rescue medication, better RRQoL scores, 75% reduction in days missed from work in patients receiving 300 mg omalizumab
Kopp et al, 2002	92 children with birch and grass pollen AR	Four treatment groups: -grass IT + omalizumab -grass IT + placebo -birch IT + omalizumab -birch IT + placebo	Symptom load was significantly reduced in both omalizumab groups compared to placebo. In vitro sulfidoleukotriene release was significantly lower with IT + omalizumab compared to IT + placebo, parallel to the reduction in symptoms and the use of rescue medication.
Kuehr et al, 2002	221 children with birch and grass pollen AR	Four treatment groups: -grass IT + omalizumab -grass IT + placebo -birch IT + omalizumab -birch IT + placebo	Significant reduction in symptom load and rescue medication use in the omalizumab + IT group compared to IT alone. Omalizumab reduced symptom load regardless of IT and had a protective effect independent of the type of allergen and additional clinical benefit to IT.
Chervinsky et al, 2003	289 patients with perennial AR	comparison omalizumab-placebo	Significantly lower NSSS and rescue antihistamines; improved RRQoL in the omalizumab group patient evaluation of efficacy significantly favored omalizumab.

Study	Patients and type of AR	Type of study	Comments
Nayak et al, 2003	287 patients with ragweed AR	retreatment with omalizumab	Decrease in serum free IgE levels.
Bez et al, 2004	225 children with birch and grass pollen AR	Four treatment groups: -grass IT + omalizumab -grass IT + placebo -birch IT + omalizumab -birch IT + placebo	Combination of IT and omalizumab: no pollen-induced increase in ECP and decrease in tryptase in nasal secretions; significantly lower tryptase levels in the omalizumab group.
Rolinck-Werninghaus et al, 2004	Further analyses during grass pollen season after previous study (Van Cauwenberge, 2005)	Four treatment groups: -birch IT + placebo -birch IT + omalizumab -grass IT + placebo -grass IT + omalizumab	Significantly diminished rescue medication use and reduction in the number of symptomatic days with omalizumab monotherapy. Superior efficacy of the omalizumab + IT combination on symptom severity compared to IT or omalizumab alone.
Vignola et al, 2004	405 patients with asthma and persistent AR	comparison omalizumab-placebo	Significant improvement in RRQoL in the omalizumab-treated patients
Casale et al, 2006	159 patients with ragweed AR	Four treatment groups: -omalizumab − placebo -omalizumab − RIT -placebo + placebo -placebo + RIT	Significant improvement in severity scores during the ragweed season with omalizumab + IT compared to IT alone

ECP = eosinophilic cationic protein; NSSS = nasal symptom severity scores; RIT = rush immunotherapy; RRQoL = rhinitis-related quality of life.

Table 1. Clinical studies with "omalizumab" and combination "omalizumab-specific immunotherapy" in allergic rhinitis.

6. Allergen-specific Immunotherapy

Two stages have been defined in AR immune pathophysiology. The first stage is named sensitization phase reaction, and is initiated by preferential activation and polarization of the immune response to environmental antigens, that culminates with a generation of a predominant Th2 immune response and production of IgE antibodies; the second stage, named effector phase reaction, is initiated with a second encounter with antigen (Ag) leading to activation of effector mechanisms, such as degranulation of granulocytes and release of histamine (Robles-Contreras et al, 2011). Allergen-induced cell degranulation is the key event in allergic inflammation and leads to early-phase symptoms. Early phase reaction (EPR) has been studied extensively in both humans and animals; EPR is initiated with a second encounter with the antigen by IgE previously attached to IgE receptors (FcεRI, FcεRII or CD23). Cross-linking of IgE receptors induces: a) release of preformed mediators such as histamine, proteases and chemotactic factors; b) activation of transcription factors and cytokine gene expression, and c) production of prostaglandins and leukotrienes by phospholipase A2 pathway (Figure 1).

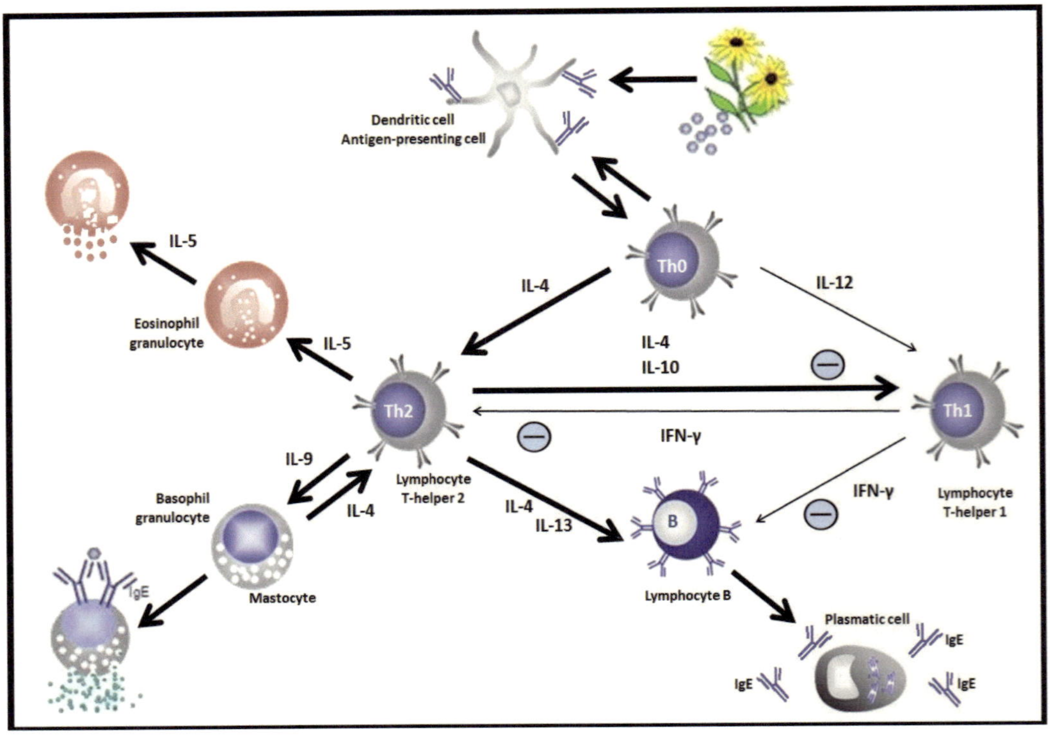

Fig. 1. Mechanism of allergic reaction.

The mechanisms of action of allergen-specific immunotherapy (SIT) include the very early desensitization effects, modulation of T-and B-cell responses and related antibody isotypes, and migration of eosinophils, basophils, and mast cells to tissues, as well as release of their mediators (Figure 2). Regulatory T (Treg) cells have been identified as key regulators of immunologic processes in peripheral tolerance to allergens. Skewing of allergen-specific effector T cells to a regulatory phenotype appears as a key event in the development of healthy immune response to allergens and successful outcome in patients undergoing allergen-specific immunotherapy (Akdis & Akdis, 2011).

Have been reported biomarkers of clinical response to IT:

a. Increase in allergen-specific serum IgG4 (Tari et al, 1990; Tari et al, 1994; Durham et al, 1999; La Rosa et al, 1999; Bufe et al, 2004; Lima et al, 2002; Smith et al, 2004; Til et al, 2004; Tonnel et al, 2004).
b. Increase in serum functional IgG responses:
   - Inhibition of basophil histamine release (Niederberger et al, 2004).
   - Inhibition of IgE-facilitated allergen binding (IgE-FAB) (Shamji et al, 2006).
c. Reduction in immediate and late-phase skin test responses to allergen (Tari et al, 1994; Durham et al, 1999; La Rosa et al, 1999; Tonnel et al, 2004).
d. Suppression of rise in Eosinophil Cationic Protein (ECP) (Gozalo et al, 1997; Passalacqua et al, 1998; Vourdas et al, 1998; Ippoliti et al, 2003) and tryptase (Marcucci et al, 2003) concentrations in nasal lavage during the pollen season

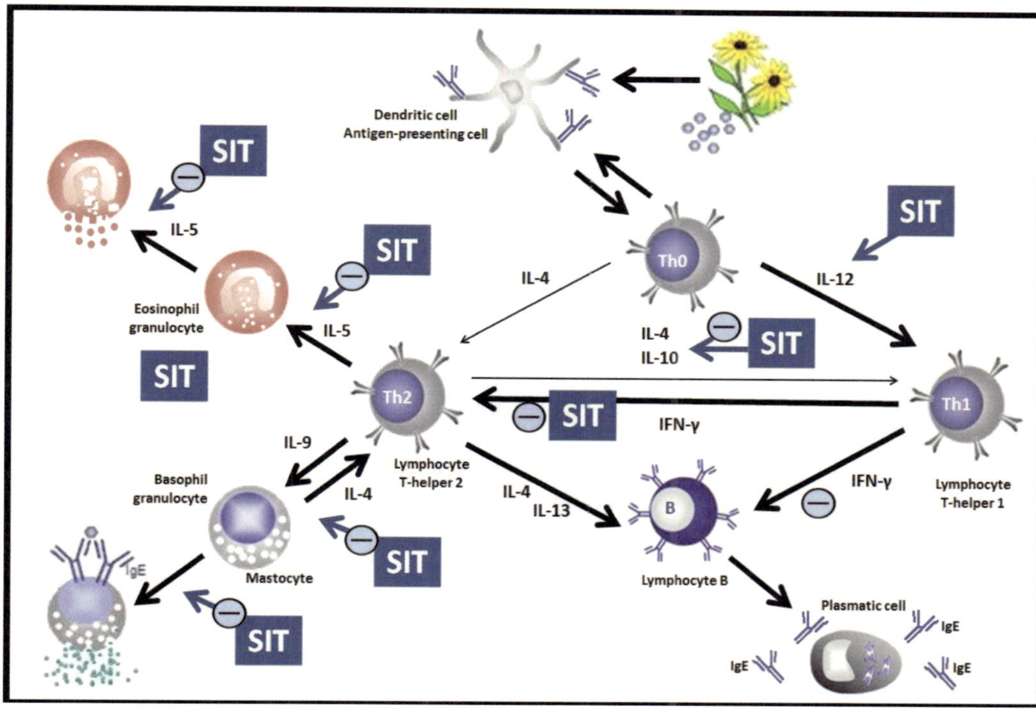

Fig. 2. Mechanisms of action of allergen-specific immunotherapy (SIT).

	Subcutaneous IT for seasonal AR (Calderon et al, 2007)	Sublingual IT for seasonal and perennial AR (Olaguibel & Álvarez-Puebla, 2005)
Participant numbers (active/placebo)	597/466	2333/2256
Symptom scores SMD random (95% CI)	-0.73 (-0.97, -0.50)	-0.49 (-0.64, -0.34)
P-value	<0.00001	<0.00001
Heterogeneity (I^2)	63%	81%
Medication scores SMD random (95% CI)	-0.57 (-0.82, -0.33)	-0.32 (-0.43, -0.21)
P-value	<0.00001	<0.00001
Heterogeneity (I^2)	64%	50%

Heterogeneity: Low = I^2 25%; Moderate = I^2 50%; High = I^2 75%;

Table 2. Efficacy of immunotherapy (IT) in AR (summary of Cochrane meta-analyses)

e. Increased in vitro IL-10 production by peripheral blood mononuclear cells (PBMC) following stimulation with allergen (Nouri-Aria et al, 2004; Francis et al, 2008).
f. Reduction in allergen-induced in vitro PBMC proliferative responses (Fanta et al, 1999).
g. Reduction in bronchial responses to allergen and methacholine challenge (Rak et al, 1988; Cirla et al, 2003).

The ARIA document clearly states that immunotherapy (IT) is considered effective in AR, and that it is the only treatment that can change the natural course of the disease and prevent its evolution into asthma (Bousquet et al, 2008).

IT, both subcutaneous and sublingual, is an effective treatment for adults and children with severe AR that does not respond to conventional pharmacotherapy and allergen avoidance measures. The efficacy of IT depends on correct patient selection, the type of allergen and the product chosen for treatment. Each vaccine requires individual assessment before recommendation for routine use. In support of the conclusions of recent meta-analyses, data have provided further evidence for the efficacy of Sublingual immunotherapy (SLIT) at least for grass pollen-induced (Table 2).

7. Therapeutic developments in the treatment of allergic rhinitis (AR)

Due to the increased prevalence of AR, its impact on quality of life, its societal costs and the fact that it is a predisposing factor for asthma, new therapeutic options are being sought. Studies are being performed with anti-leukotrienes, anti-immunoglobulin E antibodies, phosphodiesterase inhibitors, and others, which seem to confirm promising results.

Schultz et al state that, in addition to the well established therapeutic guidelines in the treatment of rhinitis with antihistamines, corticosteroids, nasal decongestants, etc., there are an increasingly number of new therapeutic alternatives, such as anti-leukotrienes, anti-immunoglobulin E antibodies, phosphodiesterase inhibitors and intranasal heparin, as well as new specific immunotherapies (recombinant). There are promising results, but more studies are needed to confirm these initial data (Schultz et al, 2003).

Bjermer and Diamant observed that, although inhaled corticosteroids are currently considered first-line drugs in the anti-inflammatory control of asthma and rhinitis, there are studies with anti-leukotrienes and anti-immunoglobulin E that are highly promising. Clinical trials are being performed with modified cytokines (Bjermer & Diamant, 2004).

Koreck et al reported on *low intensity UVB, UVA and visible light phototherapy* as treatment for AR (3 times per week for three weeks). The authors reported that there was a significant reduction in the number of eosinophils, ECP and IL-5 in the nasal lavage. They also found inhibition in the RBL-2H3 mediator release of basophils. Phototherapy is a new option in the treatment of immunologically mediated mucosal diseases, including allergic rhinitis (Koreck et al, 2005).

Kirchhoff et al used the *H1-receptor antagonist dimethindene maleate* topically on patients with seasonal allergic rhinitis for 2 weeks and compared it with placebo. With this antagonist, they achieved statistically significantly better results in the quality of life questionnaires for rhinitis than with placebo (Kirchhoff et al, 2003).

Unal et al investigated the potential benefits of the *toxin botulinum type A* on nasal symptoms of allergic rhinitis, and compared it to an isotonic saline solution as placebo. The results were significantly better in patients treated with botulinum toxin, especially in rhinorrhoea, nasal obstruction and sneezing. In selected cases, the injection of intranasal toxin botulinum may help control allergic rhinitis symptoms (Unal et al, 2003).

Monoclonal antibodies anti-IL-5 seem to be an effective treatment that reduces the number of eosinophils locally in the airway and in peripheral blood in asthmatic patients. Two monoclonal antibodies have been designed to neutralize IL-5 (mepolizumab and reslizumab). Mepolizumab is a fully humanized anti-IL-5 monoclonal IgG1 antibody that binds to free IL-5 with high affinity and specificity to prevent IL-5 from associating with the IL-5 receptor complex alpha-chain on the surface of eosinophils (Leckie et al, 2000).

There are clinical trials with recombinant soluble IL-4 receptor, and recombinant IL-12. Immunomodulatory treatments for IL-9, IL-l0, IL-12 and IL-13 are being studied, as well as immunostimulatory DNA sequences, with encouraging results.

8. Conclusions

Considering the reviewed data, and unifying the above-mentioned opinions on the treatment of AR, we provide the following guidelines:

- Inhaled corticosteroids are effective and safe for the treatment of AR, usually associated with antihistamines in persistent AR. We have found no indication for administering systemic corticosteroids unless there is another associated pathology.
- Histamine and leukotrienes are involved in the pathogenesis of allergic rhinitis. Montelukast is indicated for the prophylaxis and chronic treatment of asthma in adults and pediatric patients 12 months of age and older; for prevention of exercise-induced bronchoconstriction in patients 15 years of age and older; and for the relief of symptoms of seasonal allergic rhinitis in patients 2 years of age and older and perennial allergic rhinitis in patients 6 months of age and older
- Omalizumab represents an important clinical advance in the management of allergic diseases and can be considered to be safe in children with seasonal allergic rhinitis undergoing specific immunotherapy simultaneously.
- Immunotherapy is an effective treatment for adults and children with severe AR that does not respond to conventional pharmacotherapy and allergen avoidance measures. The efficacy of IT depends on correct patient selection, the type of allergen and the product chosen for treatment.
- Encouraging new treatments are currently being studied.

9. References

Ädelroth E, Rak S, Haahtela T, Aasand G, Rosenhall L, Zetterstrom O, et al. Recombinant humanized mAb-E25, an anti-IgE mAb, in birch pollen induced seasonal allergic rhinitis. (2000) *J Allergy Clin Immunol*, Vol.106, No.2 (August 2000), pp. 253-259, Print ISSN 0091-6749, Electronic ISSN 1097-6825.

Akdis CA, Akdis M. Mechanisms of allergen-specific immunotherapy. (2011) *J Allergy Clin Immunol*, Vol.127, No.1 (January 2011), pp. 18-27; quiz 28-29, Print ISSN 0091-6749, Electronic ISSN 1097-6825.

Allen A, Down G, Newland A, Reynard K, Rousell V, Salmon E, et al. Absolute Bioavailability of Intranasal Fluticasone Furoate in Healthy Subjects. (2007) *Clin Ther*, Vol.29, No.7 (July 2007), pp. 1415–1420, Print ISSN 0149-2918, Electronic ISSN 1879-114X.

Allen DB. Systemic effects of intranasal steroids: an endocrinologist's perspective. (2000) *J Allergy Clin Immunol*, Vol.106, No.4 Suppl (October 2000), pp. S179-S190, Print ISSN 0091-6749, Electronic ISSN 1097-6825.

Barnes PJ. New drugs for asthma. (1992) *Eur Respir J*, Vol.5, No.9 (October 1992), pp. 1126-1136, Print ISSN: 0903-1936, Electronic ISSN: 1399-3003.

Baroody FM, Shenaq D, DeTineo M, Wang J, Naclerio RM. Fluticasone furoate nasal spray reduces the nasal-ocular reflex: a mechanism for the efficacy of topical steroids in controlling allergic eye symptoms. (2009) *J Allergy Clin Immunol*, Vol.123, No.6 (June 2009), pp. 1342-1348, Print ISSN0091-6749, Electronic ISSN 1097-6825.

Baumann D, Bachert C, Högger P. Dissolution in nasal fluid, retention and anti-inflammatory activity of fluticasone furoate in human nasal tissue ex vivo. (2009) *Clin Exp Allergy*, Vol.39, No.10 (October 2009), pp. 1540-1550, Print ISSN 0954-7894, Electronic ISSN 1365-2222.

Berlucchi M, Salsi D, Valetti L, Parrinello G, Nicolai P. The role of mometasone furoate aqueous nasal spray in the treatment of adenoidal hypertrophy in the pediatric age group: preliminary results of a prospective, randomized study. (2007) *Pediatrics*, Vol.119, No.6 (June 2007), pp. e1392–e1397, Print ISSN 0031-4005, Electronic ISSN 1098-4275.

Bez C, Schubert R, Kopp M, Ersfeld Y, Rosewich M, Kuehr J, et al. Effect of anti-immunoglobulin E on nasal inflammation in patients with seasonal allergic rhinoconjunctivitis. (2004) *Clin Exp Allergy*, Vol.34, No.7 (July 2004), pp. 1079–1085, Print ISSN 0954-7894, Electronic ISSN 1365-2222.

Bjermer L, Diamant Z. Current and emerging nonsteroidal anti-inflammatory therapies targeting specific mechanisms in asthma and allergy. (2004) *Treat Respir Med*, Vol.3, No.4 (July-August 2004), pp. 235-246, Print ISSN 1176-3450.

Borish L. Allergic rhinitis: systemic inflammation and implications for management. (2003) *J Allergy Clin Immunol*, Vol.112, No.6 (December 2003), pp. 1021-1031, Print ISSN 0091-6749, Electronic ISSN 1097-6825.

Borum P, Grønborg H, Mygind N. Seasonal allergic rhinitis and depot injection of a corticosteroid. Evaluation of the efficacy of medication early and late in the season based on detailed symptom recording. (1987) *Allergy*, Vol.42, No.1 (January 1987), pp. 26-32, Print ISSN 0105-4538, Electronic ISSN: 1398-9995.

Bousquet J, Khaltaev N, Cruz AA, Denburg J, Fokkens WJ, Togias A, Zuberbier T et al. Allergic Rhinitis and its Impact on Asthma (ARIA) 2008 update (in collaboration with the World Heatlth Organization, GA(2)LEN and AllergGen). (2008) *Allergy*, Vol.63, No.86 Suppl (April 2008), pp. 8-160, Print ISSN 0105-4538, Electronic ISSN 1398-9995.

Bousquet J, Van Cauwenberge P, Khaltaev N; ARIA Workshop Group; World Health Organization. ARIA workshop group. World Health Organization. Allergic Rhinitis and its impact on asthma Workshop Report. (2001) *J Allergy Clin Immunol*, Vol.108, No.5 Suppl (November 2001), pp. S147-S334, Print ISSN 0091-6749, Electronic ISSN 1097-6825.

Bronsky EA, Druce H, Findlay SR, Hampel FC, Kaiser H, Ratner P, et al. A clinical trial of ipratropium bromide nasal spray in patients with perennial nonallergic rhinitis. (1995) *J Allergy Clin Immunol*, Vol.95, No.5 Pt 2 (May 1995), pp. 1117-1122, Print ISSN 0091-6749, Electronic ISSN 1097-6825.

Brooks CD, Karl KJ, Francom SF. Oral methylprednisolone acetate (Medrol Tablets) for seasonal rhinitis: examination of dose and symptom response. (1993) *J Clin Pharmacol,* Vol.33, No.9 (September 1993), pp. 816-822, Print ISSN: 0091-2700, Electronic ISSN: 1552-4604.

Brown EB, Seideman T, Siegelaub BA, Popovitz FACA. Depomethylprednisolone in the treatment of ragweed hay fever. (1960) *Ann Allergy,* Vol.18, No.1 (January 1960), pp. 1321-1330, Print ISSN 0003-4738.

Bryson HM, Faulds D. Intranasal fluticasone propionate. A review of its pharmacodynamic and pharmacokinetic properties, and therapeutic potential in allergic rhinitis. (1992) *Drugs,* Vol.43, No.5 (May 1992), pp. 760-775, Print ISSN 0012-6667.

Bufe A, Ziegler-Kirbach E, Stoeckmann E, Heidemann P, Gehlhar K, Holland-Letz, et al. Efficacy of sublingual swallow immunotherapy in children with severe grass pollen allergic symptoms: a double-blind placebo-controlled study. (2004) *Allergy,* Vol.59, No.5 (May 2004), pp. 498–504, Print ISSN 0105-4538, Electronic ISSN 1398-9995.

Calderon MA, Alves B, Jacobson M, Hurwitz B, Sheikh A, Durham S. Allergen injection immunotherapy for seasonal allergic rhinitis. (2007) *Cochrane Database Syst Rev,* Vol.24, No.1 (January 2007): CD001936, Print ISSN 1469-493X, Linking ISSN 1361-6137.

Casale TB, Bernstein IL, Busse WW, LaForce CF, Tinkelman DG, Stoltz RR, et al. Use of anti-IgE humanized monoclonal antibody in ragweed-induced allergic rhinitis. (1997) *J Allergy Clin Immunol,* Vol.100, No.1 (July 1997), pp. 110-121, Print ISSN 0091-6749, Electronic ISSN 1097-6825.

Casale TB, Busse WW, Kline JN, Ballas ZK, Moss MH, Townley RG, et al. Omalizumab pretreatment decreases acute reactions after rush immunotherapy for ragweed-induced seasonal allergic rhinitis. (2006) *J Allergy Clin Immunol,* Vol.117, No.1 (January 2006), pp. 134–140, Print ISSN 0091-6749, Electronic ISSN 1097-6825.

Casale TB, Condemi J, LaForce C, Nayak A, Rowe M, Watrous M, et al. Effect of omalizumab on symptoms of seasonal allergic rhinitis. A randomized controlled trial. (2001) *JAMA,* Vol.286, No.23 (December 2001), pp. 2956-2967, Print ISSN 0098-7484, Electronic ISSN 0098-3598.

Chen S T, Lu K H, Sun H L, Chang W T, Lue K H and Chou M C. Randomized placebo-controlled trial comparing montelukast and cetirizine for treating perennial allergic rhinitis in children aged 2-6 yr. (2006) *Pediatr Allergy Immunol,* Vol.17, No.1 (February 2006), pp. 49-54, Print ISSN 0905-6157, Electronic ISSN 1399-3038.

Chervinsky P, Casale TB, Townley R, Tripathy I, Hedgecock S, Fowler-Taylor A, et al. Omalizumab, an anti-IgE antibody, in the treatment of adults and adolescents with perennial allergic rhinitis. (2003) *Ann Allergy Asthma Immunol,* Vol.91, No.2 (August 2003), pp. 160-167, Print ISSN 1081-1206, Electronic ISSN 1534-4436.

Chu SY, Horton HM, Pong E, Leung IW, Chen H, Nguyen DH, et al. Reduction of total IgE by targeted coengagement of IgE B-cell receptor and FcγRIIb with Fc-engineered antibody. (2012) *J Allergy Clin Immunol,* 2012 Jan 16. [Epub ahead of print], Print ISSN 0091-6749, Electronic ISSN 1097-6825.

Ciebiada M, Gorska-Ciebiada M, Barylski M, Kmiecik T, Gorski P. Use of montelukast alone or in combination with desloratadine or levocetirizine in patients with persistent allergic rhinitis. (2011) *Am J Rhinol Allergy*, Vol.25, No.1 (January-February 2011), pp. e1-e6, Print ISSN 1945-8924, Electronic ISSN 1945-8932.

Cirla AM, Cirla PE, Parmiani S, Pecora S. A pre-seasonal birch/hazel sublingual immunotherapy can improve the outcome of grass pollen injective treatment in bisensitized individuals. A case-referent, two-year controlled study. (2003) *Allergol Immunopathol (Madr)*, Vol.31, No.1 (January-February 2003), pp. 31–43, Print ISSN 0301-0546, Electronic ISSN 1578-1267.

Cockcroft DW, MacCormack DW, Newhouse MT, Hargreave FE. Beclomethasone dipropionate aerosol in allergic rhinitis. (1976) *Can Med Assoc J*, Vol.115, No.6 (September 1976), pp. 523-526, Print ISSN 0008-4409.

Corren J. Intranasal corticosteroids for allergic rhinitis: how do different agents compare? (1999) J *Allergy Clin Immunol*, Vol.104, No.4 Pt 1 (October 1999), pp. S144-149, Print ISSN 0091-6749, Electronic ISSN 1097-6825.

DeWester J, Philpot EE, Westlund RE, Cook CK, Rickard KA. The efficacy of intranasal fluticasone propionate in the relief of ocular symptoms associated with seasonal allergic rhinitis. (2003) *Allergy Asthma Proc*, Vol.24, No.5 (September-October 2003), pp. 331-337, Print ISSN 1088-5412, Electronic ISSN 1539-6304.

Di Lorenzo G, Gervasi F, Drago A, Esposito Pellitteri M, Di Salvo A, Cosentino D, et al. Comparison of the effects of fluticasone propionate, aqueous nasal spray and levocabastine on inflammatory cells in nasal lavage and clinical activity during the pollen season in seasonal rhinitics. (1999) *Clin Exp Allergy*, Vol.29, No.10 (October 1999), pp. 1367-1377, Electronic ISSN 1365-2222.

Donnelly AL, Glass M, Minkwitz MC, Casale TB. The leukotriene D4-receptor antagonist, ICI 204,219, relieves symptoms of acute seasonal allergic rhinitis. (1995) *Am J Respir Crit Care Med*, Vol.151, No.6 (June 1995), pp. 1734-1739, Print ISSN 1073-449X, Electronic ISSN 1535-4970.

Durham SR, Varney VA, Gaga M, Jacobson MR, Varga EM, Frew AJ, et al. Grass pollen immunotherapy decreases the number of mast cells in the skin. (1999) *Clin Exp Allergy*, No.29, No.11 (November 1999), pp. 1490–1496, Print ISSN 0954-7894, Electronic ISSN 1365-2222.

Dykewicz MS, Fineman S. Executive Summary of Joint Task Force Practice Parameters on Diagnosis and Management of Rhinitis. (1998) *Ann Allergy Asthma Immunol*, Vol.81, No.5 Pt 2 (November 1998), pp. 463-468, Print ISSN 1081-1206, Electronic ISSN 1534-4436.

Edwards TB. Effectiveness and safety of beclomethasone dipropionate, an intranasal corticosteroid, in the treatment of patients with allergic rhinitis. (1995) *Clin Ther*, Vol.17, No.6 (November-December 1995), pp. 1032-1041, Print ISSN 0149-2918, Electronic ISSN 1879-114X.

Fanta C, Bohle B, Hirt W, Siemann U, Horak F, Kraft D, et al. Systemic immunological changes induced by administration of grass pollen allergens via the oral mucosa during sublingual immunotherapy. (1999) *Int Arch Allergy Immunol*, Vol.120, No.3 (November 1999), pp. 218–124, Print ISSN 1018-2438, Electronic ISSN 1423-0097.

Francis JN, James LK, Paraskevopoulos G, Wong C, Calderon MA, Durham SR, et al. Grass pollen immunotherapy: IL-10 induction and suppression of late responses precedes IgG4 inhibitory antibody activity. (2008) *J Allergy Clin Immunol*, Vol.121, No.5 (May 2008), pp. 1120–1125, Print ISSN 0091-6749, Electronic ISSN 1097-6825.

Ganderton MA, James VH. Clinical and endocrine side-effects of methylprednisolone acetate as used in hay-fever. (1970) *Br Med J*, Vol.1, No.5691 (January 1970), pp. 267-269, Print ISSN 0959-8138.

Gawchik SM, Saccar CL. A risk-benefit assessment of intranasal triamcinolone acetonide in allergic rhinitis. (2000) *Drug Saf*, Vol.23, No.4 (October 2000), pp. 309-222, Print ISSN 0114-5916.

GlaxoSmithKline. Ficha técnica de Avamys©. GlaxoSmithKline 2008. Revised: 11/11/2011.

Gozalo F, Martin S, Rico P, Alvarez E, Cortes C. Clinical efficacy and tolerance of two year Lolium perenne sublingual immunotherapy. (1997) *Allergol Immunopathol (Madr)*, Vol.25, No.5 (September-October 1997), pp. 219–227, Print ISSN 0301-0546, Electronic ISSN 1578-1267.

Hedner P, Persson G. Suppression of the hypothalamic-pituitary-adrenal axis after a single intramuscular injection of methylprednisolone acetate. (1981) *Ann Allergy*, Vol.47, No.3 (September 1981), pp. 176-179, Print ISSN 0003-4738.

Horan JD, Johnson JD. Flunisolide nasal spray in the treatment of perennial rhinitis. (1978) *Can Med Assoc J*, Vol.119, No.4 (August 1978), pp. 334-338, Print ISSN 0008-4409.

Howland WC 3rd. Fluticasone propionate: topical or systemic effects? (1996) *Clin Exp Allergy*, Vol.26, No.3 Suppl (May 1996), pp. 18-22, Print ISSN 0105-4538, Electronic ISSN: 1398-9995.

Howland WC 3rd, Hampel FC jr, Martin BG, Ratner PH, van Bavel JH, Field EA. The efficacy of fluticasone propionate aqueous nasal spray for allergic rhinitis and its relationship to topical effects. Clin Ther. 1996;18:1106-17. Print ISSN 0149-2918, Electronic ISSN 1879-114X.

International Rhinitis Management Working Group. International Consensus Report on the diagnosis and management of rhinitis. (1994) *Allergy*, Vol.49, No.19 Suppl (June 1994), pp.1-34, Print ISSN 0105-4538, Electronic ISSN: 1398-9995.

Ippoliti F, De Santis W, Volterrani A, Lenti L, Canitano N, Lucarelli S, et al. Immunomodulation during sublingual therapy in allergic children. (2003) *Pediatr Allergy Immunol*, Vol.14, No.3 (June 2003), pp. 216–221, Print ISSN 0905-6157, Electronic ISSN 1399-3038.

Kaiser HB, Findlay SR, Georgitis JW, Grossman J, Ratner PH, Tinkelman DG, et al. Long-term treatment of perennial allergic rhinitis with ipratropium bromide nasal spray 0.06%. (1995) *J Allergy Clin Immunol*, Vol.95, No.5 Pt 2 (May 1995), pp. 1128-1132, Print ISSN 0091-6749, Electronic ISSN 1097-6825.

Kamin W, Kopp MV, Erdnuess F, Schauer U, Zielen S, Wahn U. Safety of anti-IgE treatment with omalizumab in children with seasonal allergic rhinitis undergoing specific immunotherapy simultaneously. (2010) *Pediatr Allergy Immunol*, Vol.21, No.1 Pt 2 (February 2010), pp. e160-e165, Print ISSN 0905-6157, Electronic ISSN 1399-3038.

Kaszuba SM, Baroody FM, deTineo M, Haney L, Blair C, Naclerio RM. Superiority of an intranasal corticosteroid compared with an oral antihistamine in the as-needed treatment of seasonal allergic rhinitis. (2001) *Arch Int Med*, Vol.161, No.21 (November 2001), pp. 2581-2587, Print ISSN 0003-9926, Electronic ISSN 1538-3679.

Keith PK, Scadding GK. Are intranasal corticosteroids all equally consistent in managing ocular symptoms of seasonal allergic rhinitis? (2009) *Curr Med Res Opin*, Vol.25, No.8 (August 2009), pp. 2021-2041, Print ISSN 0300-7995, Electronic ISSN 1473-4877.

Keith PK, Scadding GK. Are intranasal corticosteroids all equally consistent in managing ocular symptoms of seasonal allergic rhinitis? (2010) *Curr Med Res Opin*, Vol.25, No.8 (August 2009), pp. 2021–2041, Print ISSN 0300-7995, Electronic ISSN 1473-4877 [Erratum in: (2010) *Curr Med Res Opin*, Vol.26, No.1 (January 2010), pp. 177, Print ISSN 0300-7995, Electronic ISSN 1473-4877].

Keleş N. Treatment of allergic rhinitis during pregnancy. (2004) *Am J Rhinol*, Vol.18, No.1 (January-February 2004), pp. 23-28, Print ISSN 1050-6586, Electronic ISSN 1539-6290.

Kim KT, Rabinovitch N, Uryniak T, Simpson B, O'Dowd L, Casty F. Effect of budesonide aqueous nasal spray on hypothalamic-pituitary-adrenal axis function in children with allergic rhinitis. (2004) *Ann Allergy Asthma Immunol*,Vol.93, No.1 (July 2004), pp. 61-67, Print ISSN 1081-1206, Electronic ISSN 1534-4436.

Kirchhoff CH, Kremer B, Haaf-von Below S, Kyrein HJ, Mösges R. Effects of dimethindene maleate nasal spray on the quality of life in seasonal allergic rhinitis. (2003) *Rhinology*, Vol.41, No.3 (September 2003), pp.159-166, Print ISSN 03000-0729.

Kopp MV, Brauburger J, Riedinger F, Beischer D, Ihorst G, Kamin W, et al. The effect of anti-IgE treatment on in vitro leukotriene release in children with seasonal allergic rhinitis. (2002) *J Allergy Clin Immunol*, Vol.110,No.5 (November 2002), pp. 728-735, Print ISSN 0091-6749, Electronic ISSN 1097-6825.

Koreck AI, Csoma Z, Bodai L, Ignacz F, Kenderessy AS, Kadocsa E et al. Rhinophototherapy: a new therapeutic tool for the management of allergic rhinitis. (2005) *J Allergy Clin Immunol*, Vol.115, No.3 (March 2005), pp.541-547, Print ISSN 0091-6749, Electronic ISSN 1097-6825.

Kuehr J, Brauburger J, Zielen S, Schauer U, Kamin W, Von Berg A, et al. Efficacy of combination treatment with anti-IgE plus specific immunotherapy in polysensitized children and adolescents with seasonal allergic rhinitis. (2002) *J Allergy Clin Immunol*, Vol.109, No.2 (February 2002), pp. 274-280, Print ISSN 0091-6749, Electronic ISSN 1097-6825.

La Rosa M, Ranno C, Andre C, Carat F, Tosca MA, Canonica GW. Double-blind placebo-controlled evaluation of sublingual- swallow immunotherapy with standardized *Parietaria judaica* extract in children with allergic rhinoconjunctivitis. (1999) *J Allergy Clin Immunol*, Vol.104, No.2 Pt 1 (August 1999), pp. 425–432, Print ISSN 0091-6749, Electronic ISSN 1097-6825.

LaForce CF, Dockhorn RJ, Findlay SR, Meltzer EO, Nathan RA, Stricker W, et al. Fluticasone propionate: an effective alternative treatment for seasonal allergic rhinitis in adults and adolescents. (1994) *J Fam Pract*, Vol.38, No.2 (February 1994), pp. 145-152, Print ISSN 0094-3509, Electronic ISSN 1533-7294.

Laursen LC, Faurschou P, Pals H, Svendsen UG, Weeke B. Intramuscular betamethasone dipropionate vs. oral prednisolone in hay fever patients. (1987) *Allergy*, Vol.42, No.3 (April 1987), pp. 168-172, Print ISSN 0105-4538, Electronic ISSN: 1398-9995.

Laursen LC, Faurschou P, Munch EP. Intramuscular betamethasone dipropionate vs. topical beclomethasone dipropionate and placebo in hay fever. (1988) *Allergy*, Vol.43, No.6 (August 1988), pp. 420-424, Print ISSN 0105-4538, Electronic ISSN: 1398-9995.

Leckie MJ, ten Brinke A, Khan J, Diamant Z, O'Connor BJ, Walls CM, et al. Effects of an interleukin-5 blocking monoclonal antibody on eosinophils, airway hyperresponsiveness, and the late asthmatic response. (2000) *Lancet*, Vol.356, No.9248 (December 2000), pp. 2144-2148, Print ISSN 0140-6736, Electronic ISSN 1474-547X.

Lima MT, Wilson D, Pitkin L, Roberts A, Nouri-Aria K, Jacobson M, et al. Grass pollen sublingual immunotherapy for seasonal rhinoconjunctivitis: a randomized controlled trial. (2002) *Clin Exp Allergy*, Vol.32, No.4 (April 2002), pp. 507–514, Print ISSN 0954-7894, Electronic ISSN 1365-2222.

Lipworth BJ. Leukotriene-receptor antagonists. (1999) *Lancet*, Vol.353, No.9146 (January 1999), pp. 57-62, Print ISSN 0140-6736, Electronic ISSN 1474-547X.

Lumry WR. A review of the preclinical and clinical data of newer intranasal steroids used in the treatment of allergic rhinitis. (1999) *J Allergy Clin Immunol*, Vol.194, No.4 Pt 1 (October 1999), pp. S150-S158, Print ISSN 0091-6749, Electronic ISSN 1097-6825.

Lundblad L, Sipilä P, Farstad T, Drozdziewicz D. Mometasone furoate nasal spray in the treatment of perennial non-allergic rhinitis: a nordic, multicenter, randomized, double-blind, placebo controlled study. (2001) *Acta Otolaryngol*, Vol.121, No.4 (June 2001), pp. 505-509, Print ISSN 0001-6489, Electronic ISSN 1651-2251.

Mahadevia PJ, Shah S, Leibman C, Kleinman L, O'Dowd L. Patient preferences for sensory attributes of intranasal corticosteroids and willingness to adhere to prescribed therapy for allergic rhinitis: a conjoint analysis. (2004) *Ann Allergy Asthma Immunol*, Vol.93, No.4 (October 2004), pp. 345–350, Print ISSN 1081-1206, Electronic ISSN 1534-4436.

Marcucci F, Sensi L, Frati F, Bernardini R, Novembre E, Barbato A, et al. Effects on inflammation parameters of a double-blind, placebo controlled one-year course of SLIT in children monosensitized to mites. (2003) *Allergy*, Vol.58, No.7 (July 2003), pp. 657–662, Print ISSN 0105-4538, Electronic ISSN 1398-9995.

Máspero JF, Rosenblut A, Finn A Jr, Lim J, Wu W, Philpot E. Safety and efficacy of fluticasone furoate in pediatric patient with perennial allergic rhinitis. (2008) *Otolaryngol Head Neck Surg*, Vol.138, No.1 (January 2008), pp. 30-37, Print ISSN 0194-5998, Electronic ISSN 1097-6817.

McMillin WP. Triamcinoline acetonide (kenalog) in treatment of cases of hay fever and its effect on pituitary-adrenal axis. (1971) *Ulster Med J*, Vol.40, No.2 (February 1971), pp. 176-179, Print ISSN 0041-6193.

Meltzer EO, Bachert C, Staudinger H. Treating acute rhinosinusitis: comparing efficacy and safety of mometasone furoate nasal spray, amoxicillin, and placebo. (2005) *J Allergy Clin Immunol*, Vol.116, No.6 (December 2005), pp. 1289-1295, Print ISSN 0091-6749, Electronic ISSN 1097-6825.

Meltzer EO, Berger WE, Berkowitz RB, Bronsky EA, Dvorin DJ, Finn AF et al. A dose-ranging study of mometasone furoate aqueous nasal spray in children with seasonal allergic rhinitis. (1999) *J Allergy Clin Immunol*, Vol.104, No.1 (July 1999), pp. 107-114, Print ISSN 0091-6749, Electronic ISSN 1097-6825.

Meltzer EO, Lee J, Tripathy I, Lim J, Ellsworth A, Philpot E. Efficacy and safety of once-daily fluticasone furoate nasal spray in children with seasonal allergic rhinitis treated for 2 wk. (2009) *Pediatr Allergy Immunol*, Vol.20, No.3 (May 2009), pp. 279-286, Print ISSN 0905-6157, Electronic ISSN 1399-3038.

Melzer EO, Orgel HA, Kemp JP, et al. Effect of topical intranasal fluticasone propionate on nasal mucosal cells in patients with allergic rinitis. En: Intranasal fluticasone propionate. Glaxo. 1990, pp. 2-10.

Meltzer EO, Stahlman JE, Leflein J, Meltzer S, Lim J, Dalai AA, Prillaman BA, Philpot EE. Preferences of Adult Patients with Allergic Rhinitis for the Sensory Attributes of Fluticasone Furoate Versus Fluticasone Propionate Nasal Sprays: A Randomized, Multicenter, Double-Blind, Single-Dose, Crossover Study. (2008) *Clin Ther,* Vol.30, No.2 (February 2008), pp. 271–279, Print ISSN 0149-2918, Electronic ISSN 1879-114X.

Merck Sharp & Dohme. Ficha técnica Singulair® (montelukast sodium). Merck Sharp & Dohme Corp., US Patent No.:5,565,473. Revised: 09/2011.

Minshall E, Ghaffar O, Cameron L, O Brien F, Quinn H, Rowe-Jones J et al. Assessment by nasal biopsy of long-time use of mometasone furoate aqueous nasal spray (Nasonex) in the treatment of perennial rhinitis. (1998) *Otolaryngol Head Neck Surg,* Vol.118, No.5 (May 1998), pp. 648-654, Print ISSN 0194-5998, Electronic ISSN 1097-6817.

Modgill V, Badyal DK, Verghese A. Efficacy and safety of montelukast add-on therapy in allergic rhinitis. *Methods Find Exp Clin Pharmacol,* Vol.32, No.9 (November 2010), pp. 669-674, Print ISSN 0379-0355, Electronic ISSN 2013-0155.

Mygind N, Dahl R. The rationale for use of topical corticosteroids in allergic rhinitis. (1996) *Clin Exp Allergy,* Vol.26, No.3 Suppl (May 1996), pp. 2-10, Print ISSN 0105-4538, Electronic ISSN: 1398-9995.

Mygind N, Dahl R, Nielsen LP, Hilberg O, Bjerke T. Effect of corticosteroids on nasal blockage in rhinitis measured by objective methods. (1997) *Allergy,* Vol.52, No.40 Suppl (January 1997), pp. 39-44, Print ISSN 0105-4538, Electronic ISSN: 1398-9995.

Mygind N, Laursen LC, Dahl M. Systemic corticosteroid treatment for seasonal allergic rhinitis: a common but poorly documented therapy. (2000) *Allergy,* Vol.55, No.1 (January 2000), pp. 11-15, Print ISSN 0105-4538, Electronic ISSN: 1398-9995.

Naclerio RM. Optimizing treatment options. (1998) *Clin Exp Allergy,* Vol.28, No.6 Suppl (December 1998), pp. 54-59, Print ISSN 0105-4538, Electronic ISSN: 1398-9995.

Nathan RA , Berger W, Yang W, Cheema A, Silvey MJ, Wu W, Philpot E. Effect of once-daily fluticasone furoate nasal spray on nasal symptoms in adults andadolescents with perennial allergic rhinitis. (2008) *Ann Allergy Asthma Immunol,* Vol.100, No.5 (May 2008), pp. 497–505, Print ISSN 1081-1206, Electronic ISSN 1534-4436.

Nayak A, Casale TB, Miller SD, Condemi J, McAlary M, Fowler-Taylor A, et al. Tolerability of retreatment with omalizumab, a recombinant humanized monoclonal anti-IgE antibody, during a second ragweed pollen season in patients with seasonal allergic rhinitis. (2003) *Allergy Asthma Proc,* Vol.24, No.5 (September-October 2003), pp. 323–329, ISSN Print 1088-5412, Electronic ISSN 1539-6304.

Niederberger V, Horak F, Vrtala S, Spitzauer S, Krauth MT, Valent P, et al. Vaccination with genetically engineered allergens prevents progression of allergic disease. (2004) *Proc Natl Acad Sci USA,* Vol.101, No. Suppl. 2 (October 2004), pp. 14677–1482, Print ISSN 0027-8424, Electronic ISSN 1091-6490.

Nielsen LP, Dahl R. Comparison of intranasal corticosteroids and antihistamines in allergic rhinitis: a review of randomized, controlled trials. (2003) *Am J Respir Med,* Vol.2, No.1 (January 2003), pp. 55-65, Print ISSN 1175-6365.

Nouri-Aria KT, Wachholz PA, Francis JN, Jacobson MR, Walker SM, Wilcock LK, et al. Grass pollen immunotherapy induces mucosal and peripheral IL-10 responses and blocking IgG activity. (2004) *J Immunol*, Vol.172, No.5 (March 2004), pp. 3252–3259, Print ISSN 0022-1767, Electronic ISSN 1550-6606.

Ohlander BO, Hansson RE, Karlsson KE. A comparison of three injectable corticosteroids for the treatment of patients with seasonal hay fever. (1980) *J Int Med Res*, Vol.8, No.1 (January 1980), pp. 63-69, Print ISSN 0300-0605, Electronic ISSN 1473-2300.

Olaguibel JM, Álvarez Puebla MJ. Efficacy of sublingual allergen vaccination for respiratory allergy in children. Conclusions from one meta-analysis. (2005) *J Investig Allergol Clin Immunol*, Vol.15, No.1 (January 2005), pp. 9-16, Print ISSN 1018-9068.

Passalacqua G, Albano M, Fregonese L, Riccio A, Pronzato C, Mela GS, et al. Randomised controlled trial of local allergoid immunotherapy on allergic inflammation in mite-induced rhinoconjunctivitis. (1998) *Lancet*, Vol.351, No.9103 (February 1998), pp. 629–632, Print ISSN 0140-6736, Electronic ISSN 1474-547X.

Patel P, Philip G, Yang W, Call R, Horak F, LaForce C, et al. Randomized, double-blind, placebo-controlled study of montelukast for treating perennial allergic rhinitis. (2005) *Ann Allergy Asthma Immunol*, Vol.95, No.6 (December 2005), pp. 551-557, Print ISSN 1081-1206, Electronic ISSN 1534-4436.

Patel RS, Shaw SR, Wallace AM, McGarry GW. Efficacy and systemic tolerability of mometasone furoate and betamethasone sodium phosphate. (2004) *J Laryngol Otol*, Vol.118, No.11 (November 2004), pp. 866-871, Print ISSN 0022-2151, Electronic ISSN 1748-5460.

Pelucchi A, Chiapparino A, Mastropasqua B, Marazzini L, Hernandez A, Foresi A. Effect of intranasal azelastine and beclomethasone dipropionate on nasal symptoms, nasal cytology, and bronchial responsiveness to methacholine in allergic rhinitis in response to grass pollens. (1995) *J Allergy Clin Immunol*, Vol.95, No.2 (February 1995), pp. 515-523, Print ISSN 0091-6749, Electronic ISSN 1097-6825.

Philip G, Malmstrom K, Hampel F C Jr, Weinstein S F, LaForce C F, Ratner P H, et al. Montelukast for treating seasonal allergic rhinitis: a randomized, double-blind, placebo-controlled trial performed in the spring. (2002) *Clin Exp Allergy*, Vol.32, No.7 (July 2002), pp. 1020-1028, Print ISSN 0954-7894, Electronic ISSN 1365-2222.

Pichler WJ, Klint T, Blaser M, Graf W, Sauter K, Weiss S, et al. Clinical comparison of systemic methylprednisolone acetate versus topical budesonide in patients with seasonal allergic rhinitis. (1988) *Allergy*, Vol.43, No.2 (February 1988), pp. 87-92, Print ISSN 0105-4538, Electronic ISSN: 1398-9995.

Rak S, Löwhagen O, Venge P. The effect of immunotherapy on bronchial hyperresponsiveness and eosinophil cationic protein in pollen-allergic patients. (1988) *J Allergy Clin Immunol*, Vol.82, No.3 Pt 1 (September 1988), pp. 470–480, Print ISSN 0091-6749, Electronic ISSN 1097-6825.

Robles-Contreras A, Santacruz C, Ayala J, Bracamontes E, Godinez V, Estrada-García I, et al. Allergic conjunctivitis: an immunological point of view. In: Conjunctivitis - A Complex and Multifaceted Disorder. Zdenek Pelikan (Ed.) Intech Open Access Publisher (Rijeka – Croatia) 2011, pp. 33-56, ISBN 978-953-307-750-5.

Rolinck-Werninghaus C, Hamelmann E, Keil T, Kulig M, Koetz K, Gerstner B, et al. The co-seasonal application of anti-IgE after preseasonal specific immunotherapy decreases ocular and nasal symptom scores and rescue medication use in grass pollen allergic children. (2004) *Allergy*, Vol.59, No.9 (September 2004), pp. 973–979, Print ISSN 0105-4538, Electronic ISSN 1398-9995.

Rosenblut A, Bardin PG, Muller B, Faris MA, Wu W, Caldwell MF, et al. Long-term safety of fluticasone furoate nasal spray in adults and adolescents with perennial allergic rhinitis. (2007) *Allergy*, Vol.62, No.9 (September 2007), pp. 1071–1077, Print ISSN 0105-4538, Electronic ISSN 1398-9995.

Saengpanich S, deTineo M, Naclerio RM, Baroody FM. Fluticasone nasal spray and the combination of loratadine and montelukast in seasonal allergic rhinitis. (2003) *Arch Otolaryngol Head Neck Surg*, Vol.129, No.5 (May 2003), pp. 557-562, Print ISSN 0886-4470, Electronic ISSN 1538-361X.

Salib RJ, Howarth PH. Safety and tolerability profiles of intranasal antihistamines and intranasal corticosteroids in the treatment of allergic rhinitis. (2003) *Drug Saf*, Vol.26, No.12 (November 2003), pp. 863-893, Print ISSN 0114-5916.

Scadding GK, Darby YC, Austin CE. Effect of short-term treatment with fluticasone propionate nasal spray on the response to nasal allergen challenge. (1994) *Br J Clin Pharmacol*, Vol.38, No.5 (November 1994), pp. 447-451, Print ISSN 0306-5251, Electronic ISSN 1365-2125.

Schenkel E, Skoner D, Bronsky E, Miller SD, Pearlman DS, Rooklin A et al. Absence of growth retardation in children with perennial allergic rhinitis after one year of treatment with mometasone furoate aqueous nasal spray. (2000) *Pediatrics*, Vol.105, No.2 (February 2000), pp. E22, Print ISSN 0031-4005, Electronic ISSN 1098-4275.

Schulz JI, Johnson JD, Freedman SO. Double-blind trial comparing flunisolide and placebo for the treatment of perennial rhinitis. (1978) *Clin Allergy*, Vol.8, No.4 (July 1978), pp. 313-320, Print ISSN 0009-9090.

Schultz A, Stuck BA, Feuring M, Hörmann K, Wehling M. Novel approaches in the treatment of allergic rhinitis. (2003) *Curr Opin Allergy Clin Immunol*, Vol.3, No.1 (February 2003), pp. 21-27, Print ISSN 1528-4050, Electronic ISSN 1473-6322.

Scow DT, Luttermoser GK, Dickerson KS. Leukotriene inhibitors in the treatment of allergy and asthma. (2007) Am Fam Physician, Vol.75, No.1 (January 2007), pp. 65-70, Print ISSN 0002-838X, Electronic ISSN 1532-0650.

Shamji MH, Wilcock LK, Wachholz PA, Dearman RJ, Kimber I, Wurtzen PA, et al. The IgE-facilitated allergen binding (FAB) assay: validation of a novel flow-cytometric based method for the detection of inhibitory antibody responses. (2006) *J Immunol Methods*, Vol.317, No.1-2 (December 2006), pp. 71–79, Print ISSN 0022-1759, Electronic ISSN 1872-7905.

Shiung YY, Chiang CY, Chen JB, Wu PC, Hung AF, Lu DC, et al. An anti-IgE monoclonal antibody that binds to IgE on CD23 but not on high-affinity IgE Fc receptors. (2001) *Immunobiology*, 2011 Nov 25. [Epub ahead of print], Print ISSN 0171-2985, Electronic ISSN 1878-3279.

Small CB, Hernandez J, Reyes A, Schenkel E, Damiano A, Stryszak P et al. Efficacy and safety of mometasone furoate nasal spray in nasal polyposis. (2005) *J Allergy Clin Immunol*, Vol.116, No.6 (December 2005), pp. 1275-1281, Print ISSN 0091-6749, Electronic ISSN 1097-6825.

Smith H, White P, Annila I, Poole J, Andre C, Frew A. Randomized controlled trial of high-dose sublingual immunotherapy to treat seasonal allergic rhinitis. (2004) *J Allergy Clin Immunol*, Vol.114, No.4 (October 2004), pp. 831–837, Print ISSN 0091-6749, Electronic ISSN 1097-6825.

Stjarne P, Blomgren K, Caye-Thomasen P, Salo S, Soderstrom T. The efficacy and safety of once-daily mometasone furoate nasal spray in nasal polyposis: a randomized, double-blind, placebo-controlled study. (2006) *Acta Otolaryngol*, Vol.126, No.6 (June 2006), pp. 606-612, Print ISSN 0001-6489, Electronic ISSN 1651-2251.

Storms WW. Risk-benefit assessment of fluticasone propionate in the treatment of asthma and allergic rhinitis. (1998) *J Asthma*, Vol.35, No.4 (April 1998), pp. 313-336, Print ISSN 0277-0903, Electronic ISSN 1532-4303.

Szefler SJ. Pharmacokinetics of intranasal corticosteroids. (2001) *J Allergy Clin Immunol*, Vol.108, No.1 Suppl (January 2001), pp. S26-S31. Print ISSN 0091-6749, Electronic ISSN 1097-6825.

Taramarcaz P, Gibson PG. The effectiveness of intranasal corticosteroids in combined allergic rhinitis and asthma syndrome. (2004) *Clin Exp Allergy*, Vol.34, No.12 (December 2004), pp. 1883-1889, Print ISSN 0954-7894, Electronic ISSN 1365-2222.

Tari MG, Mancino M, Madonna F, Buzzoni L, Parmiani S. Immunologic evaluation of 24 month course of sublingual immunotherapy. (1994) *Allergol Immunopathol (Madr)*, Vol.22, No.5 (September-October 1994), pp. 209–216, Print ISSN 0301-0546, Electronic ISSN 1578-1267.

Tari MG, Mancino M, Monti G. Efficacy of sublingual immunotherapy in patients with rhinitis and asthma due to house dust mite. A double-blind study. (1990) *Allergol Immunopathol (Madr)*, Vol.18, No.5 (September-October 1990), pp. 277–284, Print ISSN 0301-0546, Electronic ISSN 1578-1267.

Till SJ, Francis JN, Nouri-Aria K, Durham SR. Mechanisms of immunotherapy. (2004) *J Allergy Clin Immunol*, Vol.113, No.6 (June 2004), pp. 1025–1034, Print ISSN 0091-6749, Electronic ISSN 1097-6825.

Tonnel AB, Scherpereel A, Douay B, Mellin B, Leprince D, Goldstein N, et al. Allergic rhinitis due to house dust mites: evaluation of the efficacy of specific sublingual immunotherapy. (2004) *Allergy*, Vol.59, No.5 (May 2004), pp. 491-497, Print ISSN 0105-4538, Electronic ISSN 1398-9995.

Trangsrud AJ, Whitaker AL, Small RE. Intranasal corticosteroids for allergic rhinitis. (2002) *Pharmacotherapy*, Vol.22, No.11 (November 2002), pp. 1458-1467, Print ISSN 0277-0008, Electronic ISSN 1875-9114.

Unal M, Sevim S, Dogu O, Vayisoglu Y, Kanik A. Effect of botulinum toxin type A on nasal symptoms in patients with allergic rhinitis: a double blind, placebo-controlled clinical trial. (2003) *Acta Otolaryngol*, Vol.123, No.9 (December 2003), pp. 1060-1063, Print ISSN 0001-6489.

Van Adelsberg J, Philip G, LaForce CF, Weinstein SF, Menten J, Malice MP, et al. Randomized controlled trial evaluating the clinical benefit of montelukast for treating spring seasonal allergic rhinitis. (2003) *Ann Allergy Asthma Immunol*, Vol.90, No.2 (February 2003), pp. 214-222, Print ISSN 1081-1206, Electronic ISSN 1534-4436.

Van Cauwenberge P. ARIA: impact of compliance. (2005) *Clin Exp Allergy Rev*, Vol.5, No.1 (August 2005), pp. 3-6, Electronic ISSN 1472-9733.

Van Cauwenberge P, Bachert C, Passalacqua G, Bousquet J, Canonica G, Durham S et al. Consensus statement on the treatment of allergic rhinitis. EAACI Position paper. (2000) *Allergy*, Vol.55, No.2 (February 2000), pp. 116-134, Print ISSN 0105-4538, Electronic ISSN 1398-9995.

Van Drunen C, Meltzer EO, Bachert C, Bousquet J, Fokkens WJ. Nasal allergies and beyond: a clinical review of the pharmacology, efficacy, and safety of mometasone furoate. (2005) *Allergy*, Vol.60, No. Suppl 80(January 2005), pp. S5-S19, Print ISSN 0105-4538, Electronic ISSN 1398-9995.

Vasar M, Houle P-A, Douglass JA, Meltzer EO, Silvey MJ, Wu W, Caldwell M, Philpot E. Fluticasone furoate nasal spray: Effective monotherapy for symptoms of perennial allergic rhinitis in adults/adolescents. (2008) *Allergy Asthma Proc*, Vol.29, No.3 (May-June 2008), pp. 313-321, Print ISSN 1088-5412, Electronic ISSN 1539-6304.

Vignola AM, Humbert M, Bousquet J, Boulet L-P, Hedgecock S, Blogg M, et al. Efficacy and tolerability of anti-immunoglobulin E therapy with omalizumab in patients with concomitant allergic asthma and persistent allergic rhinitis: SOLAR. (2004) *Allergy*, Vol.59, No.7 (July 2004), pp. 709–717, Print ISSN 0105-4538, Electronic ISSN 1398-9995.

Vourdas D, Syrigou E, Potamianou P, Carat F, Batard T, André C, et al. Double-blind, placebo-controlled evaluation of sublingual immunotherapy with standardized olive pollen extract in pediatric patients with allergic rhinoconjunctivitis and mild asthma due to olive pollen sensitization. (1998) *Allergy*, Vol.53, No.7 (July 1998), pp. 662-672, Print ISSN 0105-4538, Electronic ISSN 1398-9995.

Waddell AN, Patel SK, Toma AG, Maw AR. Intranasal steroid sprays in the treatment of rhinitis: is one better than another? (2003) *J Laryngol Otol*, Vol.117, No.11 (November 2003), pp. 843-845, Print ISSN 0022-2151, Electronic ISSN 1748-5460.

Wang DY. Treatment of allergic rhinitis: H1-antihistamines and intranasal steroids. (2002) *Curr Drug Targets Inflamm Allergy*, Vol.1, No.3 (September 2002), pp. 215-220, Print ISSN 1568-010X.

Weinstein SF, Philip G, Hampel FC Jr, Malice MP, Swern AS, Dass SB, et al. Onset of efficacy of montelukast in seasonal allergic rhinitis. (2005) *Allergy Asthma Proc*, Vol.26, No.1 (January-February 2005), pp. 41-46, Print ISSN 1088-5412, Electronic ISSN 1539-6304.

Wiseman LR, Benfield P. Intranasal fluticasone propionate. A reappraisal of its pharmacology and clinical efficacy in the treatment of rhinitis. (1997) *Drugs*, Vol.53, No4 (February 1997), pp. 885-907, Print ISSN 0012-6667.

Zitt M, Kosoglou T, Hubbell J. Mometasone furoate nasal spray: a review of safety and systemic effects. (2007) *Drug Saf*, Vol.30, No.4 (March 2007), pp. 317-326, Print ISSN 0114-5916.

Section 3

Laryngology

Investigation of Experimental Wound Closure Techniques in Voice Microsurgery

C.B. Chng[1], D.P.C. Lau[2], J.Q. Choo[1] and C.K. Chui[1]
[1]Department of Mechanical Engineering,
National University of Singapore
[2]Department of Otolaryngology,
Singapore General Hospital
Singapore

1. Introduction

Microsurgery on human vocal folds typically involves the removal of benign lesions, often results in the creation of wounds in the form of epithelial micro-flaps (Benninger, Alessi et al. 1996). Conventionally, these micro-flaps are left to epithelialize without formal closure, which can result in healing by secondary intention and increased scar tissue formation (Woo 1995; Thekdi and Rosen 2002). Scar tissue in the lamina propria of the vocal fold affects its visco-elastic and vibrational properties (Bless and Welham 2010), disrupting the mucosal wave and often manifesting as hoarseness and a reduction in the phonatory capabilities of the patient (Thibeault, Gray et al. 2002). Since the precision of epithelial approximation accomplished during the surgical procedure and retained during the healing process affects the amount of scar tissue formation (Woo 1995), wound closure is of particular interest in voice microsurgery.

Extensive work has focused on improving wound closure methods to minimize scar tissue formation, ranging from micro-suturing which allows for primary healing (Woo 1995; Tsuji, Nita et al. 2009), to the use of tissue adhesives like fibrin glue (Bleach, Milford et al. 1997; Flock 2005; Kitahara, Masuda et al. 2005; Finck, Harmegnies et al. 2010; Skodacek, Arnold et al. 2011), and the use of chemical agents (Campagnolo, Tsuji et al. 2010) like Mitomycin-C (Branski, Verdolini et al. 2006; Fonseca, Malafaia et al. 2010) or stem cells (Hong, Lee et al.) to enhance the healing process of vocal fold wounds. However, various challenges faced in the execution of voice microsurgery add to the complexity of wound closure. These include limitations in instrument movement imposed by the laryngoscope, reduced tactile feedback in surgical instruments and loss of stereopsis. These are just some of the common challenges that can add to the intricacy of the closure of a simple wound, resulting in an increase in operation duration and associated risks under general anesthesia.

With this in mind, experimental evaluations of proposed microsurgical techniques are a necessary step in their development and optimization. Due to the rarity of human specimens for experimentation, different animal and synthetic models have been utilized instead. In this chapter, we discuss various vocal fold wound closure techniques as well as the models and methods used to evaluate them experimentally.

2. Background

Common causes of voice problems include benign vocal fold lesions such as nodules, polyps and cysts. While these lesions are non-cancerous, they may result in impaired vocal fold closure and vibration, and reduction of voice quality. Removal of these lesions is often carried out surgically using microlaryngoscopic techniques.

2.1 Structure of the vocal fold

Current voice microsurgery techniques are based on Hirano's discovery of the layered structure of the vocal folds (Hirano 1974; Bleach, Milford et al. 1997; James B. Snow and Ballenger 2003). Based on his microscopic work, the vocal fold was found to have three well defined layers - the epithelium, lamina propria and vocalis muscle. The lamina propria was further subdivided into 3 layers, the superficial layer of the lamina propria (SLLP), intermediate layer and deep layer.

In the SLLP, elastin and collagen fibres are loosely arranged within a matrix, whereas dense elastin fibres make up most of the intermediate layer. Collagen is densely packed in the deep layer, providing most of the support for the lamina propria (James B. Snow and Ballenger 2003). Hirano also proposed a cover-body concept, providing an explanation for the vibratory characteristics of the vocal fold. Based on his theory, the cover (consisting of stratified squamous epithelium and the underlying SLLP) is attached to the body (consisting of the vocalis and thyroarytenoid muscles) by an elastic interface or ligament (composed of the intermediate and deep layers of the lamina propria), with an increasing stiffness from superficial to deep. This allows the cover to oscillate independently due to its elastic characteristics, resulting in the mucosal wave seen on stroboscopy and most of the vibratory dynamics required for good voice production and phonation (Hirano 1974).

2.2 Wound creation

Early treatments for benign vocal fold lesions consisted of stripping (de-epithelialization) of the entire vocal fold (Sataloff, Spiegel et al. 1995). The healing process after this method of treatment often resulted in significant vocal fold scar formation which causes a change in the stiffness and viscoelastic layered structure of the lamina propria. This inhibits normal vibration of the vocal fold, and can cause significant dysphonia and possible glottic incompetence. However with the discovery by Hirano of the layered structure of the vocal fold and its implications on healing, treatment is now focused on preserving as much of the normal vocal fold structures as possible (Hochman and Zeitels 2000; Fleming, McGuff et al. 2001; Thekdi and Rosen 2002; Burns, Hillman et al. 2009). Avoiding injury to the deeper structures is important during voice microsurgery to minimize vocal fold scarring and persistent post-operative hoarseness.

Current methods in voice microsurgery are divided into two main categories based on the surgical instruments used – either laser surgery or cold surgery. In laser surgery, a CO_2 laser is used to ablate tissue and for coagulation of the target region (Yan, Olszewski et al. 2010). Together with a micro-manipulator for precise cutting, the reduced blood loss during laser surgery enables a relatively clear view of the surgical field. Although studies have found no significant difference in surgical outcomes between laser and cold surgery (Zeitels 1996; Hormann, Baker-Schreyer et al. 1999; Benninger 2000), risk of thermal damage to surrounding tissues is still dependent on familiarity with the equipment and surgical technique. This coupled with the increased cost of equipments, maintenance, additional personnel and their training (Yan, Olszewski et al. 2010), has driven the continued use of traditional "cold" voice microsurgery techniques.

Access to the vocal folds for microsurgery typically utilizes suspension laryngoscopy (Zeitels, Burns et al. 2004), where a rigid laryngoscope inserted via the patient's oral cavity provides a direct view of the vocal folds. The laryngoscope is suspended over the patient's chest, freeing the surgeon's hands for operating. A binocular operating microscope is used to provide magnification. Due to the prohibitive space constraints of laryngoscopes, microlaryngeal instruments are thin and long to access the lesion while maximizing of the surgical field. A significant level of dexterity is needed to handle the microlaryngeal tools, especially considering the fragile structure of the vocal fold. However cold surgery allows for tactile feedback and is better utilized in techniques like the micro-flap excision of benign vocal fold lesions (Zeitels 1996), which we will focus on for the course of this chapter.

2.2.1 Microflap technique

The microflap technique has been accepted as the standard approach for cold surgical removal of benign vocal fold lesions (Ford 1999; Hochman and Zeitels 2000; Lee and Chiang 2009), achieving the main principles of vocal fold surgery by minimal tissue excision, minimal trauma to SLLP and epithelium. This technique typically involves the initial creation of an epithelial incision beside the lesion. Blunt dissection is used to elevate the microflap while taking care to minimise trauma to the deeper layers of the lamina propria. Only pathologic tissue is excised and the microflap is then reapproximated (Sataloff, Spiegel et al. 1995) as seen in Figure 1.

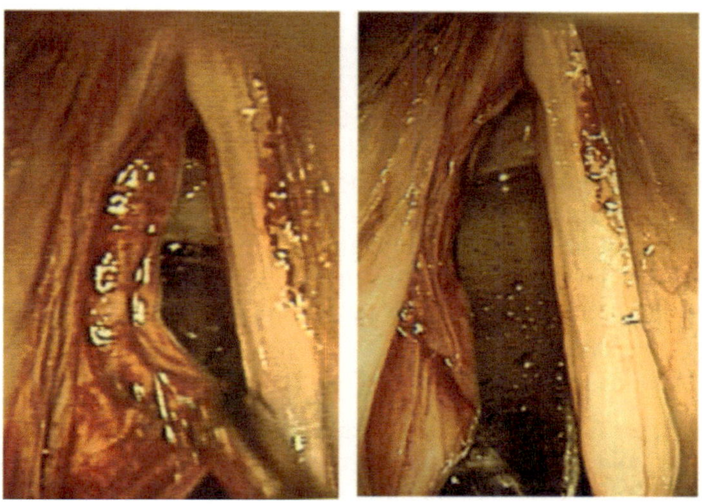

Fig. 1. Microflap technique in practise, (Left) after removal of benign lesion and (right) redraping of microflap.

2.3 Wound closure

Following excision of the lesion, the microflap is redraped to promote primary healing (Hochman and Zeitels 2000). If there is loss of epithelium or dislodgement of the microflap, then healing can occur by secondary intention. In this case granulation tissue formation and epithelial migration occur (Woo 1995), and there is correspondingly more scar tissue formation Voice rest is usually prescribed after surgery (Ishikawa and Thibeault 2010), but even with a totally compliant patient, apposition of epithelial flaps edges can be difficult to maintain. Thus various methods like micro-sutures and fibrin glue (Bleach, Milford et al. 1997; Flock 2005; Kitahara, Masuda et al. 2005; Finck, Harmegnies et al. 2010; Skodacek, Arnold et al. 2011) have been used to improve wound closure and minimize scar tissue formation.

2.3.1 Microsutures

The use of microsutures in vocal fold wound closure was proposed by Woo et al in 1995, hypothesizing that microsutures would allow precise positioning of wound edges and maintenance of the approximation (Woo 1995). This would reduce exposure of the wound site and permit primary healing to occur. They carried out the procedure in 18 patients, finding improved voice results after surgery. As there was no control group and basis for comparison in Woo et al's study, Fleming et al attempted to compare the amount of scar formation with and without microsutures in a canine model (Fleming, McGuff et al. 2001). A small sample group of 4 dogs were used, with bilateral microflap defects created in each dog. 6-0 fast absorbing gut sutures were used to close the microflap on only one side, leaving the contralateral side unclosed. The amount of scar was evaluated between 39 and 49 days post surgery. Un-sutured vocal folds were found to have at around 75% larger scar formation than sutured vocal folds, concurring with Woo et al's hypothesis that the use of microsutures improves postoperative wound healing.

Fleming et al also identified the length of time required for suture placement as the main disadvantage of this technique, suggesting that practice and familiarization with the technique using larger sutures before actual surgery could help mitigate the learning curve.

Tsuji et al recently proposed an improvement to the microsuture technique (Tsuji, Nita et al. 2009) by pre-tying a small length of 4-0 non-absorbable nylon suture to the free end of a 7-0 absorbable suture. The nylon acted as an anchor at the epithelial surface, preventing the thread from escaping and removing the need for an assistant surgeon to maintain tension on the free end of the suture. This improved the ease of performing the technique. Their new technique was tested on human cadaveric larynges for a total of 10 sutures and they reported a placement time of 5 to 7 minutes per suture.

2.3.2 Tissue adhesives

Despite good wound healing results demonstrated by micro-sutures, many surgeons prefer using adhesives to hold down epithelial flaps to achieve wound closure. Tissue adhesives such as cyanoacrylates and fibrin glue have been used (Flock 2005) and may be easier to apply than that of sutures. A potential limitation of tissue adhesives includes increased scar tissue formation if glue accumulates between the epithelial edges preventing proper approximation, or by adhering the epithelium to the underlying connective tissue without proper reformation of the intervening layered structure. Rapid curing can also restrict the surgeon from re-apposing malpositioned flaps. Lack of tensile strength of the adhesive is another concern. Fibrin glue can take several minutes for initiation of curing and several hours to develop its full strength. Especially during the curing phase it may not possess sufficient tensile strength to withstand rupture of its bond (Woo 1995). As the vocal folds vibrate at high frequencies during speech, constant shearing against the adhesive glue causes wear and the resultant debris may impede the vibratory properties of the vocal fold or result in secondary intention healing and a broader scar.

3. Selection of animal models

Experimentation on live humans is not possible or ethical in most situations. Cadaveric human larynges are also difficult or expensive to obtain. Hence, when studying a new technique or device, an animal model can provide a systematic platform for the experimentation and validation. However due to differences in vocal fold size and structure, one animal may not suit all research requirements.

Depending on the research question to be addressed and the methodological approach, these differences can limit applicability of experimental results. Selection of an appropriate animal model needs careful consideration. Practical issues like size, availability of animal, availability of the facilities to house or carry out the procedures, procurement cost and maintenance of the animal for the duration of the study can restrict researchers from acquiring their ideal animal model.

Characteristics of particular interest when considering operative techniques include the size, shape and position of the larynx and other upper airway structures to simulate surgical access. Similarity of vocal fold shape and location is essential for testing microsurgical techniques, while similar tissue composition is necessary when assessing in-vivo behaviour of implanted materials and tissue responses.

Various animal models have been used extensively in vocal fold studies with their results compared across models (Garrett, Coleman et al. 2000; Jiang, Raviv et al. 2001; Titze and Alipour 2006; Alipour and Jaiswal 2007; Alipour and Jaiswal 2008; Bless and Welham 2010; Alipour, Jaiswal et al. 2011). Three of the more commonly used models in operative studies are rabbits (Thibeault, Gray et al. 2002; Thibeault, Bless et al. 2003; Branski, Rosen et al. 2005; Carneiro and Scapini 2009; Campagnolo, Tsuji et al. 2010), dogs (Garrett, Coleman et al. 2000; Fleming, McGuff et al. 2001; Rousseau, Hirano et al. 2003; Karajanagi, Lopez-Guerra et al. 2011) and pigs (Blakeslee, Banks et al. 1995; Garrett, Coleman et al. 2000; Jiang, Raviv et al. 2001; Alipour and Jaiswal 2008; Fonseca, Malafaia et al. 2010).

3.1 Rabbit models

Due to their docile nature, relatively abundant numbers, ease of housing and management, rabbits are popular animal models. Rabbits are often used in immunological studies and exhibit similar vocal fold histology to humans. However access to rabbit vocal folds by standard suspension laryngoscopy is limited due to the smaller size of the rabbit larynx. Carneiro et al (Carneiro and Scapini 2009) used rabbits to study vocal fold grafts by exposing their vocal folds via a neck incision and laryngofissure. Branski et al (Branski, Rosen et al. 2005) studied the healing process of rabbit vocal fold after injury, using a neonatal laryngoscope to access the vocal fold. Campagnolo et al (Campagnolo, Tsuji et al. 2010) studied the healing effects of injectable corticosteroids after vocal fold surgery using a custom made laryngoscope for access.

3.2 Canine models

Canine models are used extensively in phonation studies. Comparing vocal fold structure across dogs, monkeys, pigs and human models using histology and laryngeal videostroboscopy, Garrett et al (Garrett, Coleman et al. 2000) found that unlike the human vocal fold, which has a higher elastin concentration in the deeper layers of the lamina propria, both pig and dog had a thin band of elastin concentrated just deep to the epithelial basement membrane zone. Just deep to this thin band, collagen and the elastin were less concentrated as in humans. The mucosal wave on stroboscopy was most similar between humans and canines and it was concluded that dog vocal folds were the most ideal for use in surgical studies due to its similarity in size, histology and mucosal wave. However, Fleming et al (Fleming, McGuff et al. 2001) noted that the slight differences in vocal fold structure like the thicker lamina propria and the lack of a well defined vocal ligament would have implications on its vibratory characteristics. Also, the higher cost and ethical considerations of using a companion animal for experimental studies are practical issues that need to be decided upon. Nevertheless, Fleming et al argued that as canine vocal fold healing was found to be similar to humans and similar human pathological conditions have been found to occur in canine models, they are still suitable for use in vocal fold microsurgery. Hahn et al (Hahn, Kobler et al. 2005; Hahn, Kobler et al. 2006; Hahn, Kobler et al. 2006) also compared collagen and elastin distribution in human, dog, pig and ferret larynges. They found that canine lamina propria collagen levels were most similar to those of humans, but on quantitative histology, elastin and collagen distribution in the human lamina propria was best matched by the porcine vocal fold.

3.3 Porcine models

Pigs are also common models for vocal fold studies. Based on our experience with pig models, the dimensions of the larynx in a 30 to 40 kg pig are similar to that of the adult human (Garrett, Coleman et al. 2000; Jiang, Raviv et al. 2001). The vocal folds have a similar configuration, and the intrinsic muscles and distribution of the recurrent laryngeal nerve is similar as demonstrated by detailed dissections of cadaveric porcine laryngeal neuromuscular anatomy (Knight, McDonald et al. 2005). Other phonatory characteristics such as rotational mobility of the cricothryoid joint, and relative size and innervation of the cricothyroid muscle have also been studied and found to be similar to that of humans (Jiang, Raviv et al. 2001); although these features are not of direct relevance to endoscopic laryngeal microsurgery.

An important difference between the pig and human vocal folds is that the pig has an additional fold in the vertical plane separated by a ventricle. The presence of a superior and inferior fold could relate to the thyroarytenoid muscle having two separate bellies (Knight, McDonald et al. 2005). It has been suggested that the inferior fold is the true vocal fold and the superior fold is akin to the ventricular fold in humans. However this remains a subject for debate as there is a further ventricle above the superior fold. It is suggested that vibration occurs at both folds as well as in the supraglottic structures during phonation (Kurita, Nagata et al. 1983; Alipour and Jaiswal 2008).

The pig larynx also differs in the structure of the arytenoid complex. The arytenoid cartilages have been described as fused across the posterior commissure, making laryngoscopic exposure more difficult (Garrett, Coleman et al. 2000). In addition to this, the arytenoids are also positioned more superiorly resulting in a steeper angle to the vocal folds.

However, from our experience with intubated animals, neither of these features created a significant hindrance to exposure or access to the vocal folds.

Regner used high-speed digital imaging to compare the vocal fold vibratory characteristics of ex-vivo bovine, canine, ovine, and porcine larynges with human vocal folds. By measuring amplitude, oscillation frequency, and phase difference of vocal fold vibration, it was concluded that canine and porcine larynges are the most appropriate models for vibratory or kinetic studies on phonation (Regner, Robitaille et al. 2010). Alipour also studied vibratory characteristics of excised pig, cow and sheep larynges, and concluded that the porcine larynx had the highest range of phonation frequencies, making it a good candidate for animal studies (Alipour and Jaiswal 2008).

In a similar study, Jiang et al. (Jiang, Raviv et al. 2001) concluded that pigs models provided the most similarity in vocal fold stiffness and was a reasonable alternative for phonation studies. As pigs are a common livestock, the high availability of pig larynges from local abattoirs poses less of an ethical concern for sacrificing animals for research purposes.

4. Ex-vivo experimental setups

4.1 Using animal models

Extensive ex-vivo experiments have been carried out for phonation studies (Regner and Jiang ; Jiang, Zhang et al. 2003; Skodacek, Arnold et al. 2011), for modeling the vibratory dynamics of the vocal folds. These experiments allow precise and independent control of various parameters affecting phonation, enabling systematic investigation and measurements of vocal fold vibrations.

A typical setup of such experimental systems consists of a mounting assembly, a pseudo lung, humidifiers, thermometers, flow and pressure meters. The mounting assembly where the excised larynx is housed consists of one lateral pronged micromanipulator sutured to the anterior tip of the thyroid cartilage and two other micromanipulators attached bilaterally to the arytenoid cartilages. This allows the elongation of the vocal folds to be controlled precisely. Airflow is generated by either an internal building source or a conventional compressor and is conditioned by heaters/humidifiers in order to prevent the larynges from drying out. The excised larynx is clamped directly to a tube from the pseudo lung and flowmeters and pressure meters are used to measure subglottal airflow and pressure before entry to the larynx. This experimental system can be easily adapted for use in ex-vivo surgical experimentation and can provide a platform to assess the effects of surgical procedures on vocal fold vibration.

4.2 Mechanical models

Alternatively, a mechanical model was proposed by Choo et al (Choo, Lau et al. 2010) specifically for the simulation of experiments on the vocal fold. In their design, they proposed the use of agarose as a material substitute for human vocal folds, mapping the mechanical properties of agar concentrations to that of vocal fold cover and ligament. By repeated casting of different concentrations of agarose into a mould, the phantom vocal folds were designed to mimic the layered structure of the vocal fold. In addition, vocal fold vibration was actuated externally with the use of vibrators, allowing the control of the vocal fold vibration frequency. Glottal gap and airflow could also be customized.

Using stroboscopy, Choo et al observed vibratory dynamics in their mechanically driven model similar to that of the mucosal wave in human vocal folds. After simulating a microflap and then subjecting the vocal fold phantom to vibration, cracks were found propagating radially outwards. Both these features suggested that the setup had potential for surgical experimentation.

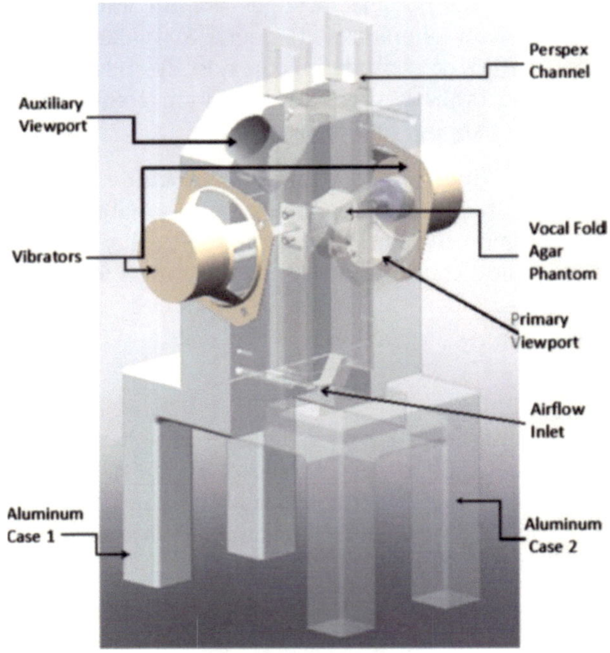

Fig. 2. Mechanical larynx setup courtesy of Choo et al (Choo, Lau et al. 2010).

5. New vocal fold wound closure device – Bioabsorbable microclips

A large part of our work is focused on the development of bioabsorable surgical microclips for vocal fold wound closure. Based on combining the ease and efficiency of using fibrin glue with the precision of microsutures, such surgical microclips have the potential to reduce vocal fold scar and procedure time, cumulating in cost savings and reduced morbidity for patients.

Surgical clips have been used in various areas of the body but have not been described previously for use on the vocal folds. This may be due to challenges facing the design of a surgical clip for application in this area, including the need for extremely small size, ability to withstand high vibration frequencies and shearing stresses during phonation, and the need for bio-absorbability. A number of materials have been studied in the design of surgical clips in other areas. Stainless steel clips and materials such as titanium and tantalum have been used for example to ligate the cystic duct and artery in laparoscopic cholecystectomy (Charara, Dion et al. 1994) However, some limitations of these materials include significant foreign body reaction, poor holding power and significant interference with roentgenologic studies like computerized tomography (CT) and magnetic resonance imaging (Klein, Jessup et al. 1994; Min Tan and Okada 1999; Pietak, Staiger et al. 2006; Rosalbino, De Negri et al. 2010). The introduction of ligating clips manufactured from novel polymers such as polydioxanone in laparoscopic cholecystectomy helped to address these limitations. These clips are completely absorbed in the process of ester bond hydrolysis over a period of 180 days and the by-products are excreted by urine. Moreover, these clips produce minimal tissue reactivity with good adhesion and are radiolucent (Klein, Jessup et al. 1994).

Earlier investigations using clips constructed from such polymers proved unsuitable for our requirements, as they could not provide adequate structural strength due to the minute size of the clips. As such, we are investigating the potential of using magnesium as the main bioabsorbable material to construct such microclips.

There are many reviews on the potential and viability of magnesium as a biomaterial (Pietak, Staiger et al. 2006; Witte, Hort et al. 2008; Zeng, Dietzel et al. 2008). Most of these studies focused on the use of magnesium in orthopaedic implants and bio-absorbable vascular stents, concentrating on improving its mechanical properties by alloying with various elements. Zhang et al. (Zhang and Yang 2008) reported significant improvement of both biocompatibility and mechanical properties with use of Zn as an additional alloying element to Mg-Si. Gu et al. (Gu, Zheng et al. 2009) reported good biocompatibility of magnesium with various alloying elements, recommending Al and Y for stents and Al, Ca, Zn, Sn, Si and Mn for orthopaedic implants. Drynda et al. (Drynda, Hassel et al. 2010) developed and evaluated fluoride coated Mg-Ca alloys for cardiovascular stents, reporting good biocompatibility and better degradation behaviour. However, as pure magnesium has been found to corrode too quickly in the low pH environment of physiological systems, much effort has also been placed into developing alloys or coatings to limit its degradation behaviour (Zeng, Dietzel et al. 2008). Rosalbino et al. (Rosalbino, De Negri et al. 2010) reported improved corrosion behaviour of Mg-Zn-Mn alloys for orthopaedic implants. Kannan et al. (Kannan and Raman 2008) studied the corrosion of AZ series (Al and Zn) magnesium alloys with the further addition of Ca, reporting significantly improved corrosion resistance with a reduction in mechanical properties (15% ultimate tensile strength and 20% elongation before fracture). Zhang et al. (Zhang, Zhang et al. 2009) reported the use of dual layer coatings of hydroxyapatite to considerably slow down the degradation of 99.9% pure magnesium substrates without heat treatment.

Based on the good biocompatibility and healing results demonstrated by these previous studies, we hypothesized that a bio-absorbable magnesium clip will be able to hold the wound site more securely and facilitate better healing as compared to surgical glue adhesives. Furthermore, with a design specifically aimed to reduce technical complexity in achieving apposition of epithelial flaps, a specifically designed prototype applicator could improve the ease of handling and speed of insertion, possibly translating to improved surgical outcomes. Due to the difficulty of simulating the vocal fold environment for both mechanical and bioabsorbability studies, in-vivo experiments were carried out to evaluate the feasibility of the clips in accordance to an approved protocol.

5.1 In-vivo evaluation of microclips

A 30-40 kg pig has upper airway dimensions that provide reasonable approximation to that of an adult human. Using this in-vivo model we were able to approach the larynx using a standard adult operating laryngoscope (Promed 222mm operating laryngoscope, Tuttlingen, Germany). To simulate endoscopic laryngeal microsurgery, the pig was positioned supine with the cervical spine slightly flexed. The laryngoscope was passed trans-orally following intubation with a size 5 endotracheal tube. As in most mammals, the epiglottis is intra-nasal and must therefore be drawn down into the oropharynx in order to access the vocal folds during laryngoscopy; if per-oral intubation is performed, this is usually accomplished during intubation. The laryngoscope was suspended on a custom made frame that enabled adjustments to be made to the position of the scope's tip, so as to optimize visualization of the vocal folds. By combining this with a 400mm focal-length binocular microscope, the setup as seen in Figure 3 was close to that expected during surgery in an adult human.

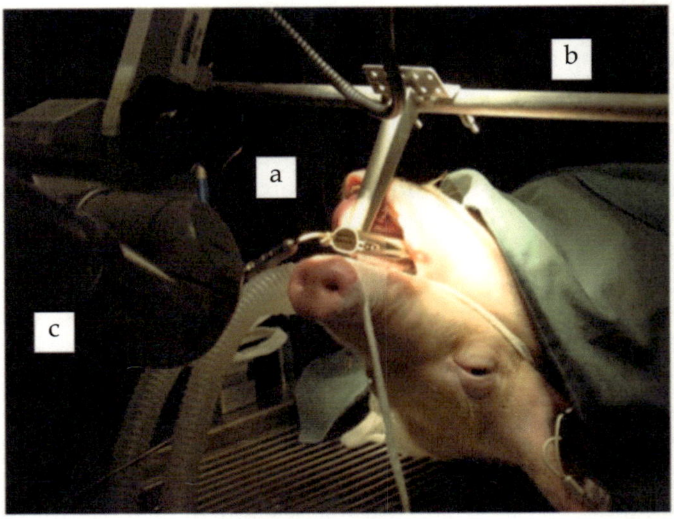

Fig. 3. Setup for endoscopic laryngeal microsurgery in the anaesthetized pig. (a) Operating laryngoscope. (b) Suspension device. (c) Binocular microscope.

A longitudinal incision was made on one or both vocal folds using a sickle knife. An epithelial flap was elevated using micro-forceps and a dissector. The flap was then replaced and secured with either micro-clips (3-6 clips on one side), microsuture or fibrin glue. The animal was monitored daily until the end of the three weeks study, after which the animal was sacrificed and its vocal fold excised for histological evaluation.

Feedback on the surgical procedure for the microclips was generally positive. Implantation time was found to be less than a minute per microclip due to the straightforward nature of the application technique. Due to the limited workspace within the laryngoscope, microsuturing was found to be more complex than applying the microclips, which greatly simplified approximation of the vocal fold wound edges. From preliminary results of the excised vocal folds after sacrificing the pigs, there was no damage found on the contra-lateral vocal folds, demonstrating the safety of the microclips. We are still awaiting histological results, but scar formation is comparable to that of using sutures based on visual inspection.

6. Conclusion

We have given an overview of the current techniques used clinically for vocal fold wound closure and an update on the potential of some microsurgical techniques proposed in current literature. Animal and artificial models have been discussed, highlighting the complexities of selecting appropriate experimental models and methods for evaluation of vocal fold microsurgery. We shared our experience in experimental microsurgery with respect to wound closure, specifically addressing the vocal fold microclip, which is a new wound closure device. The methods for testing the integrity and bio-absorption properties of such devices in vivo and the technical challenges of applying such devices accurately during microsurgery in the larynx were also discussed.

7. References

Alipour, F. and S. Jaiswal (2008). "Phonatory characteristics of excised pig, sheep, and cow larynges." *J Acoust Soc Am* 123 (6): 4572-4581.

Alipour, F., S. Jaiswal, et al. (2011). "Vocal Fold Elasticity in the Pig, Sheep, and Cow Larynges." *Journal of Voice* 25 (2): 130-136.

Alipour, J. and S. Jaiswal (2007). "Glottal airflow resistance in excised pig, sheep and cow larynges." *Journal of Voice*.

Benninger, M. S. (2000). "Microdissection or Microspot CO2 Laser for Limited Vocal Fold Benign Lesions: A Prospective Randomized Trial." *The Laryngoscope* 110 (S92): 1-1.

Benninger, M. S., D. Alessi, et al. (1996). "Vocal fold scarring: Current concepts and management." *Otolaryngology - Head and Neck Surgery* 115 (5): 474-482.

Blakeslee, D. B., R. E. Banks, et al. (1995). "Analysis of Vocal Fold Function in the Miniswine Model." *Journal of Investigative Surgery* 8 (6): 409-424.

Bleach, N., C. Milford, et al., Eds. (1997). *Operative Otorhinolaryngology*, Blackwell Science Ltd.

Bless, D. and N. Welham. (2010). "Characterization of vocal fold scar formation, prophylaxis, and treatment using animal models." 6. Retrieved 9417024, 18, from http://ovidsp.ovid.com/ovidweb.cgi?T=JS&PAGE=reference&D=ovftl&NEWS=N&AN=00020840-201012000-00003.

Branski, R. C., C. A. Rosen, et al. (2005). "Acute vocal fold wound healing in a rabbit model." *Ann Otol Rhinol Laryngol* 114 (1 Pt 1): 19-24.

Branski, R. C., K. Verdolini, et al. (2006). "Vocal Fold Wound Healing: A Review for Clinicians." *Journal of Voice* 20 (3): 432-442.

Burns, J. A., R. E. Hillman, et al. (2009). "Phonomicrosurgical treatment of intracordal vocal-fold cysts in singers." *The Laryngoscope* 119 (2): 419-422.

Campagnolo, A. M., D. H. Tsuji, et al. (2010). "Histologic study of acute vocal fold wound healing after corticosteroid injection in a rabbit model." *Ann Otol Rhinol Laryngol* 119 (2): 133-139.

Carneiro, C. d. G. and F. Scapini (2009). "The Rabbit as an Experimental Model in Laryngology." *Arq. Int. Otorrinolaringol.* 13 (2): 146-150.

Charara, J., Y. M. Dion, et al. (1994). "Mechanical characterization of endoscopic surgical staples during an experimental hernia repair." *Clinical Materials* 16 (Compendex): 81-89.

Choo, J. Q., D. P. Lau, et al. (2010). "Design of a mechanical larynx with agarose as a soft tissue substitute for vocal fold applications." *J Biomech Eng* 132 (6): 065001.

Drynda, A., T. Hassel, et al. (2010). "Development and biocompatibility of a novel corrodible fluoride-coated magnesium-calcium alloy with improved degradation kinetics and adequate mechanical properties for cardiovascular applications." *Journal of Biomedical Materials Research - Part A* 93 (Compendex): 763-775.

Finck, C. L., B. Harmegnies, et al. (2010). "Implantation of Esterified Hyaluronic Acid in Microdissected Reinke's Space After Vocal Fold Microsurgery: Short- and Long-Term Results." *Journal of Voice* 24 (5): 626-635.

Fleming, D. J., S. McGuff, et al. (2001). "Comparison of microflap healing outcomes with traditional and microsuturing techniques: initial results in a canine model." *Ann Otol Rhinol Laryngol* 110 (8): 707-712.

Flock, S., Marchitto, KS (2005). "Progress toward seamless tissue fusion for wound closure." 38 (2005).

Fonseca, V. R., O. Malafaia, et al. (2010). "Angiogenesis, fibrinogenesis and presence of synechiae after exeresis of a swine vocal fold mucosal microflap and use of topical mitomycin-C." *Acta Cir Bras* 25 (1): 80-85.

Ford, C. N. (1999). "Advances and Refinements in Phonosurgery." *The Laryngoscope* 109 (12): 1891-1900.

Garrett, C. G., J. R. Coleman, et al. (2000). "Comparative histology and vibration of the vocal folds: implications for experimental studies in microlaryngeal surgery." *Laryngoscope* 110 (5 Pt 1): 814-824.

Gu, X., Y. Zheng, et al. (2009). "In vitro corrosion and biocompatibility of binary magnesium alloys." *Biomaterials* 30 (Compendex): 484-498.

Hahn, M. S., J. B. Kobler, et al. (2006). "Quantitative and comparative studies of the vocal fold extracellular matrix. I: Elastic fibers and hyaluronic acid." *Ann Otol Rhinol Laryngol* 115 (2): 156-164.

Hahn, M. S., J. B. Kobler, et al. (2005). "Midmembranous vocal fold lamina propria proteoglycans across selected species." *Ann Otol Rhinol Laryngol* 114 (6): 451-462.

Hahn, M. S., J. B. Kobler, et al. (2006). "Quantitative and comparative studies of the vocal fold extracellular matrix II: collagen." *Ann Otol Rhinol Laryngol* 115 (3): 225-232.

Hirano, M. (1974). "Morphological structure of the vocal cord as a vibrator and its variations." *Folia Phoniatr (Basel)* 26 (2): 89-94.

Hochman, I. I. and S. M. Zeitels (2000). "Phonomicrosurgical management of vocal fold polyps: The subepithelial microflap resection technique." *Journal of Voice* 14 (1): 112-118.

Hong, S. J., S. H. Lee, et al. "Vocal fold wound healing after injection of human adipose-derived stem cells in a rabbit model." *Acta Oto-laryngologica* 0 (0): 1-7.

Hormann, K., A. Baker-Schreyer, et al. (1999). "Functional results after CO2 laser surgery compared with conventional phonosurgery." *J Laryngol Otol* 113 (2): 140-144.

Ishikawa, K. and S. Thibeault (2010). "Voice Rest Versus Exercise: A Review of the Literature." *Journal of voice : official journal of the Voice Foundation* 24 (4): 379-387.

James B. Snow, J. and J. J. Ballenger (2003). *Ballenger's Otorhinolaryngology Head and Neck Surgery*, BC Decker Inc.

Jiang, J. J., J. R. Raviv, et al. (2001). "Comparison of the phonation-related structures among pig, dog, white-tailed deer, and human larynges." *Ann Otol Rhinol Laryngol* 110 (12): 1120-1125.

Jiang, J. J., Y. Zhang, et al. (2003). "Nonlinear dynamics of phonations in excised larynx experiments." *J Acoust Soc Am* 114 (4 Pt 1): 2198-2205.

Kannan, M. B. and R. K. S. Raman (2008). "In vitro degradation and mechanical integrity of calcium-containing magnesium alloys in modified-simulated body fluid." *Biomaterials* 29 (Compendex): 2306-2314.

Karajanagi, S. S., G. Lopez-Guerra, et al. (2011). "Assessment of canine vocal fold function after injection of a new biomaterial designed to treat phonatory mucosal scarring." *Ann Otol Rhinol Laryngol* 120 (3): 175-184.

Kitahara, S., Y. Masuda, et al. (2005). "Vocal fold injury following endotracheal intubation." *J Laryngol Otol* 119 (10): 825-827.

Klein, R., G. Jessup, et al. (1994). "Comparison of titanium and absorbable polymeric surgical clips for use of laparoscopic cholecsystectomy." *Surgical Endoscopy* 8 (1994).

Knight, M. J., S. E. McDonald, et al. (2005). "Intrinsic muscles and distribution of the recurrent laryngeal nerve in the pig larynx." *Eur Arch Otorhinolaryngol* 262 (4): 281-285.

Kurita, S., K. Nagata, et al. (1983). *A comparative study of the layer structure of the vocal fold*. San Diego, College Hill.

Lee, K. W. and F. Y. Chiang (2009). "Current practice and feasibility in microlaryngeal surgery: microsurgical pressing excision technique." *Curr Opin Otolaryngol Head Neck Surg* 17 (6): 431-435.

Min Tan, T. and M. Okada (1999). "The efficiency of absorbable clips in minimally invasive surgery." *Surgery Today* 29 (8): 828-831.

Pietak, A. M., M. P. Staiger, et al. (2006). "Magnesium and its alloys as orthopedic biomaterials: A review." *Biomaterials* 27 (Copyright 2006, IEE): 1728-1734.

Regner, M. F. and J. J. Jiang "Phonation Threshold Power in Ex Vivo Laryngeal Models." *Journal of Voice* In Press, Corrected Proof.

Regner, M. F., M. J. Robitaille, et al. (2010). "Interspecies comparison of mucosal wave properties using high-speed digital imaging." *Laryngoscope* 120 (6): 1188-1194.

Rosalbino, F., S. De Negri, et al. (2010). "Bio-corrosion characterization of Mg-Zn-X (X = Ca, Mn, Si) alloys for biomedical applications." *Journal of Materials Science: Materials in Medicine* 21 (Compendex): 1091-1098.

Rousseau, B., S. Hirano, et al. (2003). "Characterization of vocal fold scarring in a canine model." *Laryngoscope* 113 (4): 620-627.

Sataloff, R. T., J. R. Spiegel, et al. (1995). "Laryngeal mini-microflap: A new technique and reassessment of the microflap saga." *Journal of Voice* 9 (2): 198-204.

Skodacek, D., U. Arnold, et al. (2011). "Chondrocytes suspended in modified fibrin glue for vocal fold augmentation: An in vitro study in a porcine larynx model." *Head & Neck*: n/a-n/a.

Thekdi, A. A. and C. A. Rosen (2002). "Surgical treatment of benign vocal fold lesions." *Current Opinion in Otolaryngology & Head and Neck Surgery* 10 (6): 492-496.

Thibeault, S. L., D. M. Bless, et al. (2003). "Interstitial protein alterations in rabbit vocal fold with scar." *Journal of Voice* 17 (3): 377-383.

Thibeault, S. L., S. D. Gray, et al. (2002). "Histologic and Rheologic Characterization of Vocal Fold Scarring." *Journal of Voice* 16 (1): 96-104.

Titze, I. and F. Alipour (2006). *The myoelastic aerodynamic theory of phonation*, National Center for Voice and Speech.

Tsuji, D. H., L. M. Nita, et al. (2009). "T-Shaped Microsuture: A New Suture Technique for Laryngeal Microsurgery." *Journal of Voice* 23 (6): 739-742.

Witte, F., N. Hort, et al. (2008). "Degradable biomaterials based on magnesium corrosion." *Current Opinion in Solid State & Materials Science* 12 (Copyright 2009, The Institution of Engineering and Technology): 63-72.

Woo, P. (1995). "Endoscopic Microsuture Repair of Vocal Fold Defects." *Journal of Voice* 9 (3): 332-339.

Yan, Y., A. E. Olszewski, et al. (2010). "Use of Lasers in Laryngeal Surgery." *Journal of Voice* 24 (1): 102-109.

Zeitels, S. M. (1996). "Laser Versus Cold Instruments for Microlaryngoscopic Surgery." *The Laryngoscope* 106 (5): 545-552.

Zeitels, S. M., J. A. Burns, et al. (2004). "Suspension laryngoscopy revisited." *Ann Otol Rhinol Laryngol* 113 (1): 16-22.

Zeng, R., W. Dietzel, et al. (2008). "Progress and challenge for magnesium alloys as biomaterials." *Advanced Engineering Materials* 10 (Copyright 2008, The Institution of Engineering and Technology): B3-B14.

Zhang, E. and L. Yang (2008). "Microstructure, mechanical properties and bio-corrosion properties of Mg-Zn-Mn-Ca alloy for biomedical application." *Materials Science and Engineering A* 497 (Compendex): 111-118.

Zhang, Y., G. Zhang, et al. (2009). "Controlling the biodegradation rate of magnesium using biomimetic apatite coating." *Journal of Biomedical Materials Research - Part B Applied Biomaterials* 89 (Compendex): 408-414.

8

Comparison Among Phonation of the Sustained Vowel /ε/, Lip Trills, and Tongue Trills: The Amplitude of Vocal Fold Vibration and the Closed Quotient

Gislaine Ferro Cordeiro, Arlindo Neto Montagnoli and Domingos Hiroshi Tsuji
University of São Paulo School of Medicine
Brasil

1. Introduction

Trill exercises are traditionally used in the clinical practice of speech-language pathology as vocal warm-ups in the treatment of dysphonia (Behlau & Pontes, 1995; Sataloff, 1991). They are also used by voice coaches (Aydos & Hanayama, 2004; Scarpel & Pinho, 2001) in the training of professional voice users, such as singers, actors (including voice actors), teachers, and lawyers. Although there are various types of trill exercises, including gargling, voiced fricatives, and simultaneous tongue/lip trills, the most commonly used exercises are tongue trills and lip trills (Scwarz & Cielo, 2009; Menezes *et al.*, 2005).

In the literature, the first reports of trill exercises date from the 1970s, at which time the tongue trill was already considered a "universal technique," i.e., a technique that can change the overall quality of the voice (Linklater, 1976). Trills are among the so-called facilitating sounds (Behlau & Pontes, 1995), and trill exercises can be used in the treatment of hyperkinetic and hypokinetic disorders (Schneider & Sataloff, 2007; Speyer, 2008); they can also be used as vocal warm-ups (Aydos & Hanayama, 2004; Speyer, 2008). Trill exercises are therefore widely disseminated among voice coaches, including speech-language pathologists, singing teachers, and drama teachers (Aydos & Hanayama, 2004). In individuals with a normal voice, tongue trills increase the amplitude of vocal fold vibration, reduce the glottal gap (Rodrigues, 2001), and improve the results of auditory-perceptual and acoustic analyses, resulting in less shimmer, a higher harmonics-to-noise ratio, increased amplitude of the harmonics, and decreased noise (Schwarz & Cielo, 2009; Rodrigues, 1995). During tongue trills, the entire laryngeal framework vibrates and there is anteroposterior constriction of the pharynx (Bueno, 2006). After the performance of tongue trills, the fundamental frequency increases, broad- and narrow-band spectrograms become clearer, and glottic closure increases, as do the amplitude and symmetry of vocal fold vibration, all of which demonstrate that tongue trills change the glottal source and vocal tract filter (Scwarz & Cielo, 2009).

Speech-language pathologists also use tongue trills, principally in individuals diagnosed with vocal nodules (Bueno, 2006). In addition, tongue trills can be used in individuals with chronic edema and in those with hyperfunctional dysphonia (Pinho & Pontes, 2008). Some authors also recommend tongue trills in cases of hypofunctional dysphonia (Behlau e Pontes, 1995). Manieka-Aleksandrovix (2006) collected data regarding 500 patients with aphonia due to psychogenic dysphonia and found that gargling is one of the exercises used on the first day of therapy for voice rehabilitation.

Casper *et al.* (1992) employed tongue trills as a therapeutic resource in individuals with vocal fold paralysis and in those having undergone laryngeal surgery (Woo *et al.*, 1994). The tongue trill is contraindicated for individuals with recent-onset acute inflammation, because the exercise can aggravate the inflammatory phase. In the immediate postoperative period, tongue trills can delay healing (Pinho & Pontes, 2008) and, in cases of papillomatosis, stimulate the dissemination of the disease (Pinho & Tsuji, 2006).

When performing trill exercises, individuals should keep the tongue (or lips) and the mandible relaxed, coordinating the airflow so that vibration can occur (Scneider & Sataloff, 2007). The tongue trill is maintained by the interaction among the firmness of the body of tongue, control of the tip of the tongue, glottic closure, and control of the exhaled air. The exercise should be performed with the sides of the body of tongue firmly pressed against the dental alveoli and the tip of the tongue positioned in the region of the incisive papilla, free to vibrate (McGowan, 1992). As a result, the entire vocal tract vibrates (Scwarz & Cielo, 2009). For lip vibration (lip trill) to occur, the lips should be held together tightly enough to promote airway occlusion and relaxed enough for air pressure to overcome the resistance (Gaskill e Erickson, 2008). During lip trills, as during tongue trills, there is interaction among the vocal tract, glottal vibration, and the exhaled air during lip trills (Titze, 2006). During all trill exercises, the vibrating organ acts as a valve and creates oscillatory differences in external pressure and in the pressure in the cavity behind the constriction. This produces differences in the pressure, speed, and volume of air in the oral cavity, causing changes in the pharyngeal wall. Therefore, for vocal fold vibration to occur concomitantly with the point of oscillation of the oral cavity, subglottic air pressure must be greater than is that during normal phonation (McGowan, 1992).

Tongue and lip vibration follow the same principle as does the vocal fold mass effect: the anterior part of the vocal tract is occluded by the tip of the tongue or the lips. Intraoral pressure becomes greater than the atmospheric pressure and therefore greater than the force that maintains the anterior part of the vocal tract closed. Therefore, the anterior part of the vocal tract opens and is subsequently "sucked out" by the speed of the airflow (McGowan, 1992).

According to Gaskill and Erickison (2008), the difference between lip trills and other exercises that focus on the anterior part of the vocal tract is that the lip trill is the only exercise that promotes lip occlusion and non-occlusion (without loss of muscle tone). This causes the lips to vibrate, although at a frequency lower than that of vocal fold vibration. Therefore, airflow and subglottic pressure must adjust in order to allow the lips and the vocal folds to vibrate, overloading the vocal folds. The variations that occur in the pharynx during lip trills can increase the force of mucosal vibration during the wavelike motion of the vocal folds (McGowan, 1992).

Because of high vocal demand, professional voice users should maintain the fitness of all of the structures involved in phonation. For professional voice users, voice training should address a wide range of issues, from breathing to voice articulation and projection. Trill exercises involve a functional balance among the vibrating organ (the tongue, the lips, or a combination of the two), the vocal tract, the larynx, and the exhaled air. Therefore, they constitute one of the principal tools for vocal warm-up and training in professional voice users (Aydos & Hanayama, 2004; Nix, 1999).

Studies involving electroglottography (EGG) and comparing the closed quotient during lip trills with that during phonation of the vowel /a/ before and after the exercise showed a reduction of approximately 50% in the closed quotient during the performance of lip trills (Gaskill & Erickson, 2008) and an increase in the value when the exercise was performed at high intensity by singers (Cordeiro *et al.*, in prelo). The change is more evident in untrained individuals. The mechanical interaction between the source and the filter plus a lower adduction of the vocal process were reported to be responsible for the results obtained(15). The closed quotient varies widely during trill exercises (Cordeiro *et al.*, in prelo).

Recent studies have attempted to determine the best exercise prescription (the most effective duration and number of repetitions per session) for each case. Menezes *et al.*. (2005) suggested that, for individuals with no complaints or dysphonia, trill exercises be performed for a maximum of three and five minutes by females and males, respectively. For females with nodules, the ideal exercise duration is five minutes, the exercise leading to signs of vocal fatigue if performed for seven minutes or more (Menezes, 2011). , According to Schwarz (2009), when prescribing the exercise, the vocal resistance of the individual should be taken into consideration. In the study conducted by Schwarz (2009), the individuals performed three series of fifteen trills with a 30-second interval of passive rest between each series, and the author reported that voice quality improved after the exercise.

In this chapter, we determine whether there are differences among tongue trills, lip trills, and phonation of the sustained vowel /ɛ/ in classically trained singers in terms of the maximum amplitude of vocal fold vibration, mean closed quotient, and standard deviation of the closed quotient, as assessed by EGG. We chose to compare the vocal fold vibration seen during lip and tongue trills with that seen during phonation of the sustained vowel /ɛ/ because that vowel is considered an open vowel, produced with minimal constriction of the vocal tract (Story, 1998; Gregio, 2006).

2. Study sample and method

2.1 Ethical aspects

The present study was approved by the Research Ethics Committee of the *Hospital das Clínicas da Faculdade de Medicina da Universidade de São Paulo* (HCFMUSP, University of São Paulo School of Medicine *Hospital das Clínicas*; Protocol no. 907/06, February 14, 2007; Appendix 1), located in the city of São Paulo, Brazil. All participating individuals gave written informed consent.

2.2 Study sample

In the present study, we evaluated 14 individuals (7 males and 7 females). We applied the following criteria:

- inclusion criteria—being a healthy, classically trained, professional singer; having laryngeal control; having mastered the techniques for performing lip and tongue trills; and presenting with no vocal fold lesions
- exclusion criteria—having been a professional singer for less than three years; presenting with singing or speaking voice complaints; presenting with incomplete glottal closure; having reported intolerance to examination of the larynx

A total of 4 individuals were excluded from the present study. Of those, 2 were male and 2 were female. Of the 2 males, 1 was excluded because he could not tolerate the examination of the larynx and 1 was excluded because he had been a professional singer for less than three years (one year and six months). Of the 2 females, 1 was excluded because she could not tolerate the examination of the larynx and 1 was excluded because she presented with speaking voice complaints.

A total of 10 singers were analyzed. Their characteristics are shown in Table 1.

Individual	Gender	Age	Years singing professionally	Voice type
1	Female	24	4	Soprano
2	Female	45	20	Soprano
3	Female	30	3	Mezzo-soprano
4	Female	30	4	Mezzo-soprano
5	Female	48	15	Contralto
6	Male	29	5	Tenor
7	Male	27	6	Tenor
8	Male	33	12	Baritone
9	Male	34	15	Baritone
10	Male	38	18	Bass

Table 1. Characteristics of the individuals included in the study sample

2.3 Method

2.3.1 Preparation for data collection

Before data collection, we measured the vocal range of each participant. Vocal range is the distance between the lowest and the highest note that an individual can produce, excluding the vocal fry register and including the falsetto.

After having measured the vocal range of the participants, we selected the 5th whole step above the lowest possible note that each individual was able to produce (Cooper, 1979). The participants were then asked to produce, in that note and with their larynx in a low position, the sustained vowel /ɛ/, lip trills, and tongue trills, as well as the voiced fricatives /v/, /z/, and /ʒ/, at the highest and lowest possible intensities of which they were capable. As shown in Table 2, we chose the lowest of the highest intensities and the highest of the lowest intensities, in order to standardize the intensities during exercise training and data collection. The voiced fricatives were used because the lowest of the highest intensities is commonly achieved during the phonation of those sounds; therefore, the participants were able to perform the tests comfortably without experiencing vocal fatigue or aperiodicity due to the use of threshold-range phonation (Jiang *et al.*, 2001) during the performance of trill exercises.

Intensity	Vowel /ɛ/	Lip trill	Tongue trill	/v/	/z/	/ʒ/
Highest (dB)	51	52	52	<50	<50	51
Lowest (dB)	85	70	71	68	70	71

Table 2. Highest and lowest intensities achieved by individual 1 during sustained phonations. The values chosen for data collection were 52 dB for the lowest intensity and 68 dB for the highest intensity

In order to measure vocal range, as well as to determine and maintain the selected note, we used a Casio VL-Tone-VL1 keyboard (Casio Computer Co., Ltd., Tokyo, Japan). Intensity was measured with a sound pressure level meter (model 33-2055, RadioShack Corporation, Fort Worth, TX, USA) placed 30 cm from the corner of the mouth of the singer.

After the abovementioned procedure, each singer practiced producing the sounds at the requested note and at the intensity selected (maximum variation, 2 dB), with minimal effort and maintaining the larynx in the same (low) position, for ≥ 10 seconds. The practice session was conducted with the aid of a speech-language pathologist specializing in voice, who instructed the singers during a meeting held before data collection. On the day of data collection, previously agreed upon by the singers and the investigators, the phonation tasks were performed again before each test.

Participants were informed of the objectives and conditions of the present study before the first evaluation was scheduled. If a participant presented with illness, sleep deprivation, vocal fatigue, or dysphonia on the day of data collection, the evaluation was rescheduled.

2.3.2 Data collection and analysis

The individuals underwent videolaryngostroboscopy by an experienced otolaryngologist of the HCFMUSP Clinical Otolaryngology Division Voice Group Outpatient Clinic and EGG at the *Centro de Especialização em Fonoaudiologia Clínica* (CEFAC, Center for Clinical Audiology and Speech-Language Pathology), both located in the city of São Paulo. The tests were performed on different days so that the singers did not experience vocal fatigue. For the tests, the individuals were asked to produce the sustained vowel /ɛ/ and perform tongue and lip trills for as long as possible at the same frequency and intensities as those used in the training sessions (5th whole step above the lowest note in their range and the lowest of the highest/highest of the lowest, respectively). Frequency was controlled by the singers. In order to do that, they used the same keyboard that was used in the training sessions. Intensity was monitored by a speech-language pathologist in the examination room, using the same sound pressure level meter that was used in the training sessions, which was again positioned at 30 cm from the corner of the mouth of the singer. We made intraindividual comparisons. Low-intensity phonations were compared only with one another, as were high-intensity phonations.

2.3.2.1 Videolaryngostroboscopy

We used videolaryngostroboscopy in order to measure the amplitude of vocal fold vibration during the exercises. The singers were instructed to sit in a chair, with both hips well supported, head held straight, and the chin at a 90° angle to the neck. In order to maintain the head of each participant fixed in position, the chair was equipped with a headrest that was adjusted to the height of the individual and a piece of foam that was covered with comfortable fabric, measuring 14 cm in width, 10 cm in height, and 7 cm in depth. In addition, their heads were secured to the headrest with a headband (Figure 1).

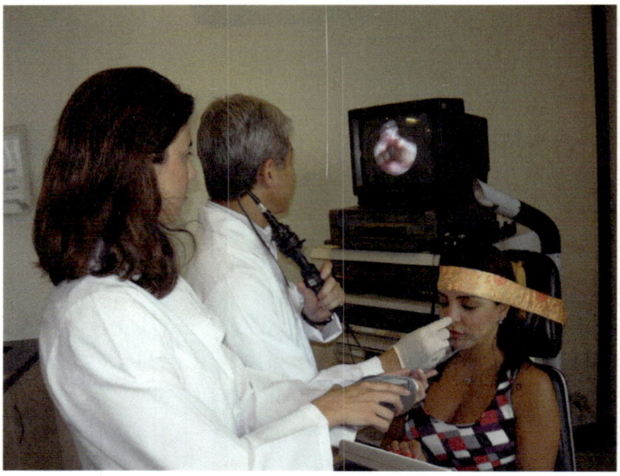

Fig. 1. Photograph of a singer undergoing videolaryngostroboscopy.

Images of vocal fold vibration were obtained with a stroboscopic light source (4914; Brüel & Kjær Sound & Vibration Measurement A/S, Nærum, Denmark) and captured with a 3.2-mm fiberoptic laryngoscope (ENT-30PIII; Machida Endoscope Co., Ltd., Tokyo, Japan), positioned so that the region of the arytenoid cartilages and the vocal folds were fully visible. In addition, we attempted to keep variations in the angle and distance of recording to a minimum. To that end, the otolaryngologist held the fiberoptic laryngoscope between the thumb and middle finger, with the index finger resting on the tip of the nose of the individual being examined (Figure 1).

The fiberoptic laryngoscope was connected to a charge-coupled device camera (IK-M41A; Toshiba, Tokyo, Japan), and the images were recorded on videotape with an NTSC videocassette recorder (NV-FS90; Panasonic Corporation, Osaka, Japan). The images were digitized on a computer (Inspiron 1525; Dell, Inc., Round Rock, TX, USA) equipped with a 1.73-GHz Pentium Duo CPU T2370 processor (Intel Corporation, Santa Clara, CA, USA), 2 GB of RAM, and a 32-bit operating system. In order to digitize the images, we used a video capture card (PCTV Pro USB; Avid Technology, Inc., Burlington, MA, USA) and the program Studio QuickStart, version 10.8 (Pinnacle/Avid Technology, Inc., Burlington, MA,

USA). The digitized images were analyzed frame by frame, and, for each individual, we obtained photographs of the following phonations at their peak amplitudes:

- low intensity—sustained vowel /ɛ/, 5 photographs; lip trills, 3 photographs; and tongue trills, 3 photographs
- high intensity—sustained vowel /ɛ/, 5 photographs; lip trills, 3 photographs; and tongue trills, 3 photographs

The photos were edited with Adobe Photoshop CS2 software, version 9.0 (Adobe Systems Incorporated, San Jose, CA, USA), which allowed better visualization of the amplitude of vocal fold vibration, as well as of the limits of the region of the right arytenoid cartilage (Figures 2a and 2b).

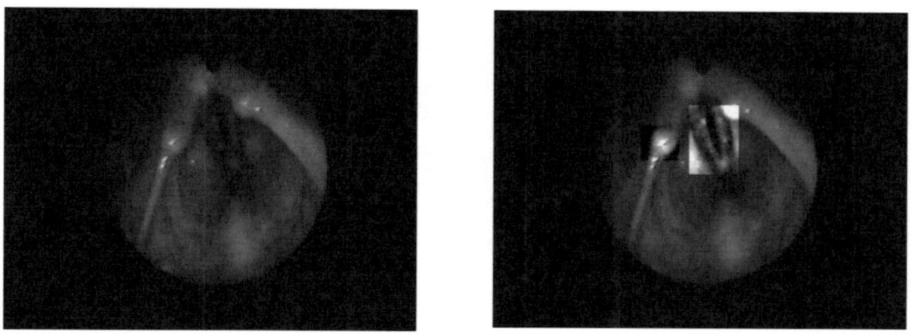

a b

Fig. 2. Photograph of the maximum amplitude of vocal fold vibration during lip trills. In a, unedited image; and in b, edited image.

In order to measure the maximum amplitude of vibration, we imported the edited images into the program X-Cade, version 2.0, specifically designed for the present study by Dr. Arlindo Neto Montagnoli, an engineer at the Federal University of São Carlos School of Electrical Engineering, located in the city of São Carlos, Brazil. Measurements were taken from a total of 220 photographs.

In order to reduce the number of measurement errors caused by variations in the position of the fiberoptic laryngoscope, we also measured the length of the anatomical structure near the arytenoid region. The structure is a cuneiform cartilage covered by the arytenoid mucosa and was used as a reference for comparison. That structure was chosen because its configuration is not changed by the phonation task being performed. We first measured the largest diameter of the abovementioned structure, which the software automatically converted into a comparative reference that was used in order to measure the amplitude of vocal fold vibration. Therefore, when we refer to the amplitude of vocal fold vibration as being 0.5, this means that the amplitude value corresponds to half the measurement of the region corresponding to the cuneiform cartilage (Figure 3).

All of the measurements were taken in a blinded fashion by the same rater, who, for each individual evaluated, adopted the following self-calibration method: before considering a measurement to be valid, the rater measured the images obtained from a given individual several times until the measurements taken from the same image were within two decimal places of each other. The images from each individual were measured without interruption. Otherwise, the calibration process was restarted, and the measurements were taken again. The data were tabulated and entered into a database for subsequent statistical analysis.

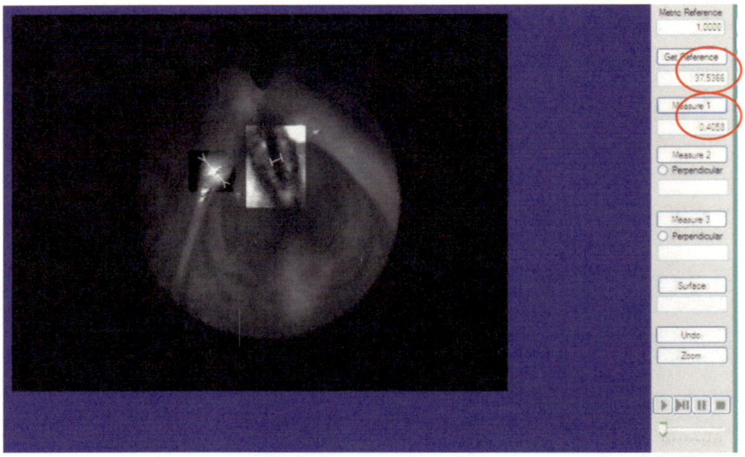

Fig. 3. X-Cade software. The amplitude measurement corresponds to 0.4 of the measurement of the arytenoid cartilage.

2.3.2.2 EGG

In order to measure the EGG signal, we referred the individuals to a sound-treated booth in a quiet room in the CEFAC Voice and Speech Laboratory. We used an EG2-Standard electroglottograph (Glottal Enterprises, Syracuse, NY, USA). The electroglottograph was connected to a computer audio interface (BCA2000; MUSIC Group Services EU GmbH, Willich, Germany), which was in turn connected to a computer equipped with a 1.66-GB Centron processor (Advanced Micro Devices, Inc., Sunnyvale, CA, USA).

The individuals were asked to remove any metal objects that they might be wearing in the head and neck region and to sit upright in a chair equipped with a headrest. To ensure the safety of the individuals, we placed a rubber mat under the chair. The neck region was cleaned with dry paper towel. We applied a thin layer of hypoallergenic electrically conductive gel (SPECTRA 360®; Parker Laboratories, Inc., Fairfield, NJ, USA) to the electrodes, which were placed over each ala of the thyroid cartilage and secured with a Velcro strap around the neck. To ensure that the electrodes were positioned correctly, we asked the participants to produce the sustained vowel and perform tongue trills. We then observed whether the green LEDs of the top LED array (Electrode Placement/Laryngeal Movement) on the front panel of the electroglottograph were on. To confirm that there was signal, we observed whether the green LEDs of the bottom LED array (Signal) were on. To record the signal, we selected the Vocal Fold Contact Area signal option, and high or low gain was determined by monitoring the LED signal indicator. The signal was saved as a .wav file and edited with the audio editing suite Sound Forge, version 7.0, (Sony Creative Software, Inc., Middleton, WI, USA) at a sampling frequency of 22,050 Hz and a resolution of 16 bits.

The EGG waveforms were submitted to high band-pass filtering with the program delay0.bat, designed by Maurílio Nunes Vieira, an engineer at the Federal University of Minas Gerais, located in the city of Belo Horizonte, Brazil. The waveforms were initially graded by two speech-language pathologists with experience in EGG and one engineer, in accordance with the grading system proposed by Vieira (1997):

- grade 1, free from gross errors
- grade 2, as accurate as possible
- grade 3, able to trace signals with irregular excitation
- grade 4, able to locate every individual glottal stop

Only grade 1 and grade 2 waveforms were included in the study. In order to take automatic measurements, we used the technique developed by Vieira (1997). We assessed the mean and standard deviation of the closed quotient for each task.

The closed quotient is the ratio between the closed phase and the complete cycle of the EGG waveform (Figure 4). The mean closed quotient is the measurement of each EGG waveform divided by the number of waveforms analyzed by the software. The standard deviation is the variation in that measurement over time.

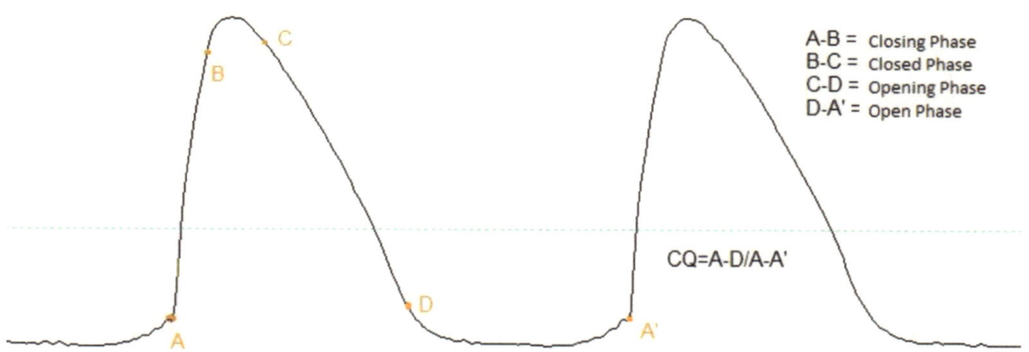

Fig. 4. Phases of the EGG waveform and the closed quotient (CQ).

2.4 Statistical analysis

In order to analyze the results, we adopted a level of significance of 5% ($p = 0.05$) for all statistical tests. The Statistical Package for the Social Sciences, version 13.0 (SPSS Inc., Chicago, IL, USA) was used for the analysis. In order to determine the differences among phonation of the sustained vowel /ɛ/, lip trills, and tongue trills, we used Friedman's test.

For the cases in which the difference was statistically significant, we used the Wilcoxon signed rank test in order to identify the types that differed.

For the presentation of the results, the measurements taken automatically by the program were considered to constitute the intraindividual means and standard deviations, whereas the values obtained by statistical analysis of those results were considered to constitute the interindividual means and standard deviations.

3. Results

3.1 Videolaryngostroboscopy

During videolaryngostroboscopy, it was occasionally difficult to synchronize the stroboscopic illumination with the vocal fold vibration during lip and tongue trills. Therefore, during those tasks, we photographed only those moments of the cycles at which the maximum opening was evident. During the phonation of the sustained vowel /ε/ task, we encountered no such difficulty.

Although the otolaryngologist maintained the fiberoptic laryngoscope in position, laryngeal movement caused variations in the distance between the larynx and the laryngoscope, which in turn caused variations in the images of the larynx. Among the 220 images analyzed in the present study, the larynx was too far from the laryngoscope in 163 (74%). Of the remaining 57 images (26%), 11 (5%) were images of sustained vowel phonation, 19 (9%) were images of lip trills, and 27 (12%) were images of tongue trills. The measurements of vocal fold vibration amplitude are presented in Tables 3 through 6 and illustrated in Figures 5 and 6.

3.1.1 Low intensity

Variable	N	Vibration amplitude					p
		Mean	SD	Minimum	Maximum	Median	
/ε/	10	0.11	0.03	0.06	0.16	0.11	
Lip trills	10	0.17	0.06	0.10	0.32	0.16	0.002*
Tngue trills	10	0.15	0.04	0.08	0.21	0.16	

*Friedman's test, among all three variables

Table 3. Maximum amplitude of vocal fold vibration during phonation of the sustained vowel /ε/ compared with that of vocal fold vibration during tongue and lip trills at low intensity

Pair	p*
Lip trills versus sustained vowel /ɛ/ phonation	0.007
Tongue trills versus sustained vowel /ɛ/ phonation	0.005
Tongue trills versus lip trills	0.677

*Wilcoxon signed rank test

Table 4. Pairwise comparisons among phonation of the sustained vowel /ɛ/, lip trills, and tongue trills at low intensity in terms of the amplitude of vocal fold vibration

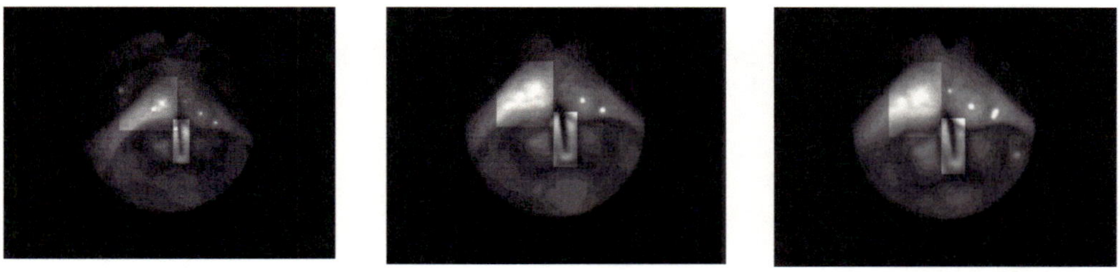

a 0.08 b 0.11 c 0.12

Fig. 5. Maximum amplitude of vocal fold vibration during phonation tasks at low intensity in relation to the cuneiform cartilage, as assessed by videolaryngostroboscopy. In a, phonation of the sustained vowel /ɛ/; in b, sustained lip trills; and in c, sustained tongue trills.

3.1.2 High intensity

Variable	N	Vibration amplitude					P
		Mean	SD	Minimum	Maximum	Median	
/ɛ/	10	0.16	0.05	0.11	0.30	0.15	
Lip trills	10	0.29	0.08	0.16	0.40	0.30	0.001*
Tongue trills	10	0.26	0.12	0.15	0.50	0.21	

*Friedman's test, among all three variables

Table 5. Maximum amplitude of vocal fold vibration during phonation of the sustained vowel /ɛ/ compared with that of vocal fold vibration during tongue and lip trills at high intensity

Pair	p*
Lip trills versus sustained vowel /ɛ/ phonation	0.005
Tongue trills versus sustained vowel /ɛ/ phonation	0.005
Tongue trills versus lip trills	0.308

*Wilcoxon signed rank test

Table 6. Pairwise comparisons among phonation of the sustained vowel /ɛ/, lip trills, and tongue trills at high intensity in terms of the amplitude of vocal fold vibration

The values obtained during phonation of the sustained vowel /ɛ/ were significantly different from those obtained during lip and tongue trills at high and low intensities ($p > 0.01$). The statistical tests revealed that the maximum amplitude of vocal fold vibration during phonation of the sustained vowel /ɛ/ was significantly different from that of vocal fold vibration during lip and tongue trills. However, there were no significant differences between lip and tongue trills in terms of the maximum amplitude of vocal fold vibration.

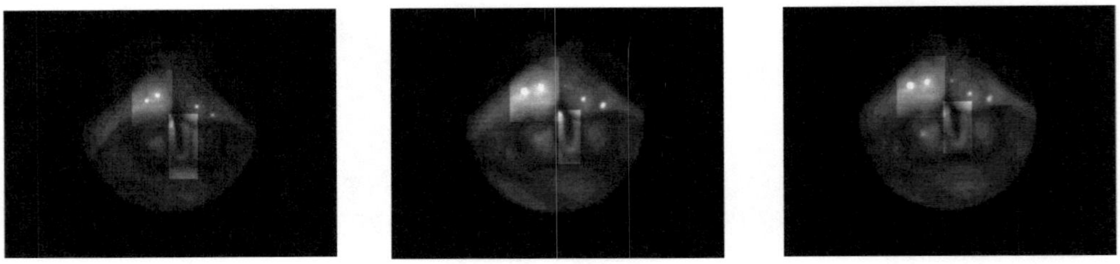

a 0.12 b 0.19 c 0.22

Fig. 6. Maximum amplitude of vocal fold vibration during phonation tasks at high intensity in relation to the cuneiform cartilage, as assessed by videolaryngostroboscopy. In a, phonation of the sustained vowel /ɛ/; in b, sustained tongue trills; and in c, lip trills.

3.2 EGG – Closed quotient

All of the EGG waveforms were either grade 1 or grade 2 in accordance with the criteria proposed by Vieira (1997) and were therefore appropriate for automatic measurements.

The measurements taken automatically by the program for analysis of the EGG waveform were considered to constitute the intraindividual means and standard deviations of the closed quotient. Those values were considered the study variables and placed on the vertical axes of the tables. The interindividual means and standard deviations of the closed quotient were obtained by statistical analysis and were placed on the horizontal axes of the tables.

Tables 7 through 10 show the results related to the intraindividual means and standard deviations of the closed quotient.

3.2.1 Low intensity

Measurement	Task	N	Mean	SD	Minimum	Maximum	Median	p*
Intraindividual mean of the closed quotient	/ε/	10	47.72	12.27	31.87	67.27	51.64	0.301
	lip trills	10	50.97	12.96	33.93	71.48	53.36	
	tongue trills	10	52.25	9.55	37.50	67.76	54.43	
Intraindividual SD of the closed quotient	/ε/	10	3.12	3.40	0.88	12.18	1.99	0.020
	lip trills	10	6.55	3.12	3.86	12.63	5.34	
	tongue trills	10	7.63	4.41	2.09	13.85	6.54	

*Friedman's test

Table 7. Closed quotient: number of samples, mean, standard deviation, minimum value, maximum value, median, and significance of the differences among phonation of the sustained vowel /ε/, lip trills, and tongue trills at low intensity

Measurement	Pairs	p*
Intraindividual SD of the closed quotient	Lip trills versus sustained vowel /ε/ phonation	0.059
	Tongue trills versus sustained vowel /ε/ phonation	0.037
	Tongue trills versus lip trills	0.508

*Wilcoxon signed rank test

Table 8. Pairwise comparisons among phonation of the sustained vowel /ε/, lip trills, and tongue trills at low intensity in terms of the automatic measurements of significant values

3.2.2 High intensity

Measurement	Task	N	Mean	SD	Minimum	Maximum	Median	p*
Intraindividual mean of the closed quotient	/ε/	10	50.71	6.90	36.47	56.07	54.52	0.007
	lip trills	10	59.21	12.57	42.85	82.73	54.68	
	tongue trills	10	54.60	9.72	40.63	72.56	52.52	
Intraindividual SD of the closed quotient	/ε/	10	1.62	0.84	0.77	3.17	1.39	0.020
	lip trills	10	6.64	5.36	1.21	15.48	4.23	
	tongue trills	10	4.75	2.78	1.68	9.50	4.15	

*Friedman's test

Table 9. Automatic measurements, as taken by EGG: number of samples, mean, standard deviation, minimum value, maximum value, median, and significance of the differences among phonation of the sustained vowel /ε/, lip trills, and tongue trills at high intensity

Measurement	Pairs	p*
Intraindividual mean of the closed quotient	Lip trills versus sustained vowel /ε/ phonation	0.013
	Tongue trills versus sustained vowel /ε/ phonation	0.139
	Tongue trills versus lip trills	0.017
Intraindividual SD of the closed quotient	Lip trills versus sustained vowel /ε/ phonation	0.017
	Tongue trills versus sustained vowel /ε/ phonation	0.013
	Tongue trills versus lip trills	0.114

*Wilcoxon signed rank test

Table 10. Pairwise comparisons among phonation of the sustained vowel /ε/, lip trills, and tongue trills at high intensity in terms of the automatic measurements of significant values

4. Discussion

Our results show that, in general, tongue trills and lip trills were similar in terms of the amplitude of vocal fold vibration. However, there were differences between tongue trills and vowel /ε/ phonation, as well as between lip trills and vowel /ε/ phonation, in terms of the amplitude of vocal fold vibration.

We measured the largest diameter of the region corresponding to the cuneiform cartilage as a reference to the maximum amplitude of vocal fold vibration in order to make the measurements more reliable. The individuals were their own controls, and the amplitude of vocal fold vibration was expressed as a fraction of the cuneiform cartilage size in order to reduce potential errors caused by movement of the laryngoscope and larynx during videolaryngostroboscopy.

Other studies have employed a similar methodology, having used the distance between the anterior commissure and the vocal process as a reference (Omori *et al.*, 1996; Tsuji *et al.*, 2003). We were unable to use that measurement in our study because we noted a change in glottal configuration during tongue trills, as reported in a study by Bueno (2006), who observed anteroposterior constriction of the laryngeal vestibule, without medialization or vibration of the vestibular vocal fold, during tongue trills.

The proximity of the distal end of the laryngoscope to the larynx can generate barrel distortion of linearity (Lee, 1980). In that type of distortion, the proportion of the measurements in the center of the image (represented in the present study as the vibration amplitude measurement) is smaller than is that of those in the periphery (represented as the cuneiform cartilage measurement) for the same millimetric measurement (Lee, 1980). Of the 220 images analyzed in the present study, 163 (74%) were indicative that the laryngoscope was far enough from the larynx to avoid that type of distortion. Of the images that were indicative that the laryngoscope was closer to the larynx and that could therefore show distortion, 21% (46/220) were obtained during the trill exercises and 5% (11/220) were obtained during the sustained vowel phonation task.

We believe that those distortions were not enough to interfere with the present study, given that the amplitude of vocal fold vibration was greater during the trill exercises than during the sustained vowel phonation task, even when the image was indicative that the laryngoscope was close to the larynx.

There were significant differences among phonation of the sustained vowel /ɛ/, lip trills, and tongue trills in terms of the maximum amplitude of vocal fold vibration at low and high intensities ($p = 0.002$ and $p = 0.001$, respectively). The Wilcoxon signed rank test revealed significant differences between lip trills and phonation of the sustained vowel /ɛ/, as well as between tongue trills and phonation of the sustained vowel /ɛ/.

For the performance of lip trills and tongue trills, pulmonary airflow has to increase in order to maintain vocal fold vibration and lip or tongue vibration (Titze, 2009; Warren *et al.*, 1992; Titze 1988, McGowan, 1992). The increase in airflow can lead to an increase in subglottic pressure, which can in turn lead to an increase in the amplitude of vocal fold vibration (Garrel *et al.*, 2008; Titze, 2009).

In the present study, during the measurement of amplitude, it was difficult to synchronize the flashes of light from the stroboscope with the vocal fold vibration during lip and tongue trills in some cases. We had no such difficulty when we measured the amplitude of vocal fold vibration during phonation of the sustained vowel /ɛ/. Therefore, during lip trills and tongue trills, we photographed only those moments of the cycles at which the maximum opening was visible.

Increased airflow can also lead to aperiodicity of vocal fold vibration (Jiang, 2001; Tao, 2007) and can destabilize the flashes of light from the stroboscope (Sercarz *et al.*, 1992). In previous studies, we found that the standard deviation of the intraindividual closed quotient was highest during lip trills and tongue trills, the values being higher at high intensities, which is due to increased airflow (Russell *et al.*, 1998; Alku, 2006). Those results might indicate differences in the periodicity of the EGG waveform during trill exercises and corroborate the abovementioned hypothesis.

Bueno (2006) observed pronounced movement of the laryngeal framework during tongue trills; such movement can make it difficult for the contact microphone to pick up the fundamental frequency. Because the cycles observed under the stroboscopic light are not the actual vocal fold vibration cycles, which require regularity in order to generate reliable images (Sercarz *et al.*, 1992; Patel *et al.*, 2008), a study involving a high-speed camera would be needed in order to have a better view of vocal fold vibration during tongue and lip trills. To that end, a device that is compatible with the laryngoscope is needed. Studies involving a qualitative analysis of both the periodicity of the EGG waveform and the amplitude of the EGG signal could also be useful in the investigation of the mechanism of vocal fold vibration during trill exercises.

The standard deviation of the closed quotient is a numerical representation of the variation in the closed quotient in the EGG waveform. Because the standard deviation of the closed quotient was higher during the trill exercises (at high or low intensity) in the present study, we can affirm that the variation in the closed quotient is greater during trill exercises than during phonation of the sustained vowel /ɛ/.

For tongue trills and lip trills to occur, the anterior part of the vocal tract has to be occluded by the tongue or the lips. Intraoral pressure increases and becomes greater than the force that maintains the anterior part of the vocal tract closed; therefore, the anterior part of the vocal tract opens and is "sucked out" by the speed of the airflow (McGowan, 1992), closing the vibration cycle, as occurs in the vocal fold vibration model. Therefore, supraglottic pressure and, consequently, vocal tract impedance oscillate.

The theory of source-filter interaction (Titze, 2008; Titze *et al.*, 2008) states that the acoustic pressure in the vocal tract changes the phonation threshold pressure and interferes with vocal fold vibration. The theory of source-filter interaction states that, when the vibratory motion of the point of articulation makes the acoustic pressure in the vocal tract oscillate, the phonation threshold pressure also oscillates, which might explain why the standard deviation of the closed quotient was higher during trill exercises in the present study.

According to Titze (2006), the objective of voice training is to promote the interaction between the source and the filter and therefore increase vocal intensity, efficiency, and economy (Titze, 2006). According to the author, lip trills and tongue trills are among the semi-occluded vocal tract exercises. Because semi-occluded vocal tract exercises promote a mechanical interaction between the source and the filter (Titze, 2008; Titze *et al.*, 2008) they change vocal fold impedance and therefore inhibit vocal fold vibration (Story *et al.*, 2000).

Vocal tract pressure during voiced fricatives must be constant, which distinguishes voiced fricatives from the exercises analyzed in the present study. New clinical studies comparing the two types of exercises should be conducted.

In our studies, the mean closed quotient was highest during lip trills at high intensity, which distinguished lip trills from tongue trills and phonation of the sustained vowel /ɛ/. According to the literature (Story *et al.*, 2000; Titze, 2006), a more anterior obstruction translates to greater vocal tract impedance. Although lip trills are slightly more anterior than are tongue trills, the influence of supraglottic and subglottic pressure on vocal fold vibration is not linear (Zhang, 2009; Titze, 2008; Hatzikirou *et al.*, 2006, Titze, 2008), meaning that the airflow changes caused by increased intensity can lead to different vocal fold vibration proportions and differentiate between high- and low-intensity vibrations (Tao *et al.*, 2007; Becker *et al.*, 2009).

Gaskill and Erikson (2008) found systematic differences between the closed quotient of lip trills and that of phonation of the sustained vowel /ɛ/; as we did in the present study, the authors argued that those differences might be due to the interaction between the source and the filter. In addition, the authors found differences between trained and untrained individuals in terms of the results obtained; the differences were attributed to the fact that trained individuals have better control over glottic closure.

Some authors have reported that the sound produced by the larynx is not linear (Jing *et all*, 2001) and depends on numerous factors. Therefore, any difference in biomechanics, structure (such as tissue geometry, density, and viscosity), airflow control, or vocal tract control can cause differences in vocal fold vibration. Trained individuals have more control over those factors, and this can actually result in differences between trained and untrained individuals, as well as between trained individuals and patients with morphological changes in the vocal folds, in terms of vocal fold vibration during a given phonation task.

Because patients with vocal fold pathologies present with structural changes (and, consequently, biomechanical changes), trill exercises probably produce different effects in those individuals than in individuals without morphological changes. According to the literature, bulging caused by vocal fold pathologies interfere with glottal flow resistance, glottal width, glottal area, and mean glottal volume velocity (Alipour & Scherer, 2000).

Studies involving vocal exercises (including tongue and lip trills) in various settings should be conducted in order to provide a deeper understanding of the physiology of vocal exercises in each of those situations and therefore assist speech-language pathologists in prescribing the exercises. The present study can support some of the theories that underlie the use of trill exercises in the clinical practice of speech-language pathology, as well as in the voice training of professional voice users. According to McGowan (1996), the variations that occur in the pharynx during lip trills can increase the force of mucosal vibration during the wavelike motion of the vocal folds.

The greater amplitude of mucosal vibration and the higher standard deviation of the closed quotient during trill exercises reflect changes in the wavelike motion of the vocal folds; this can explain, at least in part, the improvement in voice quality (Rodrigues, 1995) after the use of those exercises, as well as warranting the use of trill exercises in patients with vocal fold pathologies, such as nodules (Bueno, 2006), edema (Pinho e Pontes, 2008), and sulci. The probable need for airflow control and the source-filter interaction caused by the articulatory oscillation warrant the use of trill exercises during the training of professional voice users, as recommended by Aydos and Hanayama (2004) and Nix (1999).

However, further studies are needed in order to provide a deeper understanding of the effects of trill exercises on the vocal fold mucosa. To that end, a more in-depth analysis of the EGG waveform and, if possible, videolaryngostroboscopy with a high-speed camera are warranted.

For a better understanding of the effect of trill exercises and their indications, studies analyzing the blood flow in the region and the mechanics of laryngeal and vocal tract muscles during the exercises are needed.

5. Conclusion

On the basis of our results, we can conclude that, in professional singers, the maximum amplitude of vocal fold vibration is greater during lip and tongue trills than during natural phonation. In addition, we observed considerable variation in the closed quotient during the exercises employed. Lip trills differed from tongue trills only at higher intensities and in terms of the closed quotient.

6. References

Alku P.; Airas M.; Bjorkner E. & Sundberg J. (2006) An amplitude quotient based method to analyze changes in the shape of the glottal pulse in the regulation of vocal intensity. *J Acoust Soc Am.* 120(2):1052-62. ISSN 0001-4966

Aydos B & Hanayama M (2004). Técnicas de aquecimento vocal utilizadas por professores de teatro. *Rev CEFAC*: 6(1): 83-8. ISSN 1516-1846.

Becker S; Kniesburges S; Muller S; Delgado A; Link G; Kaltenbacher M, et al. (2009). Flow-structure-acoustic interaction in a human voice model. *J Acoust Soc Am*;125(3):1351-61. ISSN 0001-4966

Behlau M & Pontes P (1995). *Avaliação e tratamento das disfonias*: Editora Lovise. Rio de Janeiro. ISBN 8585274263

Bueno TC (2006). *Técnica de vibração sonorizada de língua: aspectos do aprendizado, dos efeitos acústicos e das imagens do trato vocal e da face* [mestrado]. São Paulo PUC-São Paulo; 2006.

Casper J; Colton R; Woo P & Brewer D. (1994) Physiological characteristics of selected voice therapy techniques: a preliminary research note. *British Voice Assoc*;1:131-41. 3873295.

Cordeiro GF; Montagnoli AN; Nemr NK; Menezes MHM & Tsuji DH. Comparative analysis of the closed quotient for lip and tongue trill in relation to the sustained vowel /ɛ/. *J Voice*. In Prelo. ISSN 0892-1997.

Garrel R; Scherer R; Nicollas R; Giovanni A & Ouaknine M (2008). Using the relaxation oscillations principle for simple phonation modeling. *J Voice*. 22:385-98. ISSN 0892-1997

Gaskill CS & Erickson ML. (2008) The effect of a voiced lip trill on estimated glottal closed quotient. *J Voice*.22(6):634-43. ISSN 0892-1997

Gregio FN. (2006) Configuração do trato vocal supraglótico na produção das vogais do Português: dados de imagem de ressonância magnética [Mestrado]. São Paulo: PUC-SP; 2006.

Hatzikirou H; Fitch WT & Herzel H. (2006) Voice Instabilities due to Source-Tract Interactions. *Acta acustica united with acustica* 92 468 – 75.

Jiang JJ, Zhang Y, Stern J. (2001) Modeling of chaotic vibrations in symmetric vocal folds. J *Acoust Soc Am*. 110(4):2120-8. ISSN 0001-4966

Lee KH. (1980) Quantitative assessment of linearity of scintillation cameras. *Radiology*. 136(3):790-2. ISSN 1527-1315.

Linklater K (1976). *Freeing the natural voice*. New York: Drama Book. ISBN 9780-0896760714.

Maniecka-Aleksandrowicz B; Domeracka-Kolodziej A; Rozak-Komorowska A & Szeptycka-Adamus A. (2006)Management and therapy in functional aphonia: analysis of 500 cases. *Otolaryngol Pol*. 2006;60(2):191-7. ISSN 0030-6657

McGowan RS. (1992) Tongue-tip trills and vocal-tract wall compliance. *J Acoust Soc Am*. 91(5):2903-10. ISSN 0001-4966.

Menezes MH; Duprat AC & Costa HO (2005). Vocal and laryngeal effects of voiced tongue vibration technique according to performance time. *J Voice* 22(5): 565-80. ISSN 0892-1997.

Nix J. (1999) Lip Trills and Raspberries: "High Spit Factor" Alternatives to the Nasal Continuant Consoants *Journal of Singing*.55(3):15-9. ISSN 1086-7732.

Omori K; Kacker A; Slavit DH & Blaugrund SM (1996). Quantitative videostroboscopic measurement of glottal gap and vocal function: an analysis of thyroplasty type I. *Ann Otol Rhinol Laryngol.* 105(4):280-5. ISSN 0196-0709.

Patel R; Dailey S & Bless D. (2008) Comparison of high-speed digital imaging with stroboscopy for laryngeal imaging of glottal disorders. *Ann Otol Rhinol Laryngol.* 117(6):413-24. . ISSN 0196-0709.

Pinho SM; Tsuji DH & Bohadana SC (2006) *Tratamento fonoaudiológico das disfonias dirigidos à fonocirurgia.* In: Pinho SM, Tsuji DH, S.C B, editors. Fundamentos em Laringologia e Voz. Rio de Janeiro: Revinter; p. 69 – 84. ISBN 9788573099879.

Rodrigues MRC. (2001) Estudo do exercício de vibração sonorizada de língua nas laringectomias frontolaterais. [Mestrado]. São Paulo: PUC-São Paulo.

Rodrigues S. (1995) Análise múltipla do efeito da técnica de vibração sonorizada de língua em indivíduos adultos sem queixa vocal. [Mestrado]. São Paulo: Universidade Federal de São Paulo.

Russell BA; Cerny FJ & Stathopoulos ET. (1998) Effects of varied vocal intensity on ventilation and energy expenditure in women and men. *J Speech Lang Hear Res.* 41(2):239-48. ISSN 1558-9192.

Sataloff RT (1991). *Professional Voice: The science and art of clinical care.* New York: Raven Press ISBN 1565937287.

Schneider SL & Sataloff RT (2007). Voice therapy for the professional voice. *Otolaringol Clin N Am* 40 1133-49. ISSN 030-6665.

Schwarz K & Cielo CA (2009) Vocal and larybgeal modifications produced by the sonorous tongue vibration techinique. *Pro Fono* 21(2): 161:6. ISSN 0104-5687

Sercarz JA, Berke GS, Gerratt BR, Kreiman J, Ming Y, Natividad M (1992). Synchronizing videostroboscopic images of human laryngeal vibration with physiological signals. *Am J Otolaryngol.* 13(1):40-4. ISSN 0196-0709.

Speyer R. (2008) Effects of voice therapy: a systematic review. *J Voice.* 22:565-80. ISSN 0892-1997

Story BH; Laukkanen AM & Titze IR. (2000) Acoustic impedance of an artificially lengthened and constricted vocal tract. *J Voice.* 14(4):455-69. ISSN 0892-1997.

Story BH; Titze IR & Hoffman EA. (1998) Vocal tract area functions for an adult female speaker based on volumetric imaging. *J Acoust Soc Am* 104(1):471-87. ISSN 0001-4966.

Tao C; Zhang Y; Hottinger DG & Jiang JJ. (2007) Asymmetric airflow and vibration induced by the Coanda effect in a symmetric model of the vocal folds. *J Acoust Soc Am.* 122(4):2270-8. ISSN 0001-4966.

Titze IR. (2006) Voice training and therapy with a semi-occluded vocal tract: rationale and scientific underpinnings. *J Speech Lang Hear Res.* 49(2):448-59. ISSN 1558-9192.

Titze IR. (2009) Phonation threshold pressure measurement with a semi-occluded vocal tract. *J Speech Lang Hear Res.* 52(4):1062-72. ISSN 1558-9192

Tsuji DH; de Almeida ER; Sennes LU; Butugan O & Pinho SM. (2003) Comparison between thyroplasty type I and arytenoid rotation: a study of vocal fold vibration using excised human larynges. *J Voice.* 17(4):596-604. ISSN 0892-1997.

Vieira MN; McInnes FR & Jack MA. (1997) Comparative assessment of electroglottographic and acoustic measures of jitter in pathological voices. *J Speech Lang Hear Res.* 40(1):170-82. ISSN 1558-9192

Warren DW; Rochet AP; Dalston RM & Mayo R. (1992) Controlling changes in vocal tract resistance. *J Acoust Soc Am.* 91(5):2947-53. ISSN 0001-4966

Woo P; Casper J; Colton R & Brewer D. (1994) Diagnosis and treatment of persistent dysphonia after laryngeal surgery: a retrospective analysis of 62 patients. *Laryngoscope.* 104(9):1084-91. ISSN 1531-4995

Zhang Z. (2009) Characteristics of phonation onset in a two-layer vocal fold model. *J Acoust Soc Am.* 125(2):1091-102. ISSN 0001-4966

Section 4

Head and Neck

9

Microtubule and Cdc42 are the Main Targets of Docetaxel's Suppression of Invasiveness of Head and Neck Cancer Cells

Yasunao Kogashiwa[1], Hiroyuki Sakurai[2] and Naoyuki Kohno[1]
[1]*Department of Otorhinolaryngology, Head and Neck Surgery, Kyorin University School of Medicine,*
[2]*Department of Pharmacology and Toxicology, Kyorin University School of Medicine, Japan*

1. Introduction

Many squamous cell carcinoma (SCC) of the head and neck presents with locally advanced disiease. In such cases, a combination chemotherapy of docetaxel, cisplatin, and 5FU, followed by radiation improved their survival (Posner et al. 2007; Vermorken et al. 2007). That is, addition of docetaxel to the combination of cisplatin and fluorouracil improves survival in head and neck squamous cell carcinoma. In a recent work to elucidate the possible mechanism, we investigated the effect of docetaxel on cell movement using head and neck cancer cell lines Hep2 and Ca9-22. Docetaxel treatment suppressed migration and invasiveness of head and neck cancer cells in vitro. We investigated the downstream effectors that control invasiveness after docetaxel administration in the present work.

2. IC_{10} and IC_{50} in HEp-2 and Ca9-22 cells

We used the same IC_{10} and IC_{50} concentrations (Table 1) (Kogashiwa et al. 2010) as our previous study. At IC_{10} concentrations, anti-proliferative effect was not observed.

Cell line		IC_{10}	IC_{50}
HEp-2	Cisplatin	2 μM	20 μM
	Docetaxel	5 nM	23 nM
Ca9-22	Cisplatin	10 μM	40 μM
	Docetaxel	6 nM	11 nM

Table 1 IC_{10} or IC_{50} values in two cells
IC_{10} or IC_{50} values after 1 hour drug exposure followed by a 96 hours incubation in two head and neck cell lines.

3. Docetaxel inhibits the migration of head and neck cancer cells

To assess cell migration a wound healing assay was employed. These results have been reported (Kogashiwa et al. 2010). Briefly, both in HEp-2 cell and CA9-22 cell, wound closure relative to no treatment condition is significantly reduced in docetaxel treatment while cisplatin treatment does not affect the cell migration (Fig.1.) (Kogashiwa et al. 2010).

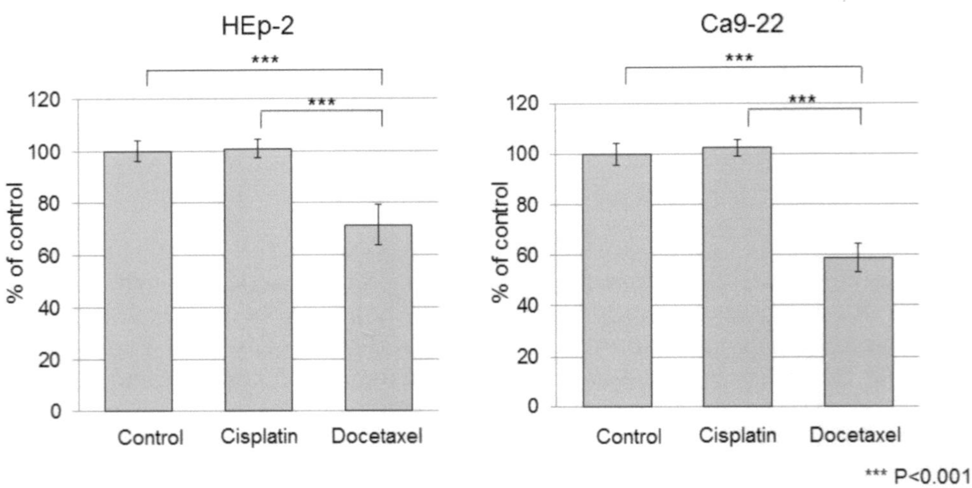

Fig. 1. Migration assay at IC10 in two head and neck cancer cell lines.
Migration rate is compared to control cell migration rate. Each data point represents mean ± SE. ***p < 0.001. 15 replicate were used in each experiments and experiments were repeated 4 times.

4. Docetaxel inhibits the invasiveness of multicellular tumor spheroids.

The similar results are obtained in three-dimensional multicellular tumor spheroid culture (Kogashiwa et al. 2010). At IC_{10} determined in monolayer culture, either cisplatin or docetaxel does not affect filopodia formation. However, at IC_{50} determined in monolayer culture, docetaxel, but not cisplatin, significantly decreases filopodia formation in HEp-2 cells in spheroid culture (Fig.2.) (Kogashiwa et al. 2010). Taken together, In the previous study, we have shown that docetaxel, but not cisplatin inhibits cell migration both in 2D and 3D culture.

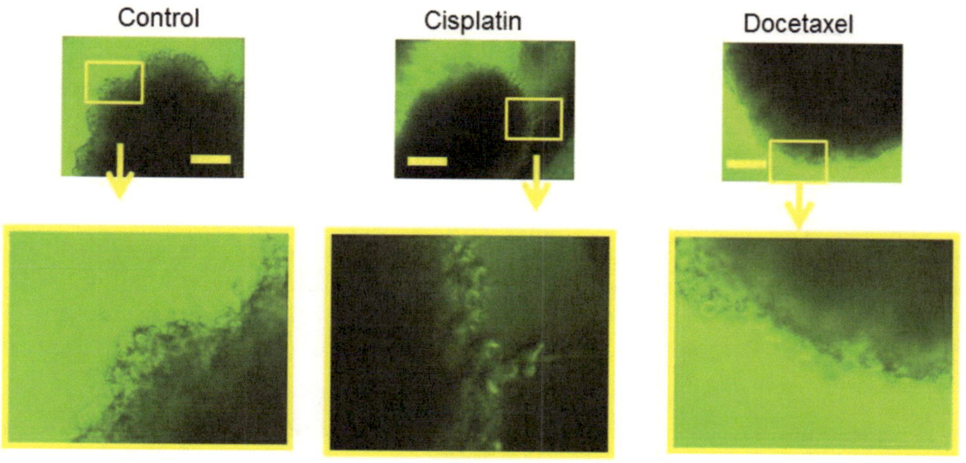

Fig. 2. 3D gel culture of HEp-2 cell spheroids at IC50 concentration.
HEp-2 cell spheroids were treated with cisplatin or docetaxel at IC50 followed by 96-hour incubation. bars= 250 μm. 4 replicate were used in each experiments and experiments were repeated 4 times.

5. Tubulin bundle was formed by docetaxel treatment

Taxanes, including docetaxel, function as a mitotic spindle toxin by inhibiting microtubule turnover. They bind to microtubules and enhance tubulin polymerization. We hypothesized that docetaxel may exert similar effect on cytosolic, non-centrisome associated microtubules resulting in decreased cell motility. We therefore examined the structure of microtubules as well as actin filaments. Consistent with previous observation, filopodia formation was less in docetaxel treatment compared to cisplatin treatment. But no gross abnormality was found in actin filament structure between the treatments. On the other hand, tubulin bundle formation was noted in docetaxel treatment but not in cisplatin treatment (Fig.3.). Then, we attempted to find the mechanism that connect deformed microtubule and decreased filopodia formation.

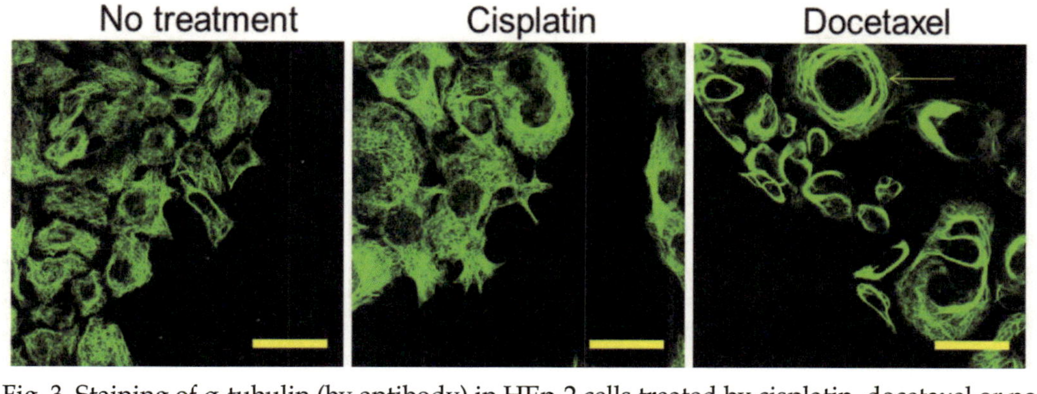

Fig. 3. Staining of α-tubulin (by antibody) in HEp-2 cells treated by cisplatin, docetaxel or no treatment at IC50. Bars=50 μm. 3 replicate were used in each experiments and experiments were repeated 4 times.

6. Docetaxel inhibited Cdc42 activity

Rho GTPases regulate many essential cellular processes, including actin dynamics, gene transcription, cell-cycle progression, cell adhesion, tumor progression and invasiveness (Hall 1998; Schmitz et al. 2000; Price et al. 2001). Among Rho-GTPases, Cdc42 is previously implicated in connecting microtubular input to actin filament organization (Cau et al. 2005). Cdc42 also promotes leading-edge extension through activation of Rac, which is implicated in formation of lamellipodia (Bishop et al. 2000). Thus, we examined activity of Cdc42, Rac and RhoA in the cells underwent cisplatin or docetaxel treatment, or no treatment. At IC_{10} concentration, docetaxel significantly decreased Cdc42 and Rac activity in HEp-2 cells, but not RhoA activity (Fig.4.; cited from (Kogashiwa et al. 2010) with modification). Total amount of Cdc42, Rac and RhoA was not significantly different among these three conditions.

It is reported that Cdc42 is activated in a thin band at cell edges extending filopodia (Nalbant et al. 2004). Consistent with the results of activity assay, Cdc42 localized at the plasma membrane was decreased after docetaxel treatment at IC_{10}. Localization of Rac1 and RhoA had no apparent changes after treatment compared to control.

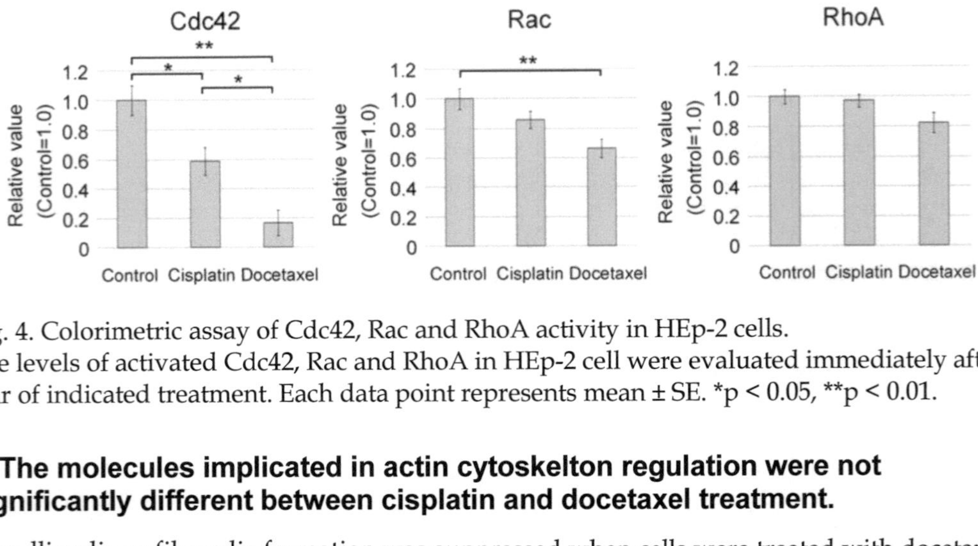

Fig. 4. Colorimetric assay of Cdc42, Rac and RhoA activity in HEp-2 cells.
The levels of activated Cdc42, Rac and RhoA in HEp-2 cell were evaluated immediately after 1 hr of indicated treatment. Each data point represents mean ± SE. $^*p < 0.05$, $^{**}p < 0.01$.

7. The molecules implicated in actin cytoskelton regulation were not significantly different between cisplatin and docetaxel treatment.

Lamellipodia or filopodia formation was suppressed when cells were treated with docetaxel (fig.5.). Ezrin/radixin/moesin (ERM) proteins link the cortical cytoskeleton to the plasma membrane. In their active conformation (i.e. phosphorylated ERM), the N-terminal ERM domain binds to the cytoplasmic tails of transmembrane proteins, and the C-terminal ERM association domain binds to actin filaments. Using a p-ERM antibody, the levels of active ERM proteins were evaluated by Western blotting after no treatment, cisplatin or docetaxel treatment at IC_{10}. There was no significant difference in the level of p-ERM among cisplatin, docetaxel and no treatment over a time course up to 48 hours (fig.6.). We also investigated the cofilin pathway as a regulator of the actin cytoskeleton. Cofilin is able to bind both G-actin and F-actin, and regulated by LIM kinase 1 and its related kinases. The levels of cofilin (fig.6.) and LIMK1 (fig.6.) were evaluated over a time course of treatment at IC_{10}. The levels of these proteins were not significantly different among cisplatin, docetaxel and no treatment, either. These results suggest that docetaxel treatment does not directly affect actin cytoskeleton remodeling.

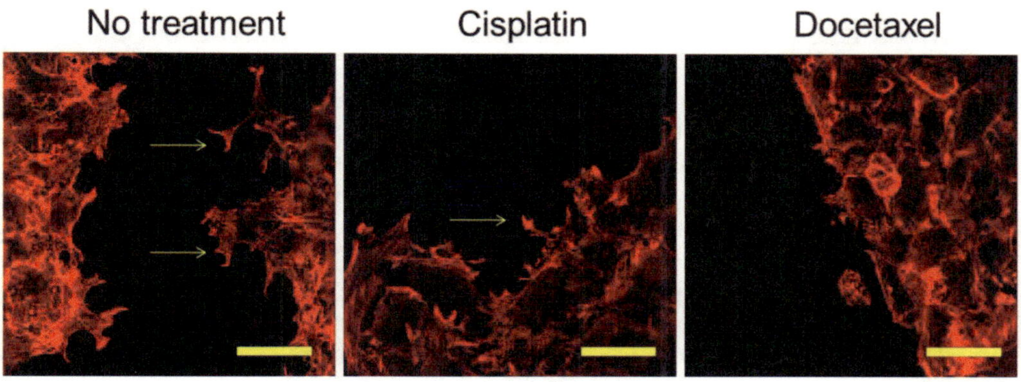

Fig. 5. Staining of F-actin (phalloidin) in HEp-2 cells treated by cisplatin, docetaxel or no treatment at IC50. Bars=50 µm. 3 replicate were used in each experiments and experiments were repeated 4 times. Arrows; filopodia

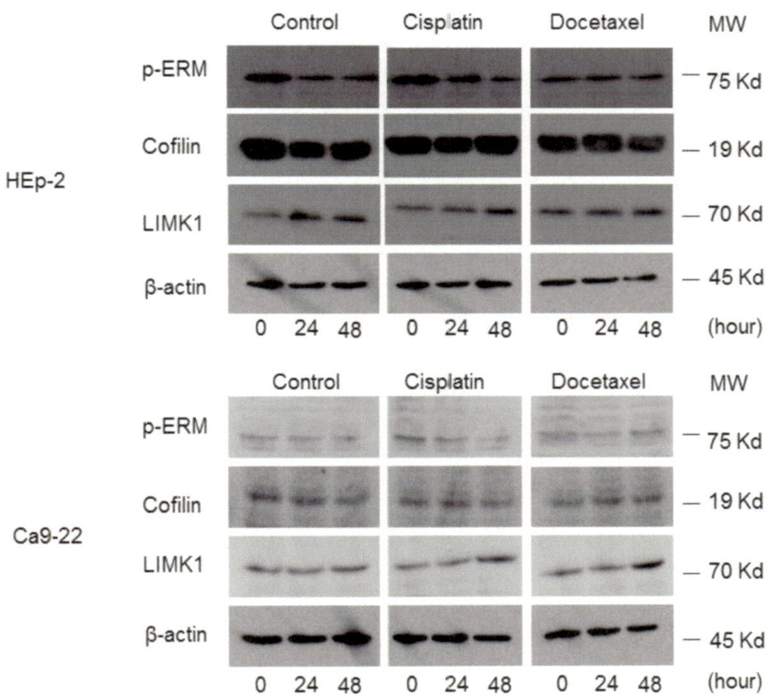

Fig. 6. Time course of the levels of p-ERM, cofilin and LIMK in HEp-2 cells and Ca9-22 cells treated with cisplatin or docetaxel.
β-actin was probed for loding control. 3 replicate were used in each experiments and experiments were repeated 3 times.

8. Docetaxel treatment did not promote epithelial-mesenchymal transition (EMT)

It has been well documented that many cancer cells lose most of their epithelial characteristics during progression and metastasis, through the process of EMT (Thiery 2002). Generally, EMT causes increased motility and invasiveness of cancer cells due to decreased cell-cell adhesion. Snail, a zinc finger transcription factor, triggers EMT through direct repression of E-cadherin transcription (Batlle et al. 2000; Cano et al. 2000). The reverse correlation of snail and E-cadherin expression has been reported for various human cancers, including SCC (Yokoyama et al. 2001). Accordingly, we investigated the snail and E-cadherin expression levels to assess whether cisplatin and/or docetaxel at IC_{10} differently influences EMT. Snail was decreasing over a time course (Fig.7.). Conversely E-cadherin was increasing over a time course (Fig.7.). But the levels of these proteins were not significantly different between cisplatin, docetaxel and no treatment. These results indicate that docetaxel treatment does not promote EMT at least in these cell lines.

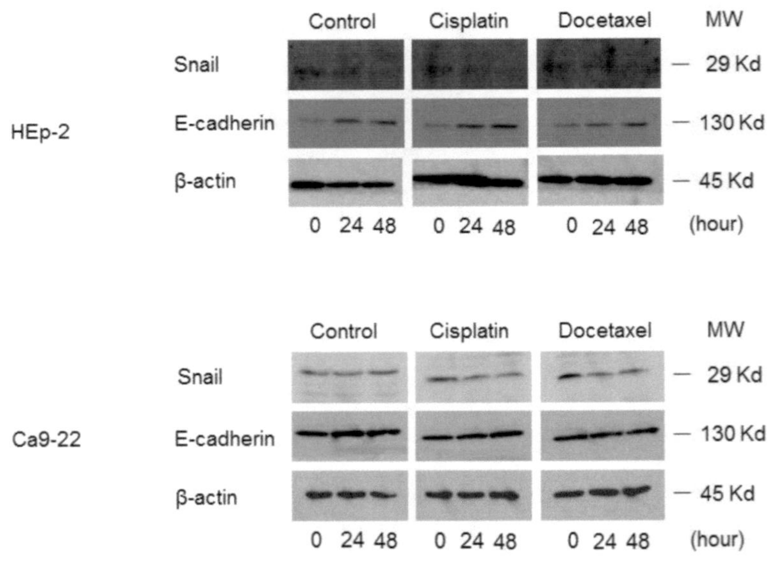

Fig. 7. Time course of snail and E-cadherin expression of HEp-2 cells and Ca9-22 cells treated with IC_{10} concentration of cisplatin or docetaxel.
β-actin was probed for loding control. 3 replicate were used in each experiments and experiments were repeated 3 times.

9. Matrix metalloproteinase (MMP) production was not significantly affected by cisplatin and docetaxel treatment

MMPs are known to play an important role in extracellular matrix remodeling during the process of tumor invasion and metastasis (Egeblad et al. 2002). Two of these enzymes, MMP-2 and MMP-9, are potent gelatinases and have been correlated with the processes of invasion and metastasis of SCC (Sheu et al. 2003; Patel et al. 2005). Gelatin zymography revealed prominent 72000 dalton bands, corresponding to MMP2 secreted from the HEp-2 and Ca9-22 cells. These bands appeared unchanged by either cisplatin or docetaxel treatment (Figure 8).

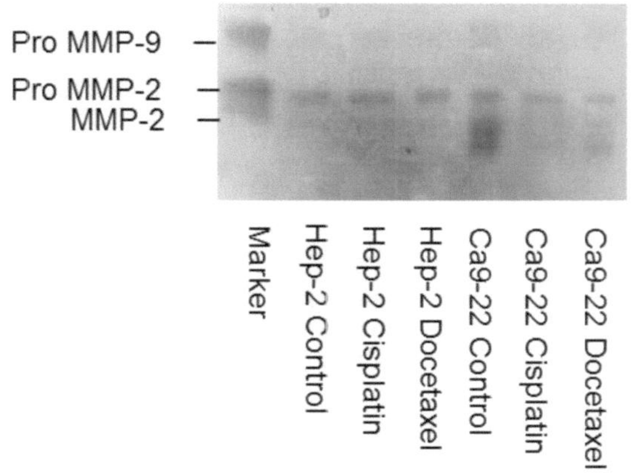

Fig. 8. Gelatin zaymograpy.
MMP secretion in HEp-2 cells and Ca9-22 cells after treatment or control were evaluated by Gelatin zymography. Gelatin zymography revealed prominent 72000 dalton bands, corresponding to MMP2 secreted from the HEp-2 and Ca9-22 cells. These bands appeared unchanged by either cisplatin or docetaxel treatment

10. Discussion

The metastatic process has traditionally been viewed as follows: (1) detachment of individual cells from the primary lesion (2) invasion of local stroma (3) entry of single cells or aggregates of tumor cells into blood vessels directly or via lymphatic channels (intravasation) (4) sticking to the vasculature distant from their origin followed by extravasation, and (5) invasion into the parenchyma of the target organ site. The newly formed lesions can themselves become the source of disseminating cells which repeat this cycle, giving rise to tertiary metastasis. Thus, Inhibition of invasion in the primary lesion should result in preventing the distant metastasis. From this point of view, our results suggest that docetaxel, which decreased local invasiveness, may prevent distant metastasis. Although the effect of docetaxel on cell migration or invasiveness of ovary cancer cells (Bijman et al. 2008) and umbilical vein endothelial cells (Bijman et al. 2006) have been described, its effect on head and neck cancer cells has not been evaluated.

Actin cytoskeleton provides the driving force for cell migration, while microtubules are required to establish cell polarity during motility in fibroblasts (Bershadsky et al. 1991). Actin is regulated by Rho family small GTPases, and it is indicated that microtubules may influence actin cytoskeleton through modulation of the activity of Rho GTPases (Wittmann et al. 2001). Among Rho GTPases, cdc42 was reported to control the polarity of actin and microtubule through distinct signal transduction pathways (Cau et al. 2005). It is possible that the abnormal tubulin bundle induced by docetaxel lead to suppression of cdc42 activity. This decreased cdc42 activity could affect actin filament and decrease the migration of the head and neck cancer cells.

In contrast, we could not find definitive evidence for docetaxel to directly affect actin cytoskeleton regulation. It did not affect EMT processes or MMP production of these head and neck cancer cell lines.

11. Conclusion

In conclusion, it is likely that docetaxel suppresses SCC migration through inhibition of microtubule turnover, which affects cdc42 activity and its subcellular localization leading to decreased filopodia formation. We propose that effect on cancer cell migration should be assessed together with anti-proliferative activity when evaluating a cancer chemotherapeutic agent. Along this line, we are now evaluating anti-migratory effect of EGFR tyrosine kinase inhibitors, another class of promising treatment for head and neck cancer.

12. References

Posner, M. R., D. M. Hershock, C. R. Blajman, E. Mickiewicz, E. Winquist, V. Gorbounova, S. Tjulandin, D. M. Shin, K. Cullen, T. J. Ervin, B. A. Murphy, L. E. Raez, R. B. Cohen, M. Spaulding, R. B. Tishler, B. Roth, C. Viroglio Rdel, V. Venkatesan, I. Romanov, S. Agarwala, K. W. Harter, M. Dugan, A. Cmelak, A. M. Markoe, P. W. Read, L. Steinbrenner, A. D. Colevas, C. M. Norris, Jr. and R. I. Haddad (2007). "Cisplatin and fluorouracil alone or with docetaxel in head and neck cancer." N Engl J Med 357(17): 1705-1715.

Vermorken, J. B., E. Remenar, C. van Herpen, T. Gorlia, R. Mesia, M. Degardin, J. S. Stewart, S. Jelic, J. Betka, J. H. Preiss, D. van den Weyngaert, A. Awada, D. Cupissol, H. R. Kienzer, A. Rey, I. Desaunois, J. Bernier and J. L. Lefebvre (2007). "Cisplatin, fluorouracil, and docetaxel in unresectable head and neck cancer." N Engl J Med 357(17): 1695-1704.

Kogashiwa, Y., H. Sakurai, T. Kimura and N. Kohno (2010). "Docetaxel suppresses invasiveness of head and neck cancer cells in vitro." Cancer Sci 101(6): 1382-1386.

Hall, A. (1998). "Rho GTPases and the actin cytoskeleton." Science 279(5350): 509-514.

Schmitz, A. A., E. E. Govek, B. Bottner and L. Van Aelst (2000). "Rho GTPases: signaling, migration, and invasion." Exp Cell Res 261(1): 1-12.

Price, L. S. and J. G. Collard (2001). "Regulation of the cytoskeleton by Rho-family GTPases: implications for tumour cell invasion." Semin Cancer Biol 11(2): 167-173.

Cau, J. and A. Hall (2005). "Cdc42 controls the polarity of the actin and microtubule cytoskeletons through two distinct signal transduction pathways." J Cell Sci 118(Pt 12): 2579-2587.

Bishop, A. L. and A. Hall (2000). "Rho GTPases and their effector proteins." Biochem J 348 Pt 2: 241-255.

Nalbant, P., L. Hodgson, V. Kraynov, A. Toutchkine and K. M. Hahn (2004). "Activation of endogenous Cdc42 visualized in living cells." Science 305(5690): 1615-1619.

Thiery, J. P. (2002). "Epithelial-mesenchymal transitions in tumour progression." Nat Rev Cancer 2(6): 442-454.

Batlle, E., E. Sancho, C. Franci, D. Dominguez, M. Monfar, J. Baulida and A. Garcia De Herreros (2000). "The transcription factor snail is a repressor of E-cadherin gene expression in epithelial tumour cells." Nat Cell Biol 2(2): 84-89.

Cano, A., M. A. Perez-Moreno, I. Rodrigo, A. Locascio, M. J. Blanco, M. G. del Barrio, F. Portillo and M. A. Nieto (2000). "The transcription factor snail controls epithelial-mesenchymal transitions by repressing E-cadherin expression." Nat Cell Biol 2(2): 76-83.

Yokoyama, K., N. Kamata, E. Hayashi, T. Hoteiya, N. Ueda, R. Fujimoto and M. Nagayama (2001). "Reverse correlation of E-cadherin and snail expression in oral squamous cell carcinoma cells in vitro." Oral Oncol 37(1): 65-71.

Egeblad, M. and Z. Werb (2002). "New functions for the matrix metalloproteinases in cancer progression." Nat Rev Cancer 2(3): 161-174.

Sheu, B. C., H. C. Lien, H. N. Ho, H. H. Lin, S. N. Chow, S. C. Huang and S. M. Hsu (2003). "Increased expression and activation of gelatinolytic matrix metalloproteinases is associated with the progression and recurrence of human cervical cancer." Cancer Res 63(19): 6537-6542.

Patel, B. P., P. M. Shah, U. M. Rawal, A. A. Desai, S. V. Shah, R. M. Rawal and P. S. Patel (2005). "Activation of MMP-2 and MMP-9 in patients with oral squamous cell carcinoma." J Surg Oncol 90(2): 81-88.

Bijman, M. N., M. P. van Berkel, G. P. van Nieuw Amerongen and E. Boven (2008). "Interference with actin dynamics is superior to disturbance of microtubule function in the inhibition of human ovarian cancer cell motility." Biochem Pharmacol 76(6): 707-716.

Bijman, M. N., G. P. van Nieuw Amerongen, N. Laurens, V. W. van Hinsbergh and E. Boven (2006). "Microtubule-targeting agents inhibit angiogenesis at subtoxic concentrations, a process associated with inhibition of Rac1 and Cdc42 activity and changes in the endothelial cytoskeleton." Mol Cancer Ther 5(9): 2348-2357.

Bershadsky, A. D., E. A. Vaisberg and J. M. Vasiliev (1991). "Pseudopodial activity at the active edge of migrating fibroblast is decreased after drug-induced microtubule depolymerization." Cell Motil Cytoskeleton 19(3): 152-158.

Wittmann, T. and C. M. Waterman-Storer (2001). "Cell motility: can Rho GTPases and microtubules point the way?" J Cell Sci 114(Pt 21): 3795-3803.

10

A Review of Tonsillectomy Techniques and Technologies

S. K. Aremu
Federal Medical Centre, Azare, Bauchi State, Nigeria

1. Introduction

1.1 Anatomy

The circular band of lymphoid tissue within the pharynx consisting of the adenoids, the palatine tonsils (Figure 1), and lingual tonsils is known as Waldeyer's ring. The palatine tonsils are lymphoid tissue with prominent germinal centers and the palatine tonsils, in contrast to the lingual tonsils and adenoids, have a distinct capsule[1]which separates the tonsils from the lateral pharyngeal walls. The tonsil lies within a bed of three muscles that make up the tonsillar fossa. Forming the anterior pillar is the palatoglossus muscle and the posterior pillar is the palatopharyngeus muscle, while the superior constrictor muscle makes up the bed of the fossa. Medially, the tonsil crypts lay exposed to the oropharynx with specialize stratified squamous epithelium.

The tonsils are well vascularized with the majority of the blood supply arising from the tonsillar branch of the facial artery.[1]The nerve supply of the tonsils arise from the ninth cranial nerve and descending branches from the lesser palatine nerves and the tympanic branch of CN IX is thought to account for the referred ear pain found in some cases of tonsillitis. The tonsils have no afferent lymphatic vessels. Their efferent lymph drainage is through the upper cervical nodes, especially to the jugulodigastric group. Tonsils and adenoids are immunologically most active between the ages of 4 and 10 years, and tend to involutes after puberty.[2]

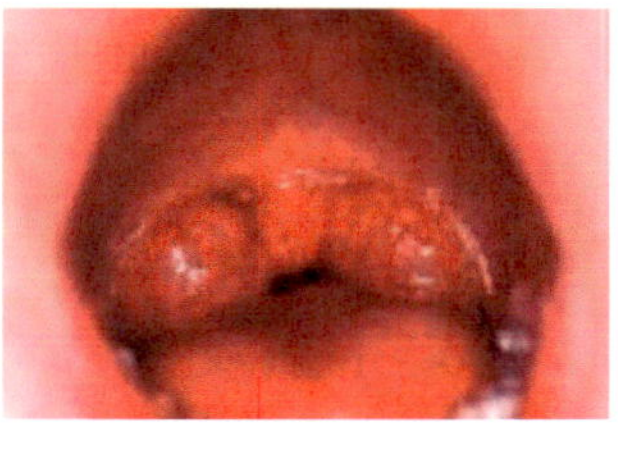

Fig. 1. Orophaynx with Palatine Tonsils.

1.2 Indications for tonsillectomy

1.2.1 Absolute[3]

1. Obstructive sleep apnea
2. Cardiopulmonary complications secondary to airway obstruction (e.g., cor pulmonale, alveolar hypoventilation)
3. Suspected malignancy (asymmetric Tonsillar Hypertrophy) [4]
4. Hemorrhagic tonsillitis
5. Tonsillitis causing febrile seizures

1.2.2 Relative[3]

1. Recurrent acute tonsillitis meeting one or more of the following criteria:
   - Seven episodes in 1 year
   - Five episodes/year for 2 consecutive years
   - Three episodes/year for 3 consecutive years
   - Two weeks of missed school or work in 1 year
2. Chronic tonsillitis refractory to antimicrobial therapy
3. Tonsillolithiasis with associated halitosis and pain, unresponsive to conservative measures
   - Peritonsillar abscess
   - Dysphagia due to tonsillar hypertrophy.

The indications for tonsillectomy have dramatically changed and are today more clearly defined. Geographical variations in the incidence of tonsillectomy are recognized and, although most of this variation may only reflect varying attitudes between physicians, there is little doubt that geographical variations in pathology are partly responsible[5].In adults, the most common indication is recurrent acute tonsillitis[5]. However the most common indication in children is obstructive sleep apnea. Patients with a prior history of recurrent tonsillitis and prior peritonsillar abscess may be more likely to develop another peritonsillar abscess and are candidates for tonsillectomy.

2. History

Tonsillectomy has been performed by otolaryngologists, general surgeons, family practitioners and general practitioners. However, in the past 30 years the recognition for the need of standardization of surgical technique resulted in a shift in practice patterns so that it is almost exclusively performed by the otolaryngologists.

The first known removal of tonsils dates back to the first century AD, when Cornelius Celsius in Rome used his own finger to perform it[6].The earliest description of the procedure was by Paul of Aegina in 625. The early instruments that were used for tonsillectomy were actually first developed for removal of the uvula. Phillip Syng invented what would become the forerunner for the modern tonsillotome.Not until the mid 18th century did Caque of Rheims performs tonsillectomies on a regular basis. Since then several different techniques have been used for tonsillectomy.

However, the difficulties encountered by surgeons, especially in controlling the peri-operative bleeding, were a major drawback .It was only 1909,when Cohen adopted suture ligation of bleeding vessels to control the hemorrhage, that tonsillectomy became a common practice in hospitals [7].

Sixty years later Haase and Noguera[8], introduced the use of diathermy and the concept of electro-dissection was first described by Goycolea6 in 1982 using monopolar diathermy.10 years later Pang[9] reported the first electro-dissection tonsillectomy using the bipolar forceps technique.

3. Preoperative evaluation

Adequate history and physical examination are essential in the preoperative diagnosis and evaluation of the patient being worked up for tonsillectomy. History alone is the most common method for diagnosing obstructive sleep apnea.[10] When the diagnosis is at all in question, the child is younger than 2 years, or there is concern about the severity of the sleep apnea, a polysomnogram should be recommended.[11]Preoperative electrocardiogram and chest x-ray are not necessary unless there is a history of heart disease.[12] Other preoperative evaluation needs to be decided based on the medical conditions of each individual patient. For example, a child with von Willebrand disease should have the input of a hematologist regarding the use of desmopressin to minimize the risk of bleeding during the intra-operative and post-operative periods.

4. General technique

4.1 Exposure

For a successful surgery, adequate exposure, of the oro-pharyn must be achieved. Also knowledge of the relevant anatomy and tissue tension is important. With the aid of a mouth gag, e.g, Boyle -Davis (Figure 2), the oropharynx is exposed. Dentition may be protected by a plastic or rubber athletic mouth guard and careful mouth gag placement. Care is taken not to allow the lateral flanges of the tongue blade of the gag to scratch dental enamel. Protection of the mucosa from electrical and thermal conductivity is achieved by interposing a gloved finger between the instrument metal and the patient.[13]

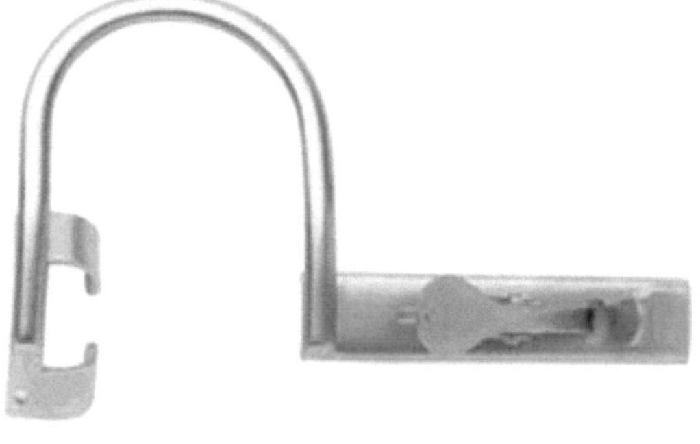

Fig. 2. Open-sided mouth gag (Davis Mouth Gag).

4.2 Surgical procedure

The method anesthesia induction and patients' positioning is similar for most patients undergoing tonsillectomy, regardless of which technique is used to remove the tonsils. The patient is placed in the supine position and orally intubated.The endotracheal tube is taped to the patient's chin in the midline. Alternatively, some practitioners prefer to use a laryngeal mask airway.[14,15]The bed is turned 90°-180° so that the surgeon can sit or stand at the head of the bed. The patient is positioned at the edge of the bed, and a small shoulder roll is placed. Either a Crowe-Davis, McIvor, or Dingman mouth gag is inserted and expanded to keep the mouth open for the duration of the procedure.Tissue tension during complete tonsillectomy is achieved by strong medial traction of Allis clamps and torsion of the tonsils medially (Figure 3).

The tonsils are then removed using 1 of the techniques described later.

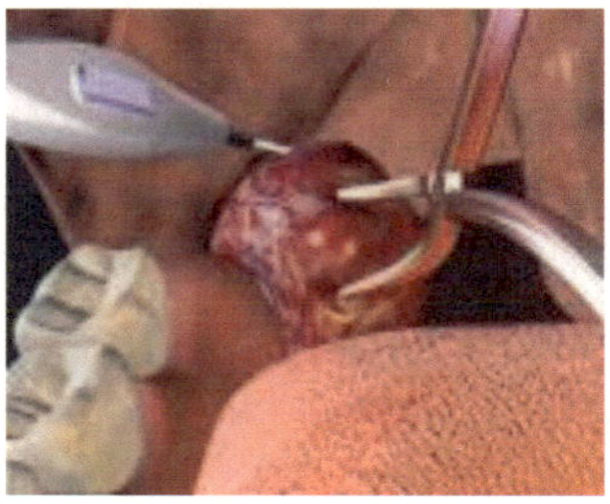

Fig. 3. Medial Traction on the Tonsil.

5. Patients and methods

50 patients (30 males, 20 females) were studied. 28(56%) had adenotonsillectomy, while 22(44%) had only tonsillectomy alone. The data was obtained by the author from three centres:University of Ilorin teaching hospital, Kwara state, IBB specialized hospital Minna, Niger state and Federal medical centre, Azare, Bauchi state.

35(70%) of the surgeries were performed using cold surgical dissection technique, while 15(30%) were done using bipolar electrocautry. All the surgeries were performed by one of two experienced surgeons. All the children were kept overnight; some were discharged the following day after they can tolerate liquid diet. Routine antibiotics and analgesics were given to all the patients.

For the 28 patients who had adenotonsillectomy, the mean operating time for the 8 bipolar electrocautries was 42.0 minutes and 47.2 minutes for the 20 cold dissection patients.

For the 22 patients who had tonsillectomy alone, the mean operating time was 31.4 minutes for the 7 bipolar electrocautries, while 34.2 minutes for the 15 cold dissections.

Complication of hemorrhage were seen in 3(6.0%) of all the patients, 2(66.7) were in cold dissection group and 1(33.3%) in bipolar electrocautry group.

6. Techniques and technologies

The techniques of Tonsillectomy can be broadly divided into 2 major categories: extracapsular (total tonsillectomy, subcapsular) and intracapsular (partial tonsillectomy). Intracapsular is also known as "subtotal," and this procedure is referred to as tonsillotomy in some literatures. Extracapsular tonsillectomy involves dissecting lateral to the tonsil in the plane between the tonsillar capsule and the pharyngeal musculature, and the tonsil is generally removed as a single unit. Partial tonsillectomy, or tonsillotomy, involves removal of most of the tonsil, while preserving a rim of lymphoid tissue and tonsillar capsule in the most recent iteration of this older technique.[16] Preservation of this margin of tissue, this "biologic dressing," may promote an easier recovery, with lower hemorrhage rates and better recovery of diet and activity reported in comparison with traditional monopolar tonsillectomy techniques.[17,18]The most common extracapsular techniques use a "cold" knife (sharp dissection), monopolar electrocautery, bipolar cautery (or bipolar scissors),or harmonic scalpel. Intracapsular techniques may use the microdebrider, bipolar radiofrequency ablation (which can also be used to remove the entire tonsil), and carbon dioxide laser. Either extracapsular or intracapsular tonsillectomy can be performed for the pediatric patient with obstructive sleep apnea, but only extracapsular techniques should be used for patients undergoing tonsillectomy as a result of tonsillitis or peritonsillar abscess. In addition, tonsils can be ablated using a laser or monopolar radiofrequency (somnoplasty) in a cooperative adult in a clinic setting.

7. "Cold" knife

A frequently used method for total tonsillectomy is the"cold"or sharp dissection technique. In this technique, the tonsil and capsule are dissected from surrounding tissue using scissors, knife, or t dissector (Figure 4) and the inferior pole is amputated with a tonsil snare.

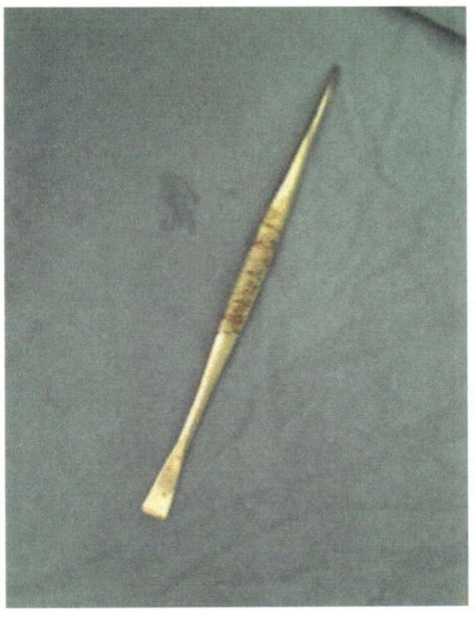

Fig. 4. Tonsil Dissector.

8. Harmonic scalpel

The harmonic scalpel (Figure 5) can be used to perform an extracapsular tonsillectomy (Ethicon Endo-Surgery Inc, Cincinnati, OH).It uses ultrasonic energy to vibrate its blade at 55,000 cycles per second. The vibration transfers energy to the tissue, providing simultaneous cutting and coagulation, so, typically, no additional instrument is needed for haemostasis. The components of the device include a generator, a hand piece, and a disposable blade. A high-frequency power supply provides energy to the hand piece. The blade oscillations dissect tissues by creating intra-cellular cavities as pressure waves are conducted through the tissues. The expansion and contraction of these cavities results in the lysis of cellular connections, resulting in tissue dissection.

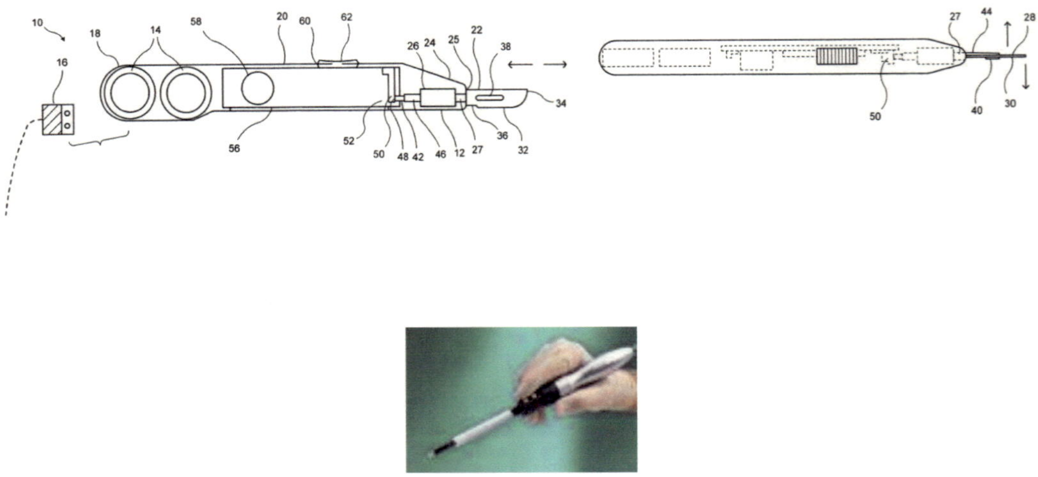

Fig. 5. Harmonic/ultrasonic scalpel.

9. Bipolar radiofrequency ablation

Bipolar radiofrequency ablation can be used to perform an extracapsular or intracapsular tonsillectomy; however, it is most commonly used to perform a partial tonsillectomy (Figure 6). The equipment includes a radiofrequency generator, foot control, saline irrigation regulator, and the coblation wand (PlasmaCare Corp, Sunnyvale, CA). During a bipolar radiofrequency ablation tonsillectomy, conductive saline solution is converted into an ionized plasma layer, resulting in molecular dissociation with minimal thermal energy transfer. Haemostasis can usually be performed with the coblation wand alone.

Fig. 6. Bipolar Probe.

10. Microdebrider tonsillectomy

This is another method for intracapsular tonsillectomy. The microdebrider is a powered rotary shaving device with continuous suction, made up of a tube, and connected to a hand piece, which, in turn, is connected to a motor with foot control and a suction device. A partial tonsillectomy is completed with the removal of approximately 90% to 95% of the tonsil, while preserving the tonsillar capsule.

11. Advantages and disadvantages of the techniques

There is great debate about the relative merits of the various tonsillectomy techniques published in many studies, with many more ongoing that compare the techniques. The existing literature consistently reports that the intracapsular (partial) techniques result in less postoperative pain, however, the degree of lessened pain continues to be much debated.[19,20,21]In addition; there is a small risk of tonsil regrowth and the necessity for an additional procedure with the intracapsular techniques. Of the extracapsular techniques, "cold" tonsillectomy results in less postoperative pain compared with an electrocautery or "hot" tonsillectomy; however, the latter procedure is typically faster and has less intraoperative blood loss.[22,23,24] Although not extensively researched thus far, a total tonsillectomy with the coblation unit may have slight advantages over electrocautery tonsillectomy.[25] The studies on outcomes of surgeries completed with the harmonic scalpel do not show any definitive advantage to the scalpel.[26,27] It is not clear which technique, if there is one, results in the lowest rate of postoperative hemorrhage.[28,29]

Most of the data available to date suggest that there is no difference in the bleeding rates between extracapsular and intracapsular tonsillectomy.[30]The equipment involved with various techniques varies in price, although the largest cost factor in any tonsillectomy is the operating time.

12. Postoperative care

A majority of children can safely be discharged home on the same day of surgery, regardless of the surgical technique used.[10,30]Children younger than 2 years or who live far from a hospital should be kept overnight for observation. Pain medication should be recommended, and most physicians prescribe either acetaminophen or acetaminophen with codeine postoperatively.[31] Some physicians recommend a soft diet postoperatively, others recommend "diet as tolerated."[10] In our centres we commence the child on firstly on cold ice cream and subsequently on liquid diet.

Studies have not shown any difference in recovery between children who have a restricted versus those who have non-restricted diets postoperatively.[32,33]

13. Long-term follow-up

Typically, the patient will be seen in the office in 2 weeks, then 1 month of the tonsillectomy to confirm adequate healing, although it is also acceptable to follow-up with a phone call only.[10,34]

14. Conclusions

Appreciation of the indications and the use of new tonsillectomy techniques and technologies, as well as an awareness of the economic ramifications of their adoption, will ultimately provide the best care for tonsillectomy patients.

15. References

[1] Casselbrant ML: What is wrong in chronic adenoiditis/tonsillitis anatomical considerations? *Int J Pediatr Otorhinolaryngol* 49:S133-135,1999.

[2] Richtsmeier WJ, Shikhani AH. The physiology and immunology of the pharyngeal lymphoid tissue. *Otolaryngol Clin North Am* 20(2):219-28, May 1987.

[3] Paradise JL: Tonsillectomy and adenoidectomy. In Bluestone CD, Stool SE, Alper CM,et al (eds): *Pediatric Otolaryngology* 4th ed. Philadelphia,W.B Saunders:1210-1222, 2002.

[4] Hoddeson EK, Gourin CG: Adult Tonsillectomy: Current Indications and Outcomes *Otolaryngol Head Neck Surg* 140(1):19-22, jan 2009.

[5] B.C.Okafo. Tonsillectomy: An Appraisal of Indications in Developing Countries. *Laryngoscope* 96(5 & 6):517 -522,July 1983.

[6] J. McAuliffe-Curtain, The history of tonsil and adenoid surgery. *Otolaryngol. Clin. North Am.* 20:415–419,1987.

[7] H. Feldman, Two hundred year history of tonsillectomy. Images from the history of otorhinolaryngology, highlighted by instruments from the collection of the German Medical History Museum in Ingolstadt. *Laryngorhinootologie* 76:751–760, 1997.

[8] F.R. Haase and J.T. Noguera, Hemostasis in tonsillectomy. *Arch. Otolaryngol.* 75:125, 1962.

[9] Y.T. Pang, H. El-Hakim and M.P. Rothera, Bipolar diathermy tonsillectomy. *Clin. Otolaryngol.*19:355–357, 1992.

[10] Kay DJ, Mehta V, Goldsmith AJ: Perioperative adeno-tonsillectomy management in children:Current practices. *Laryngoscope* 113:592-597,2003.

[11] Messner AH: Evaluation of obstructive sleep apnea by polysomnography prior to pediatric adenotonsillectomy. *Arch Otolaryngol Head Neck Surg* 125:353-356, 1999.

[12] James AL, Runciman M, Burton MJ, et al: Investigation of cardiac function in children with suspected obstructive sleep apnea. *J Otolaryngol* 32:151-154, 2003.

[13] Shah UK: Letter to editor, "A simple suggestion to reduce perioral burns during adenotonsillectomy,"inre:NauraMJ et al.Perioral burns after adenotonsillectomy. *Arch Otolaryngol Head Neck Surg* 134:673,2008.

[14] Hatcher IS,Stack CG:Postal survey of the anaesthetic techniques used for paediatric tonsillectomy surgery. *Paediatr Anaesth* 9:311-315,1999.

[15] Hern JD, Jayaraj SM, Sidhu VS, et al: The laryngeal mask airway in tonsillectomy: The surgeon's perspective. *Clin Otolaryngol* 24:122-125, 1999.

[16] Koltai PJ, Solares CA, Mascha EJ, et al: Intracapsular partial tonsillectomy for tonsil hypertrophy in children. *Laryngoscope* 112:17-19, 2002.

[17] Solares CA, Koempel JA, Hirose K, et al: Safety and efficacy of powered intracapsular tonsillectomy in children: A multi-center retrospective case series. *Int J Pediatr Otorhinolaryngol* 69:21-26, 2005.

[18] Schmidt R, Herzog A, Cook S, et al: Complications of tonsillectomy: A comparison of techniques. *Arch Otolaryngol Head Neck Surg* 133:925-928, 2007.

[19] Chan KH, Friedman NR, Allen GC, et al: Randomized, controlled, multisite study of intracapsular tonsillectomy using low-temperature plasma excision. *Arch Otolaryngol Head Neck Surg* 130:1303-1307, 2004.

[20] Chang K: Randomized controlled trial of Coblation versus electrocautery tonsillectomy. *Otolaryngol Head Neck Surg* 132:273-280, 2005.

[21] Hall MDJ, Littlefield CPD, Birkmire-Peters DP, et al: Radiofrequency ablation versus electrocautery in tonsillectomy. *Otolaryngol Head Neck Surg* 130:300-305, 2004.

[22] Leinbach RF, Markwell SJ, Colliver JA, et al: Hot versus cold tonsillectomy: A systematic review of the literature. *Otolaryngol Head Neck Surg* 129:360-364, 2003.

[23] Hanasono MM, LalakeaML, Mikulec AA,etal: Perioperative steroids in tonsillectomy using electrocautery and sharp dissection techniques. *Arch Otolaryngol Head Neck Surg* 130:917-921, 2004.

[24] Perkins J, Dahiya R: Microdissection needle tonsillectomy and postoperative pain: A pilot study. *Arch Otolaryngol Head Neck Surg* 129:1285-1288, 2003.

[25] Stoker KE, Don DM, Kang DR, et al: Pediatric total tonsillectomy using coblation compared to conventional electrosurgery: a prospective,controlled single-blind study. *Otolaryngol Head Neck Surg* 130:666-675, 2004.

[26] Shinhar S, Scotch BM, Belenky W, et al: Harmonic scalpel tonsillectomy versus hot electrocautery and cold dissection: An objective comparison. *Ear Nose Throat J* 83:712-715, 2004.

[27] Willging JP,Wiatrak B:Harmonic scalpel tonsillectomy in children:A randomized prospective study. *Otolaryngol Head Neck Surg* 128: 318-325, 2003.

[28] O'Leary S, Vorrath J: Postoperative bleeding after diathermy hage:Cold versus hot dissection.*Otolaryngol Head Neck Surg131*:833-836,2004.

[29] Lee MS, Montague ML, Hussain SS: Post-tonsillectomy hemorrhage:Cold versus hot dissection.*Otolaryngol Head Neck Surg131*:833-836,2004.

[30] Mills N, Anderson BJ, Barber C, et al: Day stay pediatric tonsillectomy—A safe procedure. *Int J Pediatr Otorhinolaryngol* 68:1367-1373,2004.

[31] Moir MS, Bair E, Shinnick P, et al: Acetaminophen versus acetaminophen with codeine after pediatric tonsillectomy. *Laryngoscope* 110: 1824-1827, 2000.

[32] Brodsky L, Radomski K, Gendler J: The effect of post-operative instruction on recovery after tonsillectomy and adenoidectomy. In J Pediatr Otorhinolaryngol 25:133-140,1993

[33] Hall MD, Brodsky L: The effect of post-operative diet on recovery in the first twelve hours after tonsillectomy and adenoidectomy. Int J Pediatric Otorhinolaryngol 31:215-220, 1995.

[34] RosbeKW,JonesD,JalisiS,etal:Efficacy of postoperative follow-up telephone calls for patients who underwent adenotonsillectomy. Arch Otolaryngol Head Neck Surg 126:718-721, 2000.

11

Management of Early Glottic Cancer

Luke Harris, Danny Enepekides and Kevin Higgins
Sunnybrook Health Sciences Centre, Toronto
Canada

1. Introduction

The management of early glottic cancer has evolved significantly over the past decade, with transoral laser (TOL) surgery and radiotherapy emerging as the two most prevalent treatment modalities. The selection of one modality over another continues to generate controversy. With both modalities showing similar efficacy with regard to survival and oncologic outcomes, the selection of one modality over another hinges upon vocal function, quality of life, and cost-effectiveness as the main outcomes of interest. This chapter will begin with a brief overview of the epidemiology and presentation of glottic cancer and will follow with a comprehensive overview of the contemporary literature comparing both treatment modalities.

2. Epidemiology and clinical presentation of glottic cancer

Laryngeal cancer is the most common malignancy of the upper aerodigestive tract (Fowler, 1997) with Surveillance Epidemiology and End Results (SEER) data estimating that 12,720 men and women (10,110 men and 2,610 women) were diagnosed with laryngeal cancer in 2010. This data estimated that 3600 men and women will die as a result of the disease. The age-adjusted incidence rate was 3.4 per 100,000 men and women per year, and the median age at diagnosis was 65 years of age (SEER, 2011). Squamous cell carcinoma constitutes the overwhelming majority of laryngeal malignancies, with smoking and alcohol abuse as the two most robust etiologic factors.

Malignancy most commonly affects the glottic subsite of the larynx, and the glottis accounts for two thirds of primary laryngeal cancers. Carcinomas of the glottis produce dysphonia at an early stage, and because of poor lymphatic drainage tend not to present with nodal disease (Bouqet, 1988; Groome et al., 2001; Shah et al., 1997). Both of these features allow for single modality therapy of glottic carcinoma in the majority of patients.

3. Management

Radiotherapy and conservation surgery are the two viable treatment modalities employed in the management of early glottic cancer, with concurrent chemoradiotherapy and radical surgery reserved for advanced disease. The controversy in early glottic carcinoma management lies in which modality to select.

Intensity modulated radiotherapy (IMRT) revolutionized radiation delivery to the head and neck in the early 1990s (Webb, 2003). IMRT has now become commonplace for radiation delivery to the larynx, allowing for precision targeting of glottic tumours and the avoidance of nearby critical structures. Surgical options for early glottic carcinoma include transoral laser (TOL) surgery, transoral robotic surgery (TORS), and open partial laryngeal surgery. TOL surgery is the most widely employed surgical option for early glottic carcinoma. TOL surgery was first reported by Strong and Jako (Strong & Jako, 1972) in 1972, and was further developed by others for the management of glottic carcinoma (Eckel et al., 2000). Centres with a significant experience with TOL surgery have expanded the indication to include select T3 and even T4 lesions (Steiner, 1993; Grant et al., 2007; Motta et al., 2005; Blanch et al., 2010). In the last decade TORS has evolved as a new technology for endolaryngeal surgery. The main advantage over TOL surgery is the enhanced surgical exposure, which is not restricted to direct line of sight. The main disadvantages are the increased operative time (which has been shown to improve with greater surgical experience (Genden et al., 2009)), and the significant financial cost of the surgical robot, its maintenance, and its per-case disposables. Currently there is no evidence demonstrating improved oncologic or functional outcomes with TORS compared to conventional TOL surgery. Open partial laryngeal surgery for early glottic carcinoma is on the decline (Silver et al., 2009). This is due to the growing availability of laser technology, the growing experience with TOL surgery, and the decreased morbidity and length of hospital stay with TOL surgery (Silver et al., 2009). Our institution restricts open partial laryngeal surgery to small, localized laryngeal carcinomas that have recurred after primary radiation or concurrent chemoradiation therapy (rT1, rT2).

Selection of one modality over another, be it TOL surgery or radiotherapy, is controversial because both modalities are similarly efficacious with respect to oncologic and survival outcomes. Because of this, many contemporary studies have focussed on vocal function, quality of life, and cost-effectiveness as important secondary considerations.

3.1 Oncologic and survival outcomes

A host of studies, largely consisting of case series, have reported oncologic and mortality outcomes with TOL surgery and radiotherapy. This led our group to publish a meta-analysis (Higgins et al., 2009) comparing laser excision to radiotherapy for the treatment of early carcinomas of the glottic larynx. The meta-analysis included over 7600 patients and compared local control, laryngectomy-free survival, and overall survival between modalities. No significant difference between TOL surgery and radiotherapy was found for local control (OR 0.81, 95% CI 0.51-1.3) and laryngectomy-free survival (OR 0.73, 95% CI 0.39-1.35). However, the analysis showed a significant increase in overall survival in favour of TOL surgery (OR 1.48, 95% CI 1.19-1.85).

Three recent single-arm series on radiotherapy for early glottic carcinoma have been published after our 2009 meta-analysis. New series by Tateya et al (Tateya et al., 2010) (150 patients with T1 and T2 disease) and Sjogren et al (Sjogren et al., 2009) (316 patients with T1 disease) noted excellent local control and overall survival rates with radiotherapy, and these results were in keeping with the published literature. Hafidh et al (Hafidh et al., 2009) reported a recent 150-patient Canadian series with 5-year T1 and T2 local control rates of 71.0% and 63.3%, respectively. The pooled T1 and T2 local control rate observed in this study was lower than those observed in the single-arm radiotherapy case series included in our meta-analysis[15], which ranged from 77.4% to 88.0%.

TOL surgery has since been studied in two single-arm series. A series by Rucci et al (Rucci et al., 2010) included 81 patients. Over one third of tumours involved the anterior commissure, a known poor prognosticator for local control with either TOL surgery or radiotherapy. The reported local control rate was 74.1% and was out of the 75.1% to 93.7% range observed in our meta-analysis (Higgins et al, 2009). Another recent series by Ansarin et al (Ansarin et al., 2010) looked specifically at patients aged 70 years or older, and documented excellent local control and overall survival rates in keeping with the published literature.

Most importantly, three studies published after our 2009 meta-analysis compared TOL surgery and radiotherapy head-to-head. Two of these studies (Mahler et al., 2010; Schrijvers et al., 2009) demonstrated a significant increase in laryngectomy-free survival (LFS) in the TOL surgery groups. The third study (Kujath et al., 2011) found a trend for increased LFS with TOL surgery.

Overall, recent single-arm series may serve to strengthen existing data which demonstrate excellent local control and survival for both modalities, but offer little new information. Two of the three head-to-head comparison studies (Mahler et al., 2010; Schrijvers et al., 2009) have demonstrated that laryngectomy-free survival may be better with TOL surgery than with radiotherapy.

3.2 Voice and quality of life

A recent systematic review (Spielmann et al., 2010) sought to determine whether there was a difference in voice outcomes and quality of life between TOL surgery and radiotherapy. The authors determined that voice outcomes and global quality of life (QOL) outcomes were comparable between modalities and stressed the need for uniform use of specific voice and QOL measurement tools to reliably make comparisons between studies. Of the fifteen studies included in the objective voice outcome analysis of the Spielmann et al review, only three demonstrated significantly better objective voice outcomes with radiotherapy. Each of these three studies used electroacoustic analysis, the criticism being that this form of objective analysis may not correlate well with subjective vocal function and QOL. Of the nine studies in the review that reported QOL outcomes, four used the Voice Handicap Index (VHI). One of these studies (Peeters et al., 2004) reported a significant improvement in the overall VHI score with TOL surgery. The remaining three studies demonstrated no significant difference in overall VHI scores between modalities. Looking again at the Spielman et al review, two of the nine studies included in the QOL analysis employed the European Organisation for Research and Treatment of Cancer (EORTC) QLQ C30 and QLQ H&N 35 questionnaires. One of the two studies (Stoeckli et al., 2001) demonstrated improved swallowing, salivary function, and dental health with TOL surgery.

Two recent Canadian studies (Kujath et al., 2011; Osborn et al., 2011) have compared voice outcomes between TOL surgery and radiotherapy. The study by Kujath et al was discussed previously with regard to oncologic outcomes, but also looked at subjective voice outcomes in a subset of 79 patients. Two tools were used to measure voice outcome. Patients who underwent TOL surgery were less likely to have an understandability score of 100 or more

(Performance Status Scale for Head and Neck Cancer Patients), and were more likely to have a Voice Handicap Index (VHI-10) score of 10 or more. However, another Canadian study by Osborn et al demonstrated a non-significant trend for increased voice-related quality of life (V-RQOL) among patients who underwent radiotherapy as opposed to TOL surgery.

Our meta-analysis (Higgins et al., 2009) demonstrated a trend for improved voice quality with radiotherapy, yet this was a non-significant finding. Currently, the major argument in favour of radiotherapy is improved voice quality, but this has yet to be born out in large-scale systematic studies. It is also difficult to link electroacoustic analytic outcomes with subjective vocal function and QOL outcomes.

3.3 Cost effectiveness

Our group (Higgins, 2011) recently published a cost-utility analysis comparing TOL surgery to radiotherapy and demonstrated an almost two-fold increase in cost with radiotherapy. The TOL surgery cost $2475.65 CAD/case, generating 1.663 QALYs, whereas radiation cost $4965.85 CAD/case, generating 1.506 QALYs. Another Canadian cost analysis was reported by Philips et al (Philips et al., 2009) and concluded that radiotherapy was four times as costly as TOL surgery. A recent Dutch study (Goor et al., 2007) also demonstrated the increased cost of radiotherapy. The total cost of radiotherapy and TOL surgery was 8322 euros and 4434 euros, respectively. In addition, an American study by Brandenburg et al (Brandenburg et al., 2001) demonstrated increased costs associated with radiotherapy compared to TOL surgery. In contrast, a single Belgian study (Gregoire et al., 1999) documented an increased cost of TOL surgery compared to radiotherapy. However, this study reported a 30% positive margin rate in the TOL surgery group, and positive margins were managed with adjuvant radiotherapy instead of re-excision.

Overall, the majority of studies point to an increased cost with radiotherapy compared to TOL surgery. However, it is worthwhile to note that each of these five studies did not include patients undergoing robotic TOL surgery, which may impact significantly on cost effectiveness.

4. Conclusion

The management of early glottic cancer is controversial, with no head to head randomized controlled trials comparing oncologic/survival or functional/QOL outcomes between modalities. The majority of studies in the literature consist of single arm retrospective series, with few head to head retrospective series. A meta-analysis by our group (Higgins et al., 2009) showed a significant increase in overall survival with TOL surgery, and similar local control and laryngectomy-free survival between modalities. Voice outcomes were similar between modalities, but with an overall tendency for improved voice outcomes with radiotherapy. Three recent head-to-head studies have been published since our analysis, with two of these studies (Mahler et al., 2010; Schrijvers et al., 2009) showing a significant increase in LFS with TOL surgery. A recent systematic review (Spielmann et al., 2010) was unable to find clear differences in voice outcomes and QOL measures between modalities. The review demonstrated improved electroacoustic scores in some patients treated with radiotherapy, but did not demonstrate improvement in voice QOL. The most striking difference between treatment modalities is financial, with four of five recent studies

(Higgins, 2011; Philips et al., 2009; Goor et al., 2007;, Brandenburg et al., 2001) showing TOL surgery to be more cost-effective. It is also worthwhile to note that TOL surgery is less time consuming for patients. Patients undergoing TOL surgery convalesce over a matter of days while patients undergoing radiotherapy are treated over four or more weeks. In summary, it is our view that although TOL surgery and radiotherapy may share similar oncologic, voice, and QOL outcomes, TOL surgery offers the distinct advantages of reduced health care costs and shorter duration of treatment.

5. References

Ansarin M, Cattaneo A, Santoro L, Massaro MA, Zorzi SF, Grosso E et al. Laser surgery of early glottic cancer in elderly. Acta Otorhinolaryngol Ital. 2010 Aug;30(4):169.

Blanch JL, Vilaseca I, Caballero M, Moragas M, Berenguer J, Bernal-Sprekelsen M. Outcome of transoral laser microsurgery for T2-T3 tumors growing in the laryngeal anterior commissure. Head Neck. 2010 Oct 27.

Bouquet J. Pathology of the head and neck New York: Churchill Livingstone; 1988. Epidemiology; p. 263-314.In: Gnepp DR, editor.

Brandenburg JH. Laser cordotomy versus radiotherapy: an objective cost analysis. Ann Otol Rhinol Laryngol. 2001 Apr;110(4):312-8.

Eckel HE, Thumfart W, Jungehülsing M, Sittel C, Stennert E. Transoral laser surgery for early glottic carcinoma. Eur Arch Otorhinolaryngol 2000;257:221–6.

Fowler JF. Fractionation and glottic carcinoma. Int J Radiat Oncol Biol Phys 1997;39:1–2.

Genden EM, Desai S, Sung CK. Transoral robotic surgery for the management of head and neck cancer: a preliminary experience. Head Neck. 2009 Mar;31(3):283-9.

Goor KM, Peeters AJ, Mahieu HF, Langendijk JA, Leemans CR, Verdonck-de Leeuw IM et al. Cordectomy by CO2 laser or radiotherapy for small T1A glottic carcinomas: costs, local control, survival, quality of life, and voice quality. Head Neck. 2007 Feb;29(2):128-36.

Grant DG, Salassa JR, Hinni ML, Pearson BW, Hayden RE, Perry WC. Transoral laser microsurgery for untreated glottic carcinoma. Otolaryngol Head Neck Surg. 2007 Sep;137(3):482-6.

Gregoire V, Hamoir M, Rosier JF, Counoy H, Eeckhoudt L, Neymark N et al. Cost-minimization analysis of treatment options for T1N0 glottic squamous cell carcinoma: comparison between external radiotherapy, laser microsurgery and partial laryngectomy. Radiother Oncol. 1999 Oct;53(1):1-13.

Groome PA, O'Sullivan B, Irish JC, Rothwell DM, Math KS, Bissett RJ et al. Glottic cancer in Ontario, Canada and the SEER areas of the United States. Do different management philosophies produce different outcome profiles? J Clin Epidemiol 2001;54:301–15.

Hafidh M, Tibbo J, Trites J, Corsten G, Hart RD, Nasser J et al. Radiotherapy for T1 and T2 laryngeal cancer: the Dalhousie University experience. J Otolaryngol Head Neck Surg. 2009 Aug;38(4):434-9.

Higgins KM. What treatment for early-stage glottic carcinoma among adult patients: CO2 endolaryngeal laser excision versus standard fractionated external beam radiation is superior in terms of cost utility? Laryngoscope. 2011 Jan;121(1):116-34.

Higgins KM, Shah MD, Ogaick MJ, Enepekides D. Treatment of early-stage glottic cancer: meta-analysis comparison of laser excision versus radiotherapy. J Otolaryngol Head Neck Surg. 2009 Dec;38(6):603-12.

Kujath M, Kerr P, Myers C, Bammeke F, Lambert P, Cooke A, Sutherland D. Functional outcomes and laryngectomy-free survival after transoral CO_2 laser microsurgery for stage 1 and 2 glottic carcinoma. J Otolaryngol Head Neck Surg. 2011 Feb; Suppl 1:S49-58.

Mahler V, Boysen M, Brøndbo K. Radiotherapy or CO(2) laser surgery as treatment of T1a glottic carcinoma? Eur Arch Otorhinolaryngol. 2010 May;267(5):743-50.

Motta G, Esposito E, Motta S, Tartaro G, Testa D. CO(2) laser surgery in the treatment of glottis cancer. Head Neck. 2005 Jul;27(7):566-73; discussion 573-4.

Osborn HA, Hu A, Venkatesan V, Nichols A, Franklin JH, Yoo JH et al. Comparison of endoscopic laser resection versus radiation therapy for the treatment of early glottic carcinoma. J Otolaryngol Head Neck Surg. 2011 Jun 1;40(3):200-4.

Peeters AJ, van Gogh CD, Goor KM, Verdonck-de Leeuw IM, Langendijk JA, Mahieu HF. Health status and voice outcome after treatment for T1a glottic carcinoma. Eur Arch Otorhinolaryngol. 2004 Nov;261(10):534-40.

Phillips TJ, Sader C, Brown T, Bullock M, Wilke D, Trites JR et al. Transoral laser microsurgery versus radiation therapy for early glottic cancer in Canada: cost analysis. J Otolaryngol Head Neck Surg. 2009 Dec;38(6):619-23.

Rucci L, Romagnoli P, Scala J. CO(2) laser therapy in Tis and T1 glottic cancer: indications and results. Head Neck. 2010 Mar;32(3):392-8.

Schrijvers ML, van Riel EL, Langendijk JA, Dikkers FG, Schuuring E, van der Wal JE et al. Higher laryngeal preservation rate after CO2 laser surgery compared with radiotherapy in T1a glottic laryngeal carcinoma. Head Neck. 2009 Jun;31(6):759-64.

Shah JP, Karnell LH, Hoffman HT, Ariyan S, Brown GS, Fee WE et al. Patterns of care for cancer of the larynx in the United States. Arch Otolaryngol Head Neck Surg 1997;123:475–83.

Silver CE, Beitler JJ, Shaha AR, Rinaldo A, Ferlito A. Current trends in initial management of laryngeal cancer: the declining use of open surgery. Eur Arch Otorhinolaryngol. 2009 Sep;266(9):1333-52.

Sjögren EV, Wiggenraad RG, Le Cessie S, Snijder S, Pomp J, Baatenburg de Jong RJ. Outcome of radiotherapy in T1 glottic carcinoma: a population-based study. Eur Arch Otorhinolaryngol. 2009 May;266(5):735-44.

Spielmann PM, Majumdar S, Morton RP. Quality of life and functional outcomes in the management of early glottic carcinoma: a systematic review of studies comparing radiotherapy and transoral laser microsurgery. Clin Otolaryngol. 2010 Oct;35(5):373-82.

Steiner W. Results of curative laser microsurgery of laryngeal carcinomas. Am J Otolaryngol 1993;14:116–21.

Stoeckli SJ, Guidicelli M, Schneider A, Huber A, Schmid S. Quality of life after treatment for early laryngeal carcinoma. Eur Arch Otorhinolaryngol. 2001 Feb;258(2):96-9.

Strong M, Jako G. Laser surgery in the larynx: early clinical experience with continuous CO2 laser. Ann Otol Rhinol Laryngol 1972;81:791–8.

[SEER] Surveillance Epidemiology and End Results. 2011. Cancer of the Larynx. Available from: http://seer.cancer.gov/statfacts/html/laryn.html. Accessed 2011 Sep 26.

Tateya I, Hirano S, Kitamura M, Kada S, Ishikawa S, Kanda T et al. Management and pitfalls of stage I/II glottic cancer. J.Acta Otolaryngol Suppl. 2010 Nov;(563):62-7.

Webb 2003. The physical basis of IMRT and inverse planning. Br J Radiol. 2003 Oct;76(910):678-89.

12

Epigenetics in Head and Neck Squamous Cell Carcinoma

Magdalena Chirilă
"Iuliu Hațieganu" University of Medicine and Pharmacy Cluj-Napoca, Romania

1. Introduction

In addition to the genetic information required to establish an organism, recent decades have unveiled a previously unknown type of chromatin modification, known as epigenetic, which is defined as heritable DNA changes that are not encoded in the sequence itself. Unlike genetic modifications, the epigenetic ones are reversible, and increasingly appear to serve fundamental roles in cell differentiation and development.

It is increasingly evident that genetics alone cannot explain the complexity of phenotypes in the living world. Heritable phenotypic characteristics that are not caused by DNA sequence alterations represent the object of epigenetics and include potentially reversible changes such as histone modifications, DNA methylation, and imprinting. At the interface between epigenetics and genomics, a new discipline that is emerging, epigenomics, promises to profoundly change the way we envision phenomena in the biological and medical sciences. Epigenetic modifications can provide an astronomic number of distinct signatures, with huge diagnostic and prognostic value, but it is essential to consider all the different sources of information.

Epigenomics-based diagnostic tools for early cancer detection represent an exciting development. Tumors shed their DNA into the blood, and epigenetic changes that occur early during tumorigenesis, sometimes even in premalignant lesions, can provide valuable biomarkers. Previous research at Epigenomics identified Septin 9 as a single gene in which DNA methylation changes occur very early in colorectal cancer development and are present in the vast majority of tumors of all stages. In most tissues, CpG (cytosine 5-phosphorylated guanine) islands around transcription start sites are largely unmethylated, but their methylation has been described in many tumors and can serve as potential biomarkers. One of the advantages of using epigenomic biomarkers is that, in most cases, DNA methylation changes precede clinical symptoms.

Stephen B. Baylin, M.D., professor of cancer research and deputy director of The Sidney Kimmel Comprehensive Cancer Center at Johns Hopkins University and colleagues recently presented a molecular model to explain how DNA methylation causes gene silencing in mammalian cells. They used the GATA-4 gene as a model to investigate how polycomb protein complexes and DNA methylation maintain the chromatin in its silent state. They found that polycomb protein occupancy at genomic regions enriched in trimethylated histone H3 lysine 27 marks establishes long-range interactions by chromatin looping. This finding promises to significantly improve our understanding of higher order chromatin organization and gene silencing both in stem cells and in cancer cells, which share intriguing similarities with respect to chromatin organization.

In addition to the work on acetylation and methylation in the context of cancer epigenetics another interest focuses on the involvement of heat shock proteins (Hsp) as molecular chaperones in cancer. Cancer cell metabolism creates a considerable amount of stress, and one of the main categories, known as proteotoxic stress, is mediated by the misfolded or unfolded protein response. Heat shock proteins are essential in maintaining the correctly folded conformation and activity of oncoproteins, and thus allow cancer cells to survive the stress response. The use of molecular chaperones as therapeutic targets for malignant tumors emerges as an exciting idea, and several Hsp90 inhibitors are currently being investigated as potential anticancer agents.

"Our individual life history is inscribed in our epigenome," states Toshikazu Ushijima, Ph.D., chief of the carcinogenesis division at the National Cancer Center Research Institute, Tokyo. Dr. Ushijima and collaborators screened genes that were silenced in esophageal squamous cell carcinomas and demonstrated that methylation levels in five promoters are significantly correlated with the duration of tobacco smoking, indicating that chronic smoking induces methylation changes in many of these genes. This finding supports the idea that smoking induces an epigenetic field of cancerization, a term that was previously described for breast, colon, liver, and stomach cancers, and is used to denote epigenetic modifications that occur during the early stages of carcinogenesis. The use of molecular chaperones as therapeutic targets for malignant tumors emerges as an exciting idea, and several Hsp90 inhibitors are currently being investigated as potential anticancer agents.

Increasingly, new revelations about epigenetic modifications promise to transform all facets of cancer biology and to provide prophylactic, diagnostic, and therapeutic benefits. Epigenetic modifications could, in addition, become one of the missing links between infectious diseases and cancer. The ability of certain viruses, bacteria, parasites, and protozoa to cause malignant transformation represents one of the most fascinating topics in life sciences. This connection was regularly re-discovered throughout the past century, it repeatedly fell into oblivion and, historically, demonstrating causality often proved challenging. It is currently estimated that approximately 20% of all cancers worldwide are linked to pathogens, and the involvement of epigenetic changes in shaping this connection could soon lead to new chapters in cancer biology, establishing links that we never would have thought could exist.

2. DNA methylation and gene dysregulation in oral carcinogenesis

Oral squamous cell carcinoma (OSCC) encompasses all the malignancies that originate in the oral tissues, which include cancer of the lip, tongue, gingiva, floor of the mouth, buccal mucosa, palate, and the retromolar trigone. It is the largest group of cancers that fall into the head and neck squamous cell cancer (HNSCC) category, making it the 6th most common cancer in the world (Silverman, 1998).

Oral cancer begins as a focal clonal overgrowth of altered progenitor cells near the basement membrane, expanding upward and laterally, replacing the normal epithelium.

Carcinogenesis in human OSCC is a multistep phenomenon (Scully et al, 2000), which is usually associated with or preceded by potentially malignant oral disorders. A series of genetic hits are required for a cell to progress through dysplasia, carcinoma in situ, invasion, and metastasis. Crucial genetic events that trigger carcinogenesis include the activation of oncogenes and inactivation of tumor suppressor genes. The current understanding in the molecular pathogenesis of oral cancer suggests that both the genetic and epigenetic alterations are implicated in this multistep process as they are known to complement each other during successive stages of oral carcinogenesis. A change in gene expression profiles is evident in cancer cells at the epigenetic level via transcriptional inactivation owing to DNA methylation (Jones,2003). Among the various epigenetic alterations that lead to altered gene expression, the most important are believed to be DNA methylation and chromatin remodeling by histone modification (Baylin & Herman, 2000). DNA methylation markers stand out for their potential to provide a unique combination of specificity, sensitivity, high information content, and applicability to a wide variety of clinical specimens. Methylation markers are particularly suited for situations where sensitive detection is necessary, such as when tumor DNA is either scarce or contaminated by excess normal DNA.

While the effects of genotoxic agents such as tobacco smoke and alcohol are the most important risk factors for the development of oral cancers, the interaction of epigenetic factors and genotoxic agents may synergistically increase the risk of oral carcinogenesis. It may be argued that an epigenetic disruption in progenitor cells might be a common event in human cancer and the epigenome is a logical target for early events in carcinogenesis. The presence of methylated CpG islands in the promoter region of human genes can suppress their expression because of the presence of 5-methylcytosine, which interferes with the binding of transcription factors or other DNA-binding proteins repressing transcription activity. Inactivation of some tumor suppressor genes, such as p16, is an initial event in head and neck cancers (Von Zeidler et al, 2004), which is frequent during early oral carcinogenesis and more so in the later stages (Lopez et al, 2003). Although many important genes and gene products have been identified through DNA methylation changes, no single unifying pathway has been identified that accounts for all OSCC. Aberrant promoter hypermethylation of tumor-associated gene leads to their inactivation, as it may inactivate one or both the alleles of the proven tumor suppressor genes in sporadic cancers and can potentially act as a second hit during the development of hereditary cancer.

Cell cycle regulation, which is coordinated by cyclin-dependent kinases, its binding partners, and the inhibitory molecules such as p16, pRb, and p15 have been widely studied in oral cancer (Chang et al, 2004; Nakahara et al, 2001; Lee et al, 2004; Soni et al, 2005). Cellular signal transduction involves the conversion of one signal or stimulus (mechanical or chemical) to another. The transduction process is usually performed by enzymes in association with second messengers (Oshiro et al, 2005; Mhaweck, 2005; Nakajima et al, 2003; Gasco et al, 2002). Wnt signaling pathway is a network of proteins best known for their role in embryogenesis and cancer. E-cadherin, Adenomatosis polyposis coli APC, ß-catenin, CDH3, SFRP family, WIF1, and DKK3 are some of the genes of Wnt pathway, which are epigenetically silenced in cancer. Wnt pathway is also involved in calcium-dependent cell adhesion through the interaction of E-cadherin and ß-catenin (Nakayama et al, 2001; Uesugi et al, 2005; Gao et al, 2005). One of the hallmarks of cancer is the down-regulation of genes involved in DNA repair pathways. O-6-methylguanine-DNA methyltransferase (MGMT), MutL homolog 1 (MLH1), and fragile histidine triad (FHIT) are most widely studied in oral cancer. Frequent inactivation of some of these repair genes in cancer has been reported to be due to promoter hypermethylation (Mikami et al, 2007; Murakami et al, 2004; Rohatgi et al, 2005; Kato et al, 2006; Rodriguez et al, 2007; Kim et al, 2004; Paradiso et al, 2004; Baer-Desurmont et al, 2007).

Failure of cells to undergo apoptosis is a common and frequent event in carcinogenesis. Resistance to apoptosis of cancer cells has great clinical significance as these cells are resistant to chemo-and radiotherapies. Thus, identifying the checkpoints of apoptosis in cancer may offer newer therapeutic modalities for the treatment of cancer. The genes, which are involved in the apoptosis, such as Death-associated protein kinase 1, p73, and RASSF2, have shown to be down-regulated in oral cancer because of promoter hypermethylation (Hasegawa et al, 2002). In head and neck cancers, a statistically significant correlation was detected between the presence of DAP kinase gene promoter hypermethylation, lymph node involvement, and advanced disease stage. Tobacco smoking was slated to play an important role in the occurrence of promoter methylation and in delineating the precise pathway that eventually resulted in a tumorigenic phenotype (Araki et al, 2002). Some of the molecular changes characteristic of early oral cancer development have been identified in immortal oral dysplasia cultures and are associated with the loss of the expression of RAR-beta and the cell cycle inhibitor p16INK4A. RAR-beta and / or p16 reexpression could be reinduced by treatment with 5-aza-2¢-deoxycytidine in some immortal dysplasias, and the possibility of reversing the immortal phenotype of some dysplasias by 5-aza-2¢-deoxycytidine was considered to be of clinical usefulness (McGregor et al, 2002).

The ability to determine methylation states in primary tumors, saliva, and serum may have a potential clinical application in creating methylation gene panels for cancer screening. Gene methylation in saliva is a promising biomarker for the follow-up and early detection of still curable relapses of patients with HNSCC (Righini et al, 2007). Sanchez-Cespedes et al. (2000) studied the promoter hypermethylation patterns of the p16, MGMT, and DAP-K genes in tumor DNA of head and neck primary tumors and paired saliva samples to test whether the cells with tumor-specific aberrant DNA methylation might be found in the saliva of affected patients. Promoter methylation in saliva DNA was found in all tumor stages and more frequently in tumors located in the oral cavity. Moreover, none of the saliva from patients with methylation-negative tumors displayed methylation of any marker. This assay allowed sensitive and accurate detection of tumor DNA in saliva and may be potentially useful for detecting and monitoring recurrence in patients with head and neck cancers.

3. Human papillomavirus-16 DNA methylation patterns

This year marks a century since Francis Peyton Rous' seminal discovery that laid the foundations of a new field at the crossroads between microorganisms and human cancer. In 1911, Rous showed that cell-free filtrates from birds with sarcoma were able to cause tumors in healthy birds. The idea that viruses are causally linked to cancer was viewed at the time with skepticism, and fell into oblivion for decades, but re-emerged later. Fifty-five years after his groundbreaking discovery, Rous received the 1966 Nobel Prize in Physiology or Medicine.

A century after this major discovery, over 20% of the cancers have been causally linked to human pathogens, including viruses, bacteria, and parasites (Zur Hausen, 2009). Why an acute infectious disease is sometimes controlled, while on other occasions it progresses to malignant tumors, is still a mystery, and the mechanisms of how pathogens may accomplish this are still elusive but, for increasing numbers of pathogens, epigenetic modifications have been implicated (Paschos & Alladay, 2010).

Three of the most extensively studied oncogenic viruses, the hepatitis B virus (HBV), human papilloma viruses (HPV), and the Epstein-Barr virus (EBV) are, at the same time, major public health concerns. HBV infects over 2 billion people worldwide, and causes chronic infection in approximately 350 million of them (Fernandez & Esteller, 2010). Human papillomavirus (HPV) is thought to be the most frequent infectious agent that causes cancer. Specific human papillomavirus serotypes were causally linked to more than 70% of cervical cancers, to most anal cancers, and to respiratory papillomatosis. In addition, this virus emerges as an increasingly important causal agent of head and neck cancers, particularly in younger patients, and has also been associated with breast cancer (Westra, 2009).

To dissect the link between inflammation and cancer, Iliopoulos et al (Illiopoulos 2009, 2010) fused the estrogen receptor ligand-binding domain to the Src kinase oncoprotein to create a tamoxifen-inducible fusion protein. By using this system, the authors found that a transient inflammatory signal generated by an induction as short as 5 minutes triggered, in an NF-_B (transcription factor)-dependent manner, an epigenetic switch similar to the one that controls tissue differentiation during development. This switch established a positive feedback loop, and as a result, nontransformed human mammary epithelial cells were becoming transformed, as revealed 24 to 36 hours later. The transformed state was propagated for many generations in the absence of the initiating inflammatory signal. Subsequently, the authors found several microRNAs that are differentially regulated as part of this positive feedback loop. The 2 most up-regulated ones, miR-21 and miR-181b-1, are key regulators of tumor-suppressor genes (Stein, 2011).

Infection with HPV, notably with high-risk HPV types as HPV-16 and 18, is a necessary step in the etiology of anogenital cancers, specifically carcinoma of the cervix uteri. DNA diagnosis confirmed the presence and transcription of HPV genomes in all cervical carcinomas, and the study of HPV oncoproteins catalyzed a variety of molecular mechanisms that convert normal into malignant cells (Munoz et al, 2003). In case of head and neck squamous cell carcinomas (HNSCC), approximately 80% of all HNSCC do not contain HPV genomes, and must therefore originate from HPV independent etiological processes, likely including mutational events triggered by tobacco and alcohol consumption. Among head and neck sites, squamous cell carcinomas of the tonsils have the strongest statistical support for an HPV dependent etiology (Syrjianen, 2005). There is less strength and consistency for a linkage between HPV infection and carcinogenesis at sites of the oral mucosa such as tongue, palate, floor of mouth and gingiva. Analysis of some HPV containing oral carcinomas revealed recombination between HPV genomes and cellular DNA as well as HPV oncogene expression (Ragin et al, 2004), properties that are generally viewed as support of carcinogenic processes under the influence of HPV. On the basis of these observations one must conclude that infection with high-risk HPV plays an etiological role in at least a proportion of malignancies of the oral cavity (Balderas-Loaeza et al, 2007).

With the recent reported increase in young HNSCC cases many of them nonsmokers, the question arises as to whether these cases have the same genetic alterations as seen in the classic progression model. Toner and O'Regan (2009) studied HNSCC in young adults using array comparative genomic hybridization on a cohort of predominantly nonsmoking young adults and compared them with a cohort of mostly smoking older adults. Results from this study showed that when stratified by age the young cohort do not have the genetic alterations that are seen so consistently in older HNSCC. In fact, the mean number of aberrations in the young nonsmokers was less than 50% of that in the older smokers. Molecular alterations at the p53 gene have been documented as being the most frequent genetic alteration observed in carcinomas and has been found to be altered in over 70% of HNSCC (Gillison et al, 2000). It has been shown that p53 sequence alteration decreased in the setting of HPV infection, since there is an alternative means of p53 silencing with the production of E6 (Mork et al, 2001). Overexpression of $p16^{INK4}$ has also been reported in head and neck cancers, and it is believed that HPV infection, via inactivation of retinoblastoma gene, accounts for these high levels of $p16^{INK4}$ expression [Mork et al, 2001]. Toner and O'Regan (2009) found that p16 methylation is a more common event in those younger than 40 years in contrast to p16 deletions, which are more common in those older than 40 years. Consequently, it appears that specific modes of inactivation of p16 in HNSCC are related to specific patient risk profiles. After detailed study of p16 mRNA expression and p16 immunohistochemistry in this cohort, it was clear that all HPV mRNA positive cases showed p16 overexpression. In relation to copy gain and loss, previous studies have found only occasional chromosomal loss in HPV16 positive cases, suggesting that HPV16 infection is an early event in HNSCC development.

Inverted papillomas are benign, rare sinonasal lesions well known for their local recurrence, invasiveness and predisposition for malignant transformation. Recurrence rates for inverted papillomas range from 6 to 33% and malignant transformation occurs in 7–10% of cases (Batsakis, 2001). Endophytic sinonasal papillomas, comprising inverted papillomas and cylindrical cell papillomas according to the World Health Organization classification, show malignant progression in up to 25% of cases (Gujrathi et al, 2003).

The exact nature and biological evolution of sinonasal papillomas is not well known. The suggested hypothesis includes viral infections, chronic inflammation, and proliferation of nasal polyps, allergy, and environmental carcinogens. In view of its epitheliotropic nature and increasing evidence, Human Papilloma Virus (types 6 and 11) is postulated to be the most probable aetiological factor. Causative factor form alignant transformation in a papilloma is still unknown. It has been seen that HPV 16 and 18 are more carcinogenic than HPV 6 and 11. Over-expression of p53 & reduced expression of CD44 has been seen in carcinomas associated with inverted and exophytic papillomas. Overexpression of p53 may serve as a marker for malignant transformation of inverted papilloma (el-Deiry, 1998). Induction of p21waf1/cip1 is associated with terminal differentiation, senescence, and apoptosis in several tissues (Yook & Kim, 1998). Expression of p21waf1/cip1 has been detected in head and neck cancers, in particular oral SCCs and its precursors (Ng et al, 1999).

Epigenetic alterations of promoter hypermethylation have not been previously reported in sinonasal papillomas. Stephen et al. (2007) investigated whether epigenetic events of aberrant promoter hypermethylation in genes known to be involved in squamous head and neck cancer underlie the pathogenesis of sinonasal papillomas. Ten formalin-fixed paraffin DNA samples from three inverted papilloma cases, two exophytic (everted) papilloma cases, and two cases with inverted and exophytic components were studied. DNA was obtained from microdissected areas of normal and papilloma areas and examined using a panel of 41 gene probes, designed to interrogate 35 unique genes for aberrant methylation status (22 genes) using the methylation-specific multiplex-ligation-specific polymerase assay. Methylation-specific PCR was employed to confirm aberrant methylation detected by the methylation-specific multiplex-ligation-specific polymerase assay. All seven cases indicated at least one epigenetic event of aberrant promoter hypermethylation. The *CDKN2B* gene was a consistent target of aberrant methylation in six of seven cases. Methylation-specific PCR confirmed hypermethylation of *CDKN2B*. Recurrent biopsies from two inverted papilloma cases had common epigenetic events. Promoter hypermethylation of *CDKN2B* was a consistent epigenetic event. Common epigenetic alterations in recurrent biopsies underscore a monoclonal origin for these lesions. Epigenetic events contribute to the underlying pathogenesis of benign inverted and exophytic papillomas. As a consistent target of aberrant promoter hypermethylation, *CDKN2B* may serve as an important epigenetic biomarker for gene reactivation studies (Stephen et al, 2007).

4. Epigenetic changes in nasopharyngeal carcinoma

Nasopharyngeal carcinoma (NPC) is rare in most part of the world but prevalent in southern China, including Guangdong and Hong Kong, and Southeast Asia, with an incidence rate of 20 to 30 per 100 000 people/year (Li et al, 2011). The unique ethnic and geographic distribution of NPC indicates its unusual etiology. Three major etiologic factors, genetic, environmental, and viral factors - Epstein-Barr virus (EBV), have been identified to lead to multiple genetic and epigenetic alterations during NPC pathogenesis by either acting alone or in synergy.

EBV is a prototype of gamma herpes virus which infects >90% of the world adult population (Liebowitz, 1994). Humans are the only natural host for EBV. Primary infection with EBV normally occurs in early childhood and is usually asymptomatic in most underdeveloped countries. But when the exposure to EBV is delayed until adolescence it occasionally presents as mononucleosis. Long-term EBV coexists with most human hosts without overt serious consequences. However, in some individuals, the virus is implicated in the development of malignancy. EBV has a strong tropism for human lymphocytes and for epithelium of the upper respiratory tract (Young & Rickinson, 2004). EBV was the first human virus identified to be associated with human lymphomas as well as epithelial tumors, such as post-transplant lymphoma, AIDS-associated lymphomas, Burkitt lymphoma, Hodgkin's disease, T-cell lymphoma, nasopharyngeal carcinoma, parotid gland carcinoma, and gastric carcinoma. (Murray & Young, 2002)

Tumorigenesis of nasopharyngeal carcinoma is a multistep process. EBV may play an important role in the progression of NPC, involving activation of oncogenes and/or the inactivation of tumor suppressor genes (TSGs). Early genetic changes may predispose the epithelial cells to EBV infection or persistent maintenance of latent cycle.

Nasopharyngeal carcinoma also distinguishes itself from other tumors by the number of genes targeted for silencing by promoter methylation. The key tumor suppressor genes like p53 or Rb which are found to be mutated in 50% of all the tumors were rarely found to be mutated in nasopharyngeal carcinoma (Wensing & Farrel, 2000). On the contrary, hypermethylation of known or candidate tumor suppressor genes involved in various fundamental pathways has been reported in NPC, such as apoptosis, DNA damage repair, tumor invasion and metastasis. Many TSGs were aberrantly methylated in their 5'CpG islands: 84% of the RASSF1A, 80% of the RARβ2, 76% of the DAP-kinase, 46% of the p16, 89,7% of the CDH13, 65% of the CHFR, 50,9% of the RASSF2A (Li et al, 2011). DNA methylation may play an important role in the maintenance of specific EBV latency programmes in the nasopharyngeal carcinoma cells. Methylation of both viral and cellular genes may be involved in the transformation of nasopharyngeal epithelial cells. Induction of epigenetic alterations in certain cellular genes was proposed as one of the mechanisms for enhancing the transformation of nasopharyngeal epithelial cells by EBV infection.

Loss of heterozygosity at 3p21 is common in various cancers including nasopharyngeal carcinoma (NPC). BLU is one of the candidate tumor suppressor genes (TSGs) in this region. Ectopic expression of BLU results in the inhibition of colony formation of cancer cells, suggesting that BLU is a tumor suppressor. Qiu and colab. (2004) identified a functional BLU promoter and found that it can be activated by environmental stresses such as heat shock, and is regulated by E2F. The promoter and first exon are located within a CpG island. BLU is highly expressed in testis and normal upper respiratory tract tissues including nasopharynx. However, in all seven NPC cell lines examined, BLU expression was downregulated and inversely correlated with promoter hypermethylation. Biallelic epigenetic inactivation of BLU was also observed in three cell lines. Hypermethylation was further detected in 19/29 (66%) of primary NPC tumors, but not in normal nasopharyngeal tissues. Treatment of NPC cell lines with 5-aza-20-deoxycytidine activated BLU expression along with promoter demethylation. Although hypermethylation of RASSF1A, another TSG located immediately downstream of BLU, was detected in 20/27 (74%) of NPC tumors, no correlation between the hypermethylation of these two TSGs was observed (Qiu et al, 2004).

Aberrant "epigenetic code" of cell signaling facilitates the subsequent selection of genetic mutations of certain signaling pathways in the initiation and progression of NPC. As more epigenetic alterations of cell signaling genes are found, we will obtain systematic understanding of the molecular features of NPC. Study of epigenetically silenced cell signaling regulators in NPC will lead to the further development of clinical strategies of NPC prevention and therapy. Moreover, promoter methylation of cell signaling regulators could serve as diagnostic biomarkers for NPC risk assessment, early detection, and prognosis (Li et al, 2011).

5. Epigenetic changes in laryngeal cancer

Laryngeal cancers are the most frequent cancers of the head and neck region and their occurrence is strongly associated with the exposure to cigarette smoke and the consumption of strong alcohols. Almost all laryngeal cancers are squamous cell carcinomas (Paluszczak et al, 2011).

The chondroitin/dermatan sulfate fine chemical structure is altered in laryngeal carcinomas (Kalathas et al, 2009) as well as in most cancers. In healthy larynx, chondroitin/dermatan sulfate (C-6 and C-4 sulfated) in the cartilaginous parts is present in greater amounts compared to cancer. Moreover, the decrease in cancer is more abrupt in C-6 sulfation; C-4 sulfation is diminished gradually to the advanced stages of cancer. These alterations may be due to differential biosynthesis of core protein precursors, to differences in the substrates pool, and to differential expression of the enzymes involved in chondroitin/dermatan sulfate biosynthesis.

The purpose of Kalathas and colab. (2010) was to examine the expression of the various chondroitin/dermatan sulfate synthesizing and modifying enzymes in laryngeal cartilage in healthy, macroscopically normal and cancerous specimens by RT-PCR analysis and western blotting. Furthermore, methylation specific PCR (MSP) was used to find out if DNA methylation is a regulative mechanism of their expression in laryngeal cancer. C4ST1 gene expression was very low in healthy specimens (20 times lower compared to the GAPDH gene), and increased in patients' specimens as indicated by both RT-PCR and western blotting. Its expression seemed to be controlled via methylation of a CpG island, since hypomethylation of the gene was observed in the pathologic samples compared to the macroscopically normal samples. D4ST1 gene was about equally expressed with the GAPDH gene and possessed its highest expression in the healthy tissues. In cancer, its expression was decreased 4 to 5 times and it was about equal between normal and pathologic samples. The CpG island near the promoter region was fully unmethylated therefore it did not affect the enzyme expression. DSE expression was not detected in the macroscopically normal samples, and the highest levels of it were observed in the pathologic samples, as indicated by RT-PCR, being about 10-times more compared to healthy. DSE expression seemed to be controlled by methylation of the promoter region in certain samples; the pathologic samples were hypomethylated compared to the macroscopically normal. The differential modification of the various glycosaminoglycans during cancer reflected differential expression of the enzymes involved in their biosynthesis. In their study, the clearest observations in laryngeal cancer were the significant decrease of CHSY3, CHST3 and D4ST1, and the significant increase of DSE. DSE is responsible for the epimerization of glucuronic acid in dermatan sulfate chains, which in addition require D4ST1 for their sulfation. The differential expression of only these two enzymes, which are highly responsible for the biosynthesis of dermatan sulfate, a glycosaminoglycan with tumor-inhibitory activity, indicates that a simple imbalance in enzymes' expression may affect tumor progression.

Different environmental factors are able to modulate the epigenetic information. It is widely accepted that the aberrant DNA methylation changes can be induced by both cigarette smoke and alcohol. Alcohol consumption and smoking induced the hypermethylation of p15 in the upper respiratory tract cells (Chang et al, 2004), while the hypermethylation of MGMT, p16 and DAPK was associated with tobacco-chewing induced oral cancers (Vuillemont et al, 2004). A correlation was also found between cigarette smoking and the hypermethylation of CDH1, RARbeta and FHIT (Van Engeland et al, 2003). Alcohol consumption was associated with the methylation of APC, p14, p16, MGMT, RASSF1A and hMLH1 (Van Engeland et al, 2003). Since alcohol and tobacco are the major risk factors for the development of laryngeal squamous cell carcinomas (LSCC), one can predict the frequent occurrence of the methylome aberrations in LSCC patients.

Since Slaughter's proposal of a genetic field defect concept for the explanation of the local relapse occurrence, much evidence has accumulated for its confirmation. The last ten years brought evidence that the genetic changes in the field are frequently accompanied by epigenetic aberrations. The epigenetic field defect was observed for oesophageal (Oka et al, 2009), lung (Guo et al, 2004) or stomach (Ushijima, 2007) cancers. Similarly, epigenetic changes in normal mucosa cells derived from surgical margins were detected in head and neck carcinomas (Martone et al, 2007). However, so far such changes have not been observed specifically in laryngeal cancers. In Paluszczak's paper (2011) evidence of a wide-spread occurrence of the aberrations in the profile of DNA methylation in laryngeal cancer patients is presented. Less than ten percent of cancer cases did not show any epigenetic changes in the normal mucosa samples. Gene methylation frequency was only slightly lower in the normal epithelium of epiglottis or trachea than in tumor cells. However, it should be taken into account that all the patients were exposed to similar laryngeal cancer risk factors. As discussed earlier, tobacco and alcohol are associated with the aberrations in the DNA methylation profile. The long-term exposure of patients to these factors could be responsible for the common appearance of epigenetic defects in a large field of upper respiratory tract mucosa. The existence of the epigenetically changed field in laryngeal cancers seems to be confirmed especially by such cases where lack of gene methylation in tumor cells was accompanied by the presence of hypermethylation in the normal epithelial cells although the percentage of patients with such gene methylation pattern was rather low.

6. Epigenetics and environment exposure

For many decades, it was assumed that chemicals are able to cause cancer only if they mutate the DNA. However, a growing body of scientific evidence reveals that this "carcinogenesis equals mutagenesis" paradigm is no longer accurate. Twenty years ago, Ashby and Tennant (1991) examined 301 chemicals tested by the US National Toxicology Program, and found that from 162 (53%) that were carcinogens, 64 (40%) were not genotoxic, illustrating the importance to focus on carcinogenic mechanisms other than genotoxicity. For many chemical agents, it has become increasingly clear that biological perturbations leading to neoplastic transformation may occur even in the absence of mutagenesis, via non-genotoxic, epigenetic changes. In addition, epigenetic changes may be relevant for tumor development and progression and ways that years ago seemed unimaginable. For example, Tanemura et al. (2009) revealed, for the first time, that CpG methylation in cutaneous melanoma is associated with tumor progression, and Nobeyama et al. (2007) demonstrated that tissue factor pathway inhibitor-2 (*TFPI-2*), a encoding a protein that suppresses the invasiveness of malignant melanoma, was methylated in 29% of metastatic lesions but in none of the primary tumors examined, pointing towards differences in gene expression and phenotypic characteristics between metastatic tumors and the primary tumor they originated from, a finding with significant therapeutic applications. The risk factors for sinonasal carcinoma include wood dust esposure, occupational exposure to chromium and nickel and its organic compounds (Luce & Leclerc, 2002)

Very high relative risks have been invariably found and 10-45 fold risks have been indicated for the sinonasal adenocarcinoma cell type in association to occupational exposure to hardwood dust, the risk related to softwood dust exposure is less clear. (Demers et al, 1997) Exposure to wood dust in the occupational setting is a common occurrence. It has been estimated that in the year 2000-2003 about 3.6 million workers were occupationally exposed to inhalable wood dust in the European Union and over half a million of these workers were estimated to be exposed to high levels (exceeding $5mg/m^3$) of wood dust (Kauppinen et al,, 2006). The terms "hardwood" and "softwood" refer to the taxonomic categorization of trees and not necessarly to the hardness of the wood. Woo dust is a complex mixture of compounds including a wide variety of biologically active substances, also genotoxic and carcinogenic compounds (Hanahan & Weinbrg, 2000). The particulate nature of the wood-dust exposure plays a role in generating reactive species of oxygen (ROS) within cells and inducing DNA damage and evoking an inflammatory response (Bornholdt & Saber, 2007). Multiple mechanism of carcinogenesis have been proposes to be involved in the development of sinonasal cancer related to wood-dust exposure, but there is very little experimental or human data in the literature. The published findings have been based on a relatively limited number of cases, mostly involving adenocarcinomas. In these studies, high frequencies of DNA copy number chamges as detected by comparative genomic hybridization have been detected (Ariza et al,, 2004 and Korinth et al, 2005), while the mutation rates reported for the KRAS gene (Fratini et al, 2006 and Yom et al, 2005) and the p53 tumor suppressor gene have been lower (Perrone et al, 2003 and Licitra et al, 2004)). Initially, KRAS and HRAS mutations were found to be quite frequent in sinonasal cancer, with implications for histogenetic and prognostic significance (Yom et al, 2005), but recent studies show that tumors with KRAS mutation might represent only a small proportion of all sinanasal carcinomas (Bornholdt et al, 2008). Most of the studies having as subject p53 mutation have concentrated on the intestinal type of adenocarcinoma, and the numbers of cases studied have been rather low. In these studies, a variable occurrence of p53 mutations has been reported (18-60%) (Licitra et al, 2004 and Perrone et al, 2003). Some of the studies have also examined the accumulation of p53 in the cell nucleus in adenocarcinoma type of sinonasal carcer. The accumulation of p53 may reflect a p53 mutation.

With the exception of chromium, which forms DNA adducts, most carcinogenic metals are weak mutagens and act by epigenetic mechanisms (Arita & Costa 2009). Nickel, a metal linked to occupational and environmental exposures, has carcinogenic effects, despite the fact that it is not known to be a mutagen (Kasprzak et al, 2003; Chen et al, 2006; Ellen et al, 2009). *In vitro* and *in vivo* experiments reveal that nickel compounds silence gene expression by causing DNA methylation, an effect explained by the ability of nickel ions to substitute magnesium in the DNA phosphate backbone and to increase heterochromatin condensation (Arita & Costa 2009). The ability of Ni^{2+} ions to displace Mg^{2+} and cause chromatin condensation, establishing dense regions of heterochromatin that prevent accessibility to the respective genomic region, was also revealed by Ellen and colleagues (2009) with atomic force microscopy and circular dichroism spectropolarimetry. Chromatin condensation could in addition trigger DNA methylation in the compacted region, which also affects gene expression. When the silenced chromosomal region contains genes that are relevant to cancer initiation or progression, such as tumor suppressor genes or senescence genes, their inactivation can lead to disease (Ellen et al, 2009).

Nickel compounds also induce global changes in histone acetylation, methylation, and ubiquitylation. Kang et al. (2004) linked nickel to hypoacetylation to apoptosis for the first time, when they found hypoacetylation and demethylation of histones as potential mechanisms leading to apopotosis. Golebiowski and Kasprzak (2005) reported decreased acetylation of histones H2A, H2B, H3 and H4, in a time- and concentration-dependent manner, in human and rat cell lines exposed to nickel. Chen et al. (2006) revealed that nickel decreased a specific histone demethylase and by this mechanism, it increased global H3K9 mono- and dimethylation in several cell lines, and strongly suggested that this increased methylation causes the silencing of a transgene. This effect was dependent, *in vitro*, on iron and 2-oxoglutarate, and it is likely that it resulted from the nickel interfering with the iron moiety of the enzyme (Chen et al, 2006). In response to soluble nickel compounds at levels that had minimal cytotoxic effects, Ke et al. (2006) described three major histone modifications: H3K9 dimethylation, increased H2A and H2B ubiquitylation, and reduced histone acetylation, which was also associated with a transgene silencing.

An interesting example is provided by hexavalent chromium, to which half a million workers in the United States and several million individuals worldwide are occupationally exposed (Ali et al, 2011). Until recently, chromium was thought to cause cancer only through its ability to damage DNA (Arita & Costa 2009). Klein et al. (2002) reported for the first time that potassium chromate, a carcinogen, causes aberrant DNA methylation and silences a reported gene in a mammalian cell line. Ali et al. (2011) found higher rates of aberrant methylation in the promoters of three tumor-suppressor genes, APC (adenomatosis polyposis coli), MGMT (O_6-methylguanine-DNA methyltransferase), and hMLH1 in lung cancers of chromate workers as compared to non-chromate lung cancer controls (95% versus 52%), with concordant methylation of multiple loci observed in more chromate lung cancers than in nonchromate ones (48% versus 12%). Chromate was also linked to post-translational histone modifications. Sun et al. (2009) found that hexavalent chromium at 5-10 μM concentrations causes global and local, gene-specific histone methylation changes in lung cancer, non-cancerous bronchial epithelial cells, and all respiratory tract which could impact tumorigenesis and tumor progression.

Benzene and aromatic hydrocarbons have increasingly emerged over the past few decades as environmental hazards. Exposure to benzene can occur in occupational settings, and also non-occupationally from coal or gasoline combustion products and cigarette smoke, which also contain polycyclic aromatic hydrocarbons. In the first study to show that low levels of a common environmental carcinogen are linked to epigenetic changes that occur in malignant human tumors, Bollati et al. (2007) reported that benzene, at low-level airborne exposures that are common in Western countries, causes epigenetic changes that reproduce modifications observed in human cancers. The authors examined 155 traffic police officers and gas station attendants, and 58 unexposed control subjects from Milan, Italy. The study revealed a dose-dependent global hypomethylation in the long interspersed nuclear element-1 (*LINE-1*) and *Alu*I repetitive sequences, in addition to hypermethylation at specific promoters, such as p15, which is also hypermethylated in patients with acute myeloid leukemia, in addition to hypomethylation in *MAGE-1*, a gene that is hypomethylated in many malignant tumors.

As a group of chemicals, polycyclic aromatic hydrocarbons (PAHs) include thousands of compounds ubiquitously distributed in the environment. An interesting fact about PAHs is that for a long time, the focus has been on their ability to cause genotoxic damage while their potential to induce epigenetic modifications was largely ignored (Upham et al, 1998). Benzopyrene, a prototype PAH, is a classic carcinogen found in vehicle emissions and in cigarette smoke - the mainstream smoke of a filter cigarette contains approximately 10 ng benzpyrene (Sherer et al, 2000), and exposure can also occur occupationally. In the first study to show that benzpyerene causes epigenetic changes, Sadikovic et al. (2008) conducted a genome-wide analysis after exposure and found 775 genes that were hypoacetylated and 1456 that were hyperacetylated. These modifications occurred in genes important for fundamental cellular processes, such as DNA replication, repair, and carcinogenesis.

In the first study that examined the effects of smoking on miRNA expression, Schembri et al. (2009) found 28 differentially expressed miRNAs in smokers, 82% of which were down regulated. One of them, mir-218, is also down regulated in several cancers, and the authors revealed that modulation of miR-218 levels lead to changes in the expression of its target genes. Xi et al. (2010) found that cigarette smoke condensate causes a significant and early increase in miR-31 that was apparent within 24 hours after exposure and persisted for 20 days after removal of the exposure.

7. Challenges in epigenetic cancer therapy

Epigenetic mechanisms regulate the interpretation of genetic information. As such, our knowledge of these mechanisms is essential for understanding the phenotypic plasticity of cells, both in the context of normal cellular differentiation and in human disease (Freinberg, 2007). Research over the past two decades has identified two major levels of epigenetic modification: DNA methylation and covalent histone modifications (Strahl & Allis, 2000 and Klose & Bird, 2006). DNA methylation is mediated by a family of enzymes termed DNA methyltransferases (DNMTs) (Goll & Bestor, 2005), while histone modification patterns are established and maintained by a diverse set of enzymes that add or subtract acetyl-, methyl-, and other modifications to various amino acids of histone proteins (Kouzarides, 2007). Both regulatory mechanisms cooperate to determine the expression potential of individual genes.

For detection of cancel cells in body fluids, a high-sensitivity method is necessary. One way is mutation detection in cells because the exact location of a mutation within a gene is usually unknown, many primer sets are necessary for complete analysis. In contrast, aberrant methylation of DNA molecule of cancer cells, even in very few in number, can be sensitively detected by using Methylation-Specific PCR method (MSP), only with one set of PCR primer can be performed on chemically stable DNA, not on RNA (Herman et al,1996 and Laird, 2003).

Considering that some aberrant DNA methylation is present in early stages of carcinogenesis, there is a possibility that such demethylating agents may protect against some cancers (Laird et al, 1995). Demethylating agents are including DNMT1 inhibitors group (Azacitadine, Decitabine, Zebularine and MG98), procainamide, procain and EGCG (epigallocatechin-3-gallate) (Fang et al, 2003 and Villar-Garea et al, 2003). Inhibitors of DNMTs have been widely used in cell culture systems to reverse abnormal DNA hypermethylation and restore silenced gene expression. However, only limited success has been achieved in clinical trials with these drugs (Thibault et al, 1998 and Goffin & Eisenhouer, 2002). Also, nucleosides analog inhibitors of DNMTs may promote genomic instability and increase the risk of cancer in other tissues, because have many potential side effects such as myelotoxicity, mutagenesis and tumorigenesis (Jones &Taylor, 1980 and Gaudet et al, 2003). There is an attractive alternative for possible clinical use of non-nucleoside analog DNMT inhibitors.

The use of these drugs raises questions regarding their potential to affect non-cancerous cells epigenetically. However, normal cells divide at a slower rate than malignant cells and incorporate less of these drugs into their DNA resulting in less of an effect on DNA methylation. Azacitadine and decitabine are labil and have acute hematological toxicities. Zebularine, a next generation DNA methylation inhibitor, might possibly overcome these problems (Marquez et al, 2005 and Yoo et al, 2008). The non-nucleoside analogue inhibitors are not as potent as the nucleoside analogues and therefore this issue needs for improvement (Chuang et al, 2005).

Another prominent example for an epigenetic drug is the histone deacetylase (HDAC) inhibitor suberoylanilide hydroxamic acid (SAHA, vorinostat, Zolinza), which has been approved for the treatment of cutaneous T cell lymphoma (Marks & Breslow, 2007). Another HDAC inhibitor (Romidepsin, Istodax) has very recently been approved for the same indication. As of today, there are at least 20 structurally different HDAC inhibitors in clinical trials, either in monotherapy or in combination therapy trials for hematological and solid tumors. It should be noted that combination therapies of HDAC inhibitors with other anticancer drugs or with radiation therapy have shown a wide range of synergistic effects, both in preclinical models and in early clinical trials (Marks & Xu, 2009). The identification of tumor-specific epigenetic pathways represents a critically important step toward the establishment of targeted epigenetic cancer therapies. One possibility is the targeting of defined DNMTs with specific oncogenic functions (Linhart et al, 2007). Another possibility is the discovery of tumor-specific functions for enzymes with specific histone modification activities. A third option is the identification of tumor-specific interactions between epigenetic pathways, like interaction between DNMTs and HDACs through methyl-CpG binding proteins.

While the clinical application potential of the interaction between DNA methylation and histone hypoacetylation remains to be established, the results from preclinical experiments clearly suggest crosstalk between epigenetic silencing systems that warrants further investigation. A particular interesting finding in this context is the interaction between histone lysine methylation and DNA hypermethylation. Several independent studies have shown that genes that are marked by bivalent chromatin structures (i.e. the presence of both H3K4 and H3K27 methylation marks) in embryonic stem cells have a high probability of becoming de novo methylated in cancer (Schlesinger et al, 2007; Ohm et al, 2007; Widschwendter et al, 2007). The mechanistic details of these interactions are only beginning to be elucidated. The available data, however, raise the intriguing possibility that cancer-specific epigenetic mutations reflect the stem cell origin of tumors. As such, targeting of the interaction between bivalent chromatin structures and DNA hypermethylation might represent a highly specific approach toward erasing cancer-specific epigenetic mutations.

"Cancer has been the tip of the iceberg, but knowledge in cancer epigenetics is going to translate to other diseases. It is clear to me that there is no disease that is pure genetics, and there is no disease that is pure epigenetics. All diseases, from cancer to neurological disorders to cardiovascular conditions, are mixtures of genetics, epigenetics, and the environment" says Manuel Esteller, M.D., Ph.D., director of the Cancer Epigenetics and Biology Program in Barcelona.

Epigenomics-based diagnostic tools for early cancer detection represent an exciting development. Tumors shed their DNA into the blood, and epigenetic changes that occur early during tumorigenesis, sometimes even in premalignant lesions, can provide valuable biomarkers. More than ever, it is imperative to focus on understanding the mechanistic details of malignant transformation initiated by human pathogens, an area that promises exciting prophylactic, diagnostic, and therapeutic applications.

8. Acknowledgements

I would like to thank **Dr. Richard A. Stein**, from Department of Molecular Biology, Lewis Thomas Lab, Princeton University, Princeton, NJ, USA, for his help and for my initiation in the mystery of epigenetics.

9. References

Ali AH, Kondo K, Namura T, Senba Y, Takizawa H, Nakagawa Y, Toba H, Kenzaki K, Sakiyama S, Tangoku A. (2011) Aberrant DNA methylation of some tumor suppressor genes in lung cancers from workers with chromate exposure. *Mol Carcinog*:50;89-99.

Araki D, Uzawa K, Watanabe T, et al. (2002) Frequent allelic losses on the short arm of chromosome 1 and decreased expression of the p73 gene at 1p36.3 in squamous cell carcinoma of the oral cavity. *Int J Oncol*; 20: 355- 360.

Arita A, Costa M. Epigenetics in metal carconogenesis: nickel, arsenic, chromium and cadmium. *Metallomics* 2009:1; 222-228.

Ariza M, Llorente JL et al. (2004) Comparative genomic hybridization in primary sinonasal adenocarcinomas. *Cancer*; 100 :335-341.

Ashby, J., Tennant, R.W. (1991) Definitive relationships among chemical structure, carcinogenicity and mutagenicity for 301 chemicals tested by the U.S. NTP. *Mutation Research*; 257:229-306.

Baert-Desurmont S, Buisine MP, Bessenay E, et al. (2007) Partial duplications of the MSH2 and MLH1 genes in hereditary nonpolyposis colorectal cancer. *Eur J Hum Genet*; 15: 383–386.

Balderas-Loaeza A, Anaya-Saavedra G, Ramirez-Amador VA et al. (2007) Human papillomavirus-16 DNA methylation patterns support a causal association of the virus with oral squamous cell carcinomas. *Int J Cancer*; 120:2165-2169.

Batsakis JG, Suarez P. (2001) Schneiderian papillomas and carcinomas: a review. *Adv Anat Pathol*;8:53–64.

Baylin SB, Herman JG. (2000) DNA Hypermethylation in tumorigenesis: epigenetics joins genetics. *Trends Genet*; 16: 168–174.

Bollati V, Baccarelli A, Hou L et al. (2007) Changes in DNA methylation patterns in subjects exposed to low-dose benzene. *Cancer Res*:67;876-880.

Bornholdt J, Hansen J et al. (2008) KRAS mutation in sinonasal cancer in relation to wood dust exposure. *BMC Cancer*; 8, 53.

Bornholdt J, Saber AT. (2007) Inflammatory response and genotoxicity of seven wood dust in the human epithelial cell line A594. *Mutat Res*; 632:78-88.

Chang HW, Ling GS, Wei WI, Yuen AP. (2004) Smoking and drinking can induce p15 methylation in the upper aerodigestive tract of healthy individuals and patients with head and neck squamous cell carcinoma. *Cancer*; 101: 125–132.

Chen H, Ke Q, Kluz T, Yan Y, Costa M. (2006) Nickel ions increase histone H3 lysine 9 dimethylation and induce transgene silencing. *Mol Cell Biol*:26;3728-3737.

Chuang JC, Yoo CB, Kwan JM, Li TW et al. (2005) Camparison of biological effects of non-nucleotide DNA methylation inhibitors versus 5-aza-2deoxycytidine. *Mol Cancer Ther;* 4:1515-1520.

Demers, PA, Teschke K, Kennedy SM. (1997) What to do about softwood ? A review of respiratory effects and recommendations regarding exposure limits. *Am J Ind Med;* 31(4): 385-398.

el-Deiry WS. (1998) p21/p53, cellular growth control and genomic integrity. *Curr Top Microbiol Immunol;* 227:121–137.

Ellen TP, Kluz T, Harder ME, Xiong J, Costa M. (2009) Heterochromatinization as a potential mechanism of nickel-induced carcinogenesis. *Biochemistry*:48;4626-32.

Fang MZ, Wang Y, Ai N, Hou Z, Sun Y et al. (2003) Tea polyphenol(-)epigallocatechin-3-gallate inhibits DNA methyltransferase and reactivates methylation-silenced genes in cancer cell lines. *Cancer Rec;* 63: 7563-7570.

Feinberg AP. (2007) Phenotypic plasticity and the epigenetics of human disease. *Nature;* 447: 433–40.

Fernandez AF, Esteller M. (2010) Viral epigenomes in human tumorigenesis. *Oncogene;* 29:1405-1420.

Frattini M, Perrone F et al. (2006) Phenotype-genotype correlation: challenge of intestinal-type adenocarcinoma of the nasal cavity and paranasal sinuses. *Head Neck;* 28(6): 909-915.

Gao S, Eiberg H, Krogdahl A, Liu CJ, Sørensen JA. (2005) Cytoplasmic expression of E-cadherin and beta-Catenin correlated with LOH and hypermethylation of the APC gene in oral squamous cell carcinomas. *J Oral Pathol Med;* 34: 116–119.

Gasco M, Bell AK, Heath V, et al. (2002) Epigenetic inactivation of 14-3-3 sigma in oral carcinoma: association with p16(INK4a) silencing and human papillomavirus negativity. *Cancer Res;* 62: 2072–2076.

Gaudet F, Hodgson JG, Eden A, Jackson-Grusby L, Dausman J. (2003) Induction of tumors in mice by genomic hypomethylation. *Science;* 300:489-492.

Gillison ML, Koch WM, Capone RB, Spafford M, Westra WH, Wu L, et al. (2000) Evidence for a causal association between human papillomavirus and a subset. *J Natl Cancer Inst.;* 92(9): 709–720.

Goffin J, Eisenhauer E. (2002) DNA methyltransferase inhibitors-state of the art. *Ann Oncol,* 13:1699-1716.

Goll MG, Bestor TH. (2005) Eukaryotic cytosine methyltransferases. *Annu Rev Biochem;* 74: 481–514.

Golebiowski F, Kasprzak KS. (2005) Inhibition of core histones acetylation by carcinogenic nickel (II). *Mol Cell Biochem*:279;133-139.

Gujrathi C, Pathak I, Freeman J, *et al.* (2003) Expression of p53 in inverted papilloma and malignancy associated with inverted papilloma. *J Otolaryngol*;32:48–50.

Guo M, House MG, Hooker C, Han Y, Heath E, Gabrielson E, et al. (2004) Promoter hypermethylation of resected bronchial margins: a field defect of changes? *Clin Cancer Res;* 10:5131–6.

Hanahan D, Weinberg RA. (2000) The hallmarks of cancer. *Cell;* 100:57-70.

Hasegawa M, Nelson HH, Peters E, Ringstrom E, Posner M, Kelsey KT. (2002) Patterns of gene promoter methylation in squamous cell cancer of the head and neck. *Oncogene;* 21: 4231–4236.

Herman JG, Graff S, Myohanen BD, Nelkin and Baylin SB. (1996) Methylation specific PCR: a novel PCR assay for methylation status of CpG islands. *Proc Natl Acad Sci;* 93:9821-9826.

Iliopoulos D, Hirsch HA, Struhl K. (2009) An epigenetic switch involving NF-kappaB, Lin28, Let-7 microRNA, and IL6 links inflammation to cell transformation. *Cell.;* 139(4):693-706.

Iliopoulos D, Jaeger SA, Hirsch HA, Bulyk ML, Struhl K. (2010) STAT3 activation of miR-21 and miR-181b-1 via PTEN and CYLD are part of the epigenetic switch linking inflammation to cancer. *Mol Cell;* 39(4):493-506.

Jones PA. (2003) Epigenetics in Carcinogenesis and cancer prevention. *Ann N Y Ac Sci ;* 983: 213–219.

Jones PA, Taylor SM. (1980) Cellular differentiation, cytidine analogs and DNA methylation. *Cell;* 20:85-93.

Kalathas D, Theocharis DA, Bounias D et al. (2009) Alterations of glycosaminoglycan disaccharide content and composition in colorectal cancer: Structural and expressional studies. *Oncol Rep.;* 22:369–375.

Kalathas D, Triantaphyllidou IE, Mastronikolis NS et al. (2010) The chondroitin/dermatan sulfate synthesizing and modifying enzymes in laryngeal cancer: expressional and epigenetic studies. *Head Neck Oncol;* 2:27.

Kang J, Zhang D, Chen J, Lin C, Liu Q. (2004) Involvement of histone hypoacetylation in Ni2+-induced bcl- 2 down-regulation and human hepatoma cell apoptosis. *J Biol Inorg Chem*:9(6);713-23.

Kato K, Hara A, Kuno T, et al. (2006) Aberrant promoter hypermethylation of p16 and MGMT genes in oral squamous cell carcinomas and the surrounding normal mucosa. *J Cancer Res Clin Oncol;* 132: 735–743.

Kauppinen T, Vincent R et al. (2006) Occupational exposure to inhalable wood dust in member states of the European Union. *Ann Occup Hyg;* 50(6):549-561.

Kasprzak KS, Sunderman FW Jr, Salnikow K. (2003) Nickel carcinogenesis. *Mutat Res*:533;67-97.

Ke Q, Davidson T, Chen H, Kluz T, Costa M. (2006) Alterations of histone modifications and transgene silencing by nickel chloride. *Carcinogenesis*:27;1481-8.

Kim JS, Kim H, Shim YM, Han J, Park J, Kim DH. (2004) Aberrant methylation of the FHIT gene in chronic smokers with early stage squamous cell carcinoma of the lung. *Carcinogenesis;* 25: 2165–2171.

Klein CB, Su L, Bowser D, Leszczynska J. (2002) Chromate-induced epimutations in mammalian cells. Environ Health Perspect. Oct;110 Suppl 5:739-43.

Klose RJ, Bird AP. (2006) Genomic DNA methylation: the mark and its mediators. *Trends Biochem Sci;* 31: 89–97.

Korinth D, Pacyna-Gengelbach M et al. (2005) Chromosomal imbalances in wood dust-related adenocarcinomas of the inner nose and their associations with pathological parameters. *J Pathol;* 207:207-215.

Kouzarides T. (2007) Chromatin modifications and their function. *Cell;* 128: 693–705.

Laird, PW. (2003) The power and the promise of DNA methylation markers. *Nat Rev Cancer;* 3:253-266.

Laird PW, Jackson-Grusby L, Fazeli A, Dickinson S, Jung W, Weinberg R, Jaenisch R. (1995) Suppression of intestinal neoplasia by DNA hypomethylation. *Cell;* 81:197-205.

Lee JK, Kim MJ, Hong SP, Hong SD. (2004) Inactivation patterns of p16 / INK4A in oral squamous cell carcinomas. *Exp Mol Med;* 36: 165–171.

Li LL, Shu XS, Wang ZH, Cao Y, Tao Q. (2011) Epigenetic disruption of cell signaling in nasopharyngeal carcinoma. *Chin J Cancer;* 30(4):230-239.

Licitra L, Suardi S et al. (2004) Prediction of TP53 status for primary cisplatic, fluorouracil, and leucovirin chemotherapy in ethmoid sinus intestinal-type adenocarcinoma. *J Clin Oncol;* 22(24):4901-4906.

Liebowitz D. (1994) Nasopharyngeal carcinoma: the Epstein-Barr virus association. *Seminars oncol;* 21:376-381.

Linhart HG, Lin H, Yamada Y et al. (2007) DNMT3b promotes tumorigenesis in vivo by gene-specific de novo methylation and transcriptional silencing. *Genes Dev;* 21:3110-3122.

Lopez M, Aguirre JM, Cuevas N, et al. (2003) Gene promoter hypermethylation in oral rinses of leukoplakia patients – a diagnostic and / or prognostic tool? *Eur J Cancer;* 39: 2306–2309. Marks PA, Breslow R. Dimethyl sulfoxide to vorinostat: development of this histone deacetylase inhibitor as an anticancer drug. Nat Biotechnol 2007; 25: 84–90.

Luce D, Leclerc A. (2002) Sinonasal cancer and occupational exposures: a pooled analysis of 12 case-control studies. *Cancer Causes Control;* 13(2):147-157.

Marks PA, Xu WS. (2009) Histone deacetylase inhibitors: potential in cancer therapy. *J Cell Biochem;* 107: 600–608.

Marquez VE, Barchi JJ, kelley JA, Rao KV, Agbaria R et al. (2005) Zebularine: a unique molecule for an epigenetically based strategy in cancer chemotherapy. The magic of its chemistry and biology. *Nucleosides Nucleotides Necleic Acids;* 24:305-318.

Martone T, Gillio-Tos A, De Marco L, Fiano V, Maule M, Cavalot A, et al. (2007) Association between hypermethylated tumor and paired surgical margins in head and neck squamous cell carcinomas. *Clin Cancer Res;* 13:5089–94.

McGregor F, Muntoni A, Fleming J, et al. (2002) Molecular changes associated with oral dysplasia progression and acquisition of immortality: potential for its reversal by 5-azacytidine. *Cancer Res;* 62: 4757–4766.

Mikami T, Yoshida T, Numata Y, et al. (2007) Low frequency of promoter methylation of O6-methylguanine DNA methyltransferase and hMLH1 in ulcerative colitis-associated tumors: comparison with sporadic colonic tumors. *Am J Clin Pathol;* 127: 366–373.

Mhawech P. (2005) 14-3-3 proteins-an update. *Cell Res;* 15: 228–236.

Mork J, Lie AK, Glattre E, Hallmans G, Jellum E, Koskela P, et al. (2001) Human papillomavirus infection as a risk factor for squamous cell carcinoma of the head and neck. *N Eng J Med.;* 344:1125–1131.

Munoz N, Bosch FX, de Sanjosé S, Herrero R, Castellsagué X, Shah KV, Snijders PJF, Meijer CJLM. (2003) Epidemiological classification of human papillomavirus types associated with cervical cancer. *N Engl J Med*; 348:518–527.

Murray PG, Young LS. (2002) The role of the Epstein-Barr virus in human disease. Front Biosci; 7:519-540.

Murakami J, Asaumi J, Maki Y, et al. (2004) Influence of CpG island methylation status in O6-methylguanine-DNA methyltransferase expression of oral cancer cell lines. *Oncol Rep*; 12: 339–345.

Nakahara Y, Shintani S, Mihara M, Ueyama Y, Matsumura T. (2001) High frequency of homozygous deletion and methylation of p16(INK4A) gene in oral squamous cell carcinomas. *Cancer Lett*; 163: 221–228.

Nakajima T, Shimooka H, Weixa P, et al. (2003) Immunohistochemical demonstration of 14-3-3 sigma protein in normal human tissues and lung cancers, and the preponderance of its strong expression in epithelial cells of squamous cell lineage. *Pathol Int*; 53: 353–360.

Nakayama S, Sasaki A, Mese H, Alcalde RE, Tsuji T, Matsumura T. (2001) The E-cadherin gene is silenced by CpG methylation in human oral squamous cell carcinomas. *Int J Cancer*; 93: 667–673.

Ng IO, Lam KY, Ng M, *et al.* (1999) Expression of p21/waf1 in oral squamous cell carcinomas—correlation with p53 and mdm2 and cellular proliferation index. *Oral Oncol*;35:63–69.

Nobeyama Y, Okochi-Takada E, Furuta J, et al. (2007) Silencing of tissue factor pathway inhibitor-2 gene in malignant melanomas. *Int J Cancer*:121;301-307.

Ohm JE, McGarvey KM, Yu X, Cheng L, et al. (2007) A stem cell-like chromatin pattern may predispose tumor suppressor genes to DNA hypermethylation and heritable silencing. *Nat Genet* ; 39: 237–242.

Oka D, Yamashita S, Tomioka T, Nakanishi Y, Kato H, Kaminishi M, et al. (2009) The presence of aberrant DNA methylation in noncancerous esophageal mucosae in association with smoking history: a target for risk diagnosis and prevention of esophageal cancers. *Cancer*; 115:3412–26.

Oshiro MM, Futscher BW, Lisberg A, et al. (2005) Epigenetic regulation of the cell type-specific gene 14-3-3 sigma. *Neoplasia*; 7: 799–808.

Qiu GH, Tan LKS, Loh KS et al. (2004) The candidate tumor suppressor gene BLU, located at the commonly deleted region 3p21.3, is an E2F-regulated, stress-responsive gene and inactivated by both epigenetic and genetic mechanisms in nasopharyngeal carcinoma. *Oncogene*; 23:4793-4806.

Paluszczak J, Misiak P, Wierzbicka M, Wozniak A, Baer-Dubowska W. (2011) Frequent hypermethylation of DAPK, RARbeta, MGMT, RASSF1A and FHIT in laryngeal squamous cell carcinomas and adjacent normal mucosa. *Oral Oncol*; 47:104-107.

Paradiso A, Ranieri G, Stea B, et al. (2004) Altered p16INK4a and FHIT expression in carcinogenesis and progression of human oral cancer. *Int J Oncol*; 24: 249–255.

Paschos K, Allday M. (2010) Epigenetic reprogramming of host genes in viral and microbial pathogenesis. *Trends in Microbiology*; 18(10): 439-447.

Perrone F, Oggionni M et al. (2003) TP53, p14ARF, p16INK4a and HRAS gene molecular analysis in intestinal-type adenocarcinoma of the nasal cavity and paranasal sinuses. *Int J Cancer*; 105(2):196-203.

Ragin CC, Reshmi SC, Gollin SM. (2004) Mapping and analysis of HPV16 integration sites in a head and neck cancer cell line. *Int J Cancer*; 110:701–709.

Righini CA, de Fraipont F, Timsit JF, et al. (2007) Tumor-specific methylation in saliva: a promising biomarker for early detection of head and neck cancer recurrence. *Clin Cancer Res*; 13: 1179–85.

Rodriguez MJ, Acha A, Ruesga MT, Rodriguez C, Rivera JM, Aguirre JM. (2007) Loss of expression of DNA repair enzyme MGMT in oral leukoplakia and early oral squamous cell carcinoma. A prognostic tool? *Cancer Lett*; 245: 263–268.

Rohatgi N, Kaur J, Srivastava A, Ralhan R. (2005) Smokeless tobacco (khaini) extracts modulate gene expression in epithelial cell culture from an oral hyperplasia. *Oral Oncol*; 41: 806–820.

Sadikovic B, Andrews J, Carter D, Robinson J, Rodenhiser DI. (2008) Genome-wide H3K9 histone acetylation profiles are altered in benzopyrene-treated MCF7 breast cancer cells. *J Biol Chem*:283;4051-60.

Sanchez-Cespedes M, Esteller M, Wu L, et al. (2000) Gene promoter hypermethylation in tumors and serum of head and neck cancer patients. *Cancer Res*; 60: 892–895.

Scherer, G., Frank, S., Riedel, K., Meger-Kossien, I., and Renner, T. (2000) Biomonitoring of Exposure to Polycyclic Aromatic Hydrocarbons of Nonoccupationally Exposed Persons. *Cancer Epidemiol. Biomark.*, 9:373-380

Schembri F, Sridhar S, Perdomo C, Gustafson AM, Zhang X, Ergun A, Lu J, Liu G, Zhang X, Bowers J, Vaziri C, Ott K, Sensinger K, Collins JJ, Brody JS, Getts R, Lenburg ME, Spira A. (2009) MicroRNAs as modulators of smoking-induced gene expression changes in human airway epithelium. *Proc Natl Acad Sci U S A*:106(7);2319-24.

Schlesinger Y, Straussman R, Keshet I, Farkash S, et al. (2007) Polycomb-mediated methylation on Lys27 of histone H3 pre-marks genes for de novo methylation in cancer. *Nat Genet*; 39: 232–36.

Scully C, Field JK, Tonkawa H. (2000) Genetic aberrations in oral or head and neck squamous cell carcinoma (SCCHN). I. Carcinogen metabolism, DNA repair and cell cycle control. *Oral Oncol*; 36: 256–263.

Silverman S. (1998). Epidemiology. In *Oral cancer. 5th edition*. Silverman S Jr. (Ed), 1-6, BC Decker Inc, ISBN 1-55089-215-4. Hamilton, Ontario, USA.

Soni S, Kaur J, Kumar A, et al. (2005) Alterations of Rb pathway components are frequent events in patients with oral epithelial dysplasia and predict clinical outcome in patients with squamous cell carcinoma. *Oncology*; 68: 314–325.

Stein RA. (2011) Epigenetics-the link between infectious diseases and cancer. JAMA; 305(14):1484-1485.

Stephen JK, Vaught LE, Chen KM et al. (2007) Epigenetic events underlie the pathogenesis of sinonasal papillomas. *Modern Pathol*; 20:1019-1027.

Strahl BD, Allis CD. (2000) The language of covalent histone modifications. *Nature*; 403: 41–5.

Sun H, Zhou X, Chen H, Li Q, Costa M. (2009) Modulation of histone methylation and MLH1 gene silencing by hexavalent chromium. *Toxicol Appl Pharmacol*: 237; 258-66.

Syrjanen S. (2005) Human papillomavirus (HPV) in head and neck cancer. *J Clin Virol*; 32: S59-S66.

Toner M, O'Regan EM. (2009) Head and Neck squamous cell carcinoma in the young: a spectrum or a distinct group? Part 2. *Head Neck Pathol*; 3:249-251.

Tanemura A, Terando AM, Sim MS, van Hoesel AQ, de Maat MF, Morton DL, Hoon DS. (2009) CpG island methylator phenotype predicts progression of malignant melanoma. *Clin Cancer Res*:15;1801-1807.

Uesugi H, Uzawa K, Kawasaki K, et al. (2005) Status of reduced expression and hypermethylation of the APC tumor suppressor gene in human oral squamous cell carcinoma. *Int J Mol Med*; 15: 597–602.

Upham BL, Weis LM, Trosko JE. (1998) Modulated gap junctional intercellular communication as a biomarker of PAH epigenetic toxicity: structure-function relationship. *Environ Health Perspect*:Suppl 4;975-981.

Ushijima T. (2007) Epigenetic field for cancerization. *J Biochem Mol Biol* ; 40:142–50.

van Engeland M, Weijenberg MP, Roemen GMJM, Brink M, de Bruine AP, Goldbohm RA, et al. (2003) Effects of dietary folate and alcohol intake on promoter methylation in sporadic colorectal cancer: The Netherlands cohort study on diet and cancer. *Cancer Res*; 63:3133–7.

Villar-Garea A, Fraga MF, Espada J, Esteller M. (2003) Procaine is a DNA demethylating agent with growth-inhibitory effects in human cancer cells. *Cancer Res*; 63:4984-4989.

von Zeidler SV, Miracca EC, Nagai MA, Birman EG. (2004) Hypermethylation of the p16 gene in normal oral mucosa of smokers. *Int J Mol Med*: 14: 807–811. Thibault A, Figg WD, Bergan RC, Lush RM, Myers CE. A phase II study of 5-aza-2deoxycytidine (decitabine) in hormone independent metastatic (D2) prostate cancer. Tumori 1998; 84:87-89.

Vuillemenot BR, Pulling LC, Palmisano WA, Hutt JA, Belinsky SA. (2004) Carcinogen exposure differentially modulates RAR-beta promoter hypermethylation, an early and frequent event in mouse lung carcinogenesis. *Carcinogenesis*; 25:623–629.

Westra WH. (2009) The changing face of head and neck cancer in the 21st century: the impact of HPV on the epidemiology and pathology of oral cancer. *Head Neck Pathol.*; 3(1):78-81.

Wensing B, Farrel PJ. (2000) Regulation of cell growth and death by Epstein-Barr virus. *Microbes Infect*; 2:77-84.

Widschwendter M, Fiegl H, Egle D, Mueller-Holzner E, et al. (2007) Epigenetic stem cell signature in cancer. *Nat Genet*; 39: 157–58.

Yom SS, Rashid A et al. (2005) Genetic analysis of sinonasal adenocarcinoma phenotypes : distinct alterations of histogenetic significance. *Mod pathol*; 18(3):315-319.

Yoo CB, Chuang JC, Byun H, Egger G, Yang AS et al. (2008) Long-term epigenetic therapy with oral zebularine has minimal side effects and prevents intestinal tumors in mice. *Cancer Prev Res*; 4:233-240.

Yook JI, Kim J. (1998) Expression of p21WAF1/CIP1 is unrelated to p53 tumour suppressor gene status in oral squamous cell carcinomas. *Oral Oncol*;34:198–203.

Young LS, Rickinson AB. (2004) Epstein-Barr virus: 40 years on. *Nature reviews*; 4:757-768.

Zur Hausen H. (2009) The search for infectious causes of human cancers: where and why. *Virology* 392(1):1-10.

Xi S, Yang M, Tao Y, Xu H, Shan J, Inchauste S, Zhang M, Mercedes L, Hong JA, Rao M, Schrump DS. (2010) Cigarette smoke induces C/EBP-β-mediated activation of miR-31 in normal human respiratory epithelia and lung cancer cells. *PLoS One*:5; e13764.